# Green & Natural Antibacterial Agents

Natural ways to prevent or treat bacterial infections

Copyright 2015

Laurie Pippen

The recipes in this book contain easily obtained ingredients that are generally accepted to be safe and effective.

Individual reactions to the contained ingredients can vary. It is not possible to predict how any individual will react to a particular recipe, treatment, or ingredient.

As with any product, a user should employ common sense when creating these recipes or using the applicable ingredients. The reader should consult a qualified herbalist or physician before using any ingredient or recipe in this book.

The enclosed materials are for informational purposes only and the reader accepts all responsibility for determining the effectiveness and usefulness of all of the included items. Neither the author nor the publisher accepts and liability for the actions of the reader or for any reactions caused by the use of the contents and ingredients.

Nothing in this guide is intended to substitute for the medical expertise and advice of your primary health care provider.

You should discuss any decisions about treatment or care with your health care provider. The information contained within this guide is believed to be accurate at the time of writing but research is being undertaken daily and new information, effects, or side effects may be discovered that conflict with the materials contained herein.

No product, service, or therapy is endorsed by the author, publisher, or other individual associated with the creation of this material. The reader should remember that the U.S. Food and Drug Administration (FDA) have not evaluated the statements made in this book. The products listed are not intended to diagnose, treat, cure, or prevent any disease.

Using any medication whether prescription, over the counter, or herbal in nature may have a marked effect on your health and each medicine may interact with others. Tell your health care provider about any complementary, supplemental, or alternative practices you use including dietary substances, herbals, or oils.

Federal regulations for dietary supplements are different from the regulations applied to prescription and over the counter drugs. Dietary supplement manufacturers are not required to prove a product's safety and effectiveness.

Plant products are sometimes marketed as dietary supplements. Plant products do have a noticeable affect on the human body. The expected action of many plant products is based on traditional use and observation. Laboratory studies have been conducted to confirm the expected affect of some traditionally used plant products but others have not been researched in a laboratory setting. Most dietary supplements, herbs, and oils have not been researched for use by pregnant women, nursing women, or children. No supplement, herb, or oil in this book is recommended for use by women who are pregnant or nursing or by children.

Each person's needs and correct dosage will vary depending on a variety of factors. You should discuss your specific needs and best dosage with a qualified herbalist or physician.

# Green & Natural Antibacterial Agents
## Natural ways to prevent or treat bacterial infections

Natural Antibacterial Agents.....................................1

Using Natural Ingredients...............................173

Harvesting & Drying Herbs............................178

Delivery Mediums........................................184

External Use of Plant Products.........................197

Glossary...................................................202

References.................................................207

## Natural Antibacterial Agents

The classification antibacterial includes anything that destroys bacteria or inhibits the ability of bacteria to grow and reproduce.

Herbals approach bacterial infection from two directions. They stimulate the immune system to produce more immune cells aiding your body's ability to fight the infection and they act in direct opposition to bacteria by inhibiting their ability to grow and reproduce so they cannot survive.

The first line of defense against bacterial infection is prevention. Disinfecting surfaces with known antibacterial cleaners, maintaining good health through diet, rest, and exercise, and minimizing exposure to infectious agents is far more effective than any treatment plan in the continued battle against bacteria.

Regardless of the preventative care you take, there are always times where treating an infection will be necessary. Traditionally, bacterial infection is fought by blending herbals that support the body's own natural defenses with those that act to inhibit and kill the bacteria. Using a combination that blends both actions helps to minimize the duration and severity of any infection.

Many herbs and oils act as natural immunostimulant and antibacterial agents. Some of these natural products work as well as or even better than the products sold in your local pharmacy. Some of the items in your local pharmacy are even created based on the chemical constituents of plants you might have growing in your own yard.

This guide contains antibacterial agents that act as both disinfectants for infected air and surfaces and disease fighting agents for the body. Both categories eliminate harmful bacteria. It is important that you read the traditional uses and side effects of each plant and discuss any alternative treatment with a qualified herbalist or physician prior to choosing a natural product.

**Acacia – Gum, Gum Arabic**
**Botanical Name:** Acacia senegal

**Properties:** Antibacterial, Anti-inflammatory, Astringent, Demulcent

**Traditional Uses:** Acacia gum is chewed as a traditional dental care agent for its ability to remove dental plaque build up and combat bacteria growth in the throat and mouth.

Powdered Acacia Gum has been used in traditional topical washes, lotions, and treatments to reduce inflammation on the surface of the skin and prevent the growth of bacteria.

Acacia Gum helps to coat inflamed mucus membranes and has traditionally been used in lozenges and treatments to sooth inflamed mouth & throat surfaces while combating bacterial infections.

**Parts Used:** Gum

**Side Effects:** Acacia is not recommended for use by women who are pregnant or nursing.

Acacia may cause an allergic reaction in some people.

Additional uses and side effects may exist but further research is necessary to determine the exact properties and effects of the root.

**General:** Acacia is a deciduous shrub or tree native to the semi-desert regions of Africa, Pakistan, and India. It is propagated in other areas for its nutritional and medicinal uses as well as its ability to restore nitrogen to poor quality soil. Acacia grows easily propagated from seeds harvested before the pods are fully dried, soaked in water, and sown directly into the soil.

The bark fibers of the acacia root are used in rope making and the wood is used in a variety of woodcraft yielding darker tones as you move toward the heart of the tree. Acacia seeds are harvested and dried for use as a vegetable or animal fodder. The leaves and pods are high in digestible protein making them a valued source of nutrition in some regions. The gum resin is harvested for use as a dental care product or as a thickening agent in foods, cosmetic, or supplements preparations. Acacia bark contains high levels of tannins and it is frequently used for tanning hides or is dried and powdered for use in topical, culinary, and supplement preparations.

Acacia Gum powder is soluble in water so it can be added to creams, lotions, liquid poultices, tooth care products, food products, and other items to stabilize the liquid and improve the texture of the final product.

1 tablespoon-powdered gum to 3 tablespoons fluid creates a syrupy result.

**Acacia, Umbrella Thorn**
**Botanical Name:** Acacia tortilis

**Properties**: Anti-inflammatory, Astringent, Antibacterial, Strengthening, Vermifuge

**Traditional Use:** Powdered Umbrella Thorn bark is traditionally sprinkled over minor wounds and abrasions to aid in removing surface bacteria while maximizing the bodies healing ability.

Umbrella Thorn gum is used as a thickening alternative to Gum Arabic in many preparations giving similar thickening and antibacterial results.

**Parts Used:** Bark, Leaf, Seed – Gum

**Side Effects:** Acacia Umbrella Thorn is not recommended for use by women who are pregnant or nursing.

Umbrella Thorn may have a mild sedative effect and you should not drive or operate heavy machinery while using Umbrella Thorn.

Umbrella Thorn is recommended for topical use only.

Additional uses and side effects may exist but further research is necessary to determine the exact properties and effects.

**General:** Umbrella Thorn is a medium sized evergreen shrub or tree native to Africa that can also be found growing in the Middle East. This drought tolerant tree is easily propagated by direct seeding with light soil coverage in sandy or loamy soils with good drainage. Soaking seeds before planting increases the germination rate.

The wood of the Umbrella Thorn is valued for use in furniture making, fencing, and other woodcraft. The seedpods have been harvested for use as a vegetable and animal fodder. The bark is high in tannin and has been used as a dying product.

The bark, leaf, seed and gum is harvested, dried, and powdered for use as a food product or in traditional supplement applications.

**Adrue, Chintul, Cyperus, Flatsedge, Guinea Rush, Jointed Flat Sedge, Kajiji, Piripiri, Zacoo
Botanical Name:** Cyperus articulatus

**Properties:** Analgesic, Antibacterial, Anticonvulsant, Anti-emetic, Antifungal, Astringent, Carminative, Contraceptive, Digestive, Purgative, Sedative, Vermifuge

**Traditional Use:** Adrue had traditionally been used as an antibacterial compound in treatments designed to combat bacterial infections.

Adrue has been used as a traditional gargle to alleviate mouth, throat and tooth pain while combating bacterial infections of the mouth and throat.

**Part Used:** Leaf, Oil, Root - Rhizome

**Side Effects:** Adrue is not recommended for use by women who are pregnant or nursing.

Adrue has been used as a traditional contraceptive aid and should not be used by those trying to conceive.

Overuse of Adrue may cause digestive upset and vomiting.

Additional uses and side effects may exist but further research is necessary to determine the exact properties and effects.

**General:**  Adrue is a tall sedge grass native to the wetlands of Jamaica and Turkey and naturalized in other regions including the Southeastern United States.  Growing up to 6 feet tall, it prefers damp, bog-like areas and is often found growing wild along lakes, rivers, and streams or cultivated to aid in stopping soil erosion.  Adrue grows in clumps and is easily propagated by rhizome division.

Adrue stems have been used in weaving baskets and mats.  The nuts have been harvested and steeped with grains to make a sweetened drink.  The rhizome is harvested, dried, and powdered for use in traditional medicinal and magical teas.

Adrue leaf and oil are traditionally used in topical preparations while the root is collected in the fall for use in traditional supplement infusions given twice daily.

**African Wild Potato, Bantu Tulip, Hypoxis, South African Star Grass, Sterretjie, Yellow Star**
**Botanical Name:** Hypoxis hemerocallidea

**Properties:**  Antibacterial, Anti-inflammatory, Astringent, Cancer, Diuretic, Dye Product, Immunostimulant, Laxative, Vermifuge

**Traditional Uses:**  African Wild Potato has traditionally been used to treat bacterial infections such as those of the urinary tract.

**Parts Used:**  Tuber

**Side Effects:**  African Wild Potato is not recommended for use by women who are pregnant or nursing.

African Wild Potato may cause constipation, diarrhea, flatulence, indigestion, and nausea in some people.

Additional uses and side effects may exist but further research is necessary to determine the exact properties and effects of use.

**General:**  The African Wild Potato is a tuberous perennial with yellow star like flowers.  Native to South Africa it is cultivated in other regions of the world as a food, medicinal, and foliage plant.

The African Wild Potato is drought tolerant and frost resistant making it an easy to grow plant that only requires full sun and well-drained soil.  Bulbs can be cold stored throughout the winter and divided in the spring or the plant can be propagated by seed though seeds require a year of dormancy prior to germination.

African Wild Potato leaves are used to make rope and the leaves and tuber have been used as a black dye product for textiles and floor waxing.

4

African Wild Potato has traditionally been harvested for use as food and in supplement extracts. African Wild Potato supplement tea is traditionally given at a dosage of 20 milligrams three times daily. Alcohol extracts are being studied for use at a rate of 1200 milligrams divided into 3 doses daily for the treatment of lung cancer. The African Wild Potato is included in numerous commercial preparations currently on the market.

## Ageratum
**Botanical Name:** Ageratum houstonianum

**Properties:** Anodyne, Antibacterial, Hypoglycemic, Insect Repellant

**Traditional Use:** Ageratum leaf juice is used in traditional topical preparations to alleviate pain and minimize infection in skin sores, ulcers, & wounds.

**Part Used:** Leaf, Whole

**Side Effects:** Ageratum is not recommended for use by women who are pregnant or nursing.

Ingestion of Ageratum may lower blood sugar.

Additional uses and side effects may exist but further research is necessary to determine the exact properties and effects of use.

**General:** Ageratum is an annual native to Southwestern North America. Hardy to zone 8, it is not particular regarding soil composition but does require full sun and consistent moisture. Ageratum is easily propagated by seed and will self-sow readily if given its own place in the garden.

The leaves are harvested and juiced or the oils extracted for use in traditional topical preparations.

## Ai Ye, Japanese Wormwood Leaf, Mugwort
**Botanical Name:** Artemisia argyi

**Properties:** Antibacterial, Antiseptic, Antiviral, Aromatic, Astringent, Expectorant, Febrifuge, Styptic

**Traditional Use:** Ai Ye leaves are traditionally used in household cleaning agents designed to prevent or reduce bacteria such as staphylococcus aureus, bacillus typhi, b. dysenteriae, e. coli, b. subtilis, and pseudomonas in the environment and as a traditional internal treatment to alleviate infection.

Ai Ye leaf oil has traditionally been sprayed in the back of the throat to alleviate the constriction and congestion associated with conditions like asthma and bronchitis while helping to combat bacterial infections of the mouth, throat, or lungs.

**Part Used:** Leaf, Oil, Seed

**Side Effects:** Ai Ye is not recommended for use by women who are pregnant or nursing.

Ai Ye may cause an allergic skin reaction in some people.

Overuse of Ai Ye may cause gastrointestinal upset.

Additional uses and side effects may exist but further research is necessary to determine the exact properties and effects of use.

**General:** Ai Ye is an herbaceous perennial that spreads by rhizome. Native to China, Japan and parts of Russia, it grows easily on dry slops, wasteland and along roadways. The plants seem to grow better and produce a stronger aroma in poor, dry soil. Seeds can be direct sown or grown in greenhouse conditions and do best when a moist environment is maintained until the plant is established.

Ai Ye it is typically harvested during flowering in the late spring or early summer, shade dried, and powdered for use in traditional supplement teas.

**Ajwain, Ajava, Ajowan, Ajwon, Bishop's Flower, Bullwort, Caraway, Carom Seeds, Thymol Seeds**
**Botanical Names:** Trachyspermum ammi

**Properties:** Abortifacient, Antibacterial, Antifungal, Anti-inflammatory, Antiseptic, Antispasmodic, Aphrodisiac, Aromatic, Bronchodilator, Digestive, Diaphoretic, Diuretic (roots), Expectorant, Hepatic, Relaxant, Vermifuge

**Traditional Use:** Ajwain is traditionally used as a steam inhalant or essential oil aromatic to reduce the length and severity of the both bacterial and viral infections.

Ajwain has long been a traditional treatment for infection and is undergoing research for its ability to combat drug resistant microbial pathogens.

The high antibacterial, antifungal, and antiviral properties of Ajwain essential oil make it a traditional ingredient in air and spray based cleaning products.

Ajwain contains high levels of antifungal, antiviral, and antibacterial agents and is traditionally used to help enhance the immune system while combating infections.

**Part Used:** Leaves, Seed, Oil

**Side Effects:** Ajwain is not recommended for use by women who are pregnant or nursing. Ajwain has been used as an abortifacient in some cultures.

Ajwain is not recommended for use by diabetics due to the high sugar content.

Essential oils are for external use only and should be properly diluted prior to use.

Additional uses and side effects may exist but further research is necessary to determine the exact properties and effects of use.

**General:** Ajwain is native to the Eastern Asia and Europe but has naturalized in many other regions where it has been harvested for hundreds of years for use as a spice or dried for use in traditional supplements. Ajwain is a frost tender annual that blooms from July to August. It is not particular regarding soil composition but does prefer full sun and consistent moisture. The seeds are harvested at the end of the flowering season and direct sown in the spring after all danger of frost has passed.

Ajwain seeds are used as a flavoring and it is cultivated as a spice product in some areas of the world. The seeds are harvested when ripe and distilled as an essential oil and the leaves, seeds, and oils are used as a traditional medicinal component and in perfumery.

Indian herbalists use the Ajwain leaf to create a strong decoction that is traditionally used at a rate of 2 teaspoons 2 times daily.

## Akebia, Chocolate Vine
**Botanical Name:** Akebia trifoliata

**Properties:** Analgesic, Antibacterial, Antifungal, Anti-inflammatory, Cardio-Tonic, Diuretic, Emmenagogue, Galactogogue

**Traditional Use:** Akebia tea is traditionally used to treat gram-positive bacterial infections.

Akebia is used in traditional supplement teas to alleviate urinary tract infections and ease urinary urgency.

**Side Effects:** Akebia is not recommended for use by women who are pregnant or nursing.

Additional uses and side effects may exist but further research is necessary to determine the exact properties and effects of use.

**General:** Akebia is native to Asia but has been cultivated or naturalized to many other regions and is considered an invasive weed by some. Akebia is a semi-evergreen climbing shrub-like vine that grows at a fast rate and is hardy to zone 5. It blooms in the early spring and the seeds ripen in the late fall. Akebia grows well in any type of soil or sun conditions but does prefer moisture. It can be direct sown but seeds do best when given a month of cold stratification prior to planting. Akebia can also be propagated by cuttings or through air layering. It will self-layer readily if given enough space.

Akebia stems are pliable and have been used in weaving mats & basket products. Akebia fruits are eaten as a raw food and the leaves are used as a tea. It is harvested in the fall, dried, and powdered for use as a food and in traditional supplement teas and topical treatments.

## Alkanet, Bee Bread, Common Bugloss
**Botanical Name:** Anchusa officinalis

**Properties:** Antibacterial, Antimicrobial, Antioxidant, Astringent, Colorant, Demulcent, Expectorant, Vermifuge

**Traditional Use:** Alkanet has antimicrobial properties that make it a traditional treatment component against infectious agents like staphylococcus aureus, staphylococcus epidermis, and candida albicans

Alkanet has traditionally been included in antibacterial cleaning products and soaps.

Ointment containing Alkanet is traditionally used as a daily application to aid in preventing infection and speeding healing of skin sores, ulcers, and wounds.

**Part Used:** Root

**Side Effects:** Alkanet is not for internal use. Alkanet may have carcinogenic properties and should be used externally only.

Alkanet is not recommended for use by women who are pregnant or nursing.

Alkanet should not be used on broken skin.

Additional uses and side effects may exist but further research is necessary to determine the exact properties and effects of use.

**General:** Alkanet is a biennial native to Europe but has naturalized too much of North America where it is considered an invasive weed by some. Hardy to zone 5, it blooms from June through October with the seeds ripening in late summer or early fall. It is not particular regarding soil composition but does prefer good drainage and full sun. Alkanet is typically propagated by seed. Seeds can be started indoors during the spring or direct sown in the late fall for spring growth.

The flowers, leaves, and young shoots are eaten as a cooked vegetable. Alkanet roots yield a red toned colorant commonly used as a culinary, cosmetic, or textile dye product. Mordants and composition can alter the colorant toward brown or purple tones.

Alkanet has been used since the time of the Ancient Greeks to heal skin diseases and treat gastrointestinal ailments. Today it is used as a traditional topical ointment at a rate of 25% alkanet root to total volume applied to the skin up to 3 times daily.

**All Heal, Blue Curls, Brownwort, Carpenter's Weed, Heal All, Prunella, Self Heal, Woundwort**
**Botanical Name:** Prunella vulgaris

**Properties:** Abortifacient, Antibacterial, Antioxidant, Antiseptic, Antispasmodic, Astringent, Diuretic, Febrifuge, Hypotensive, Immunostimulant, Styptic, Sedative

**Traditional Use:** All Heal has been used as a topical ointment or skin wash to help reduce the number and severity of bacterial related acne outbreaks while the astringent properties reduce pore size and remove excess oils from the surface of the skin.

All Heal has traditionally been used to inhibit bacteria inside and outside of the body and some research indicates that it may be effective against bacterial infections like Pseudomonas, Bacillus typhi, E. coli, and Mycobacterium tuberculi.

All Heal's bruised, fresh leaves are traditionally applied directly to a wound to speed healing and prevent infection in skin sores, ulcers, and wounds.

All Heal leaves are traditionally boiled for use in sprays or gargles designed to ease the pain & inflammation of the throat while combating bacterial infections of the mouth and throat.

**Part Used:** Whole

**Side Effects:** All Heal is not recommended for use by women who are pregnant or nursing.

All Heal is not recommended for use in children's treatments without the guidance of a qualified herbalist or physician.

All Heal may cause allergic reactions in some people.

Additional uses and side effects may exist but further research is necessary to determine the exact properties and effects of use.

**General:** All-Heal is native to Asia and Europe but has naturalized in much of the world including North America. All-Heal self-seeds readily making it easy to find growing wild in fields, along the side of the road, and in other untended places. All Heal is easy to propagate from seed, division, or through air layering. Where the nodes touch the soil it will root readily, allowing the new plant to be separated from the mother. All Heal is a member of the mint family and will spread rapidly. Do not confuse All-Heal Prunella vulgaris with Prunella grandiflora.

All-Heal is harvested and the leaves and stem are washed to remove the bitter flavor and then eaten raw or the whole plant is boiled as a cooked vegetable. The aerial parts of the plant are harvested, dried, and powdered for use as a cold or warm infusion beverage.

The whole plant is harvested for use in traditional poultices where fresh leaves are bruised and applied directly to wounds or incorporated into a poultice for sprains & bruises. The plant is harvested, dried, and powdered for use in traditional supplement infusions or tinctures.

**Almond, Beach Almond, India Almond, Sea Almond, Tropical Almond, Umbrella Tree**
**Botanical Name:** Terminalia catappa

**Properties:** Anodyne, Antibacterial, Anti-inflammatory, Antioxidant, Aphrodisiac, Astringent, Cancer, Diabetic, Hepatic, Sudorific, Vermifuge

**Traditional Use:** There are numerous types of almonds and commercial almond oil may be derived from any of the nuts. Almond, Indian Almond, and Sweet Almond oil are all categorized in commercial preparations as almond oils. You should always verify the type of almond oil you are obtaining as different almonds could have different effects.

The leaves of the India Almond have traditionally been used to treat gram positive and gram-negative bacterial infections.

The India Almond bark, root, and nut are astringent and have been used as a traditional treatment for diarrhea and other loose bowel maladies, especially those relating to a bacterial infection.

**Part Used:**  Bark, Fruit, Leaf, Root

**Side Effects:**  India Almond is not recommended for use by women who are pregnant or nursing.

Almond oil should be extracted from the almond meat only.

India Almond may lower blood sugar.

Additional uses and side effects may exist but further research is necessary to determine the exact properties and effects of use.

**General:**  The India Almond tree can be found growing wild throughout India and Southeast Asia.  It is also cultivated in other warm climates as an ornamental tree and food crop.  The India Almond is frost sensitive and hardy to zone 8-11.  It is grown as a container plant in cooler zones.  The India Almond is an evergreen or semi-deciduous tree that bears fruit that tastes similar to the commercial almond.

The hard, red wood of the India Almond has a high water resistance level and is valued for its uses in construction and watercraft making.  The leaves of the India Almond are used as plates or for water treatment and purification.  The India Almond can be eaten raw.

**Aloe, Aloe Vera, Burn Plant, Elephant's Gall, Lily of the Desert, Sabila**
**Botanical Name:**  Aloe vera, Aloe barbadensis

**Properties:**  Analgesic, Anti-inflammatory, Antibacterial, Antifungal, Emollient, Healing, Hypoallergenic, Hypoglycemic, Laxative

**Traditional Use:**  Aloe is traditionally used to treat minor skin wounds and abrasions.  Aloe is believed speed wound healing by improving blood circulation, stimulating collagen regeneration, and preventing cell death while reducing inflammation and combating bacterial infection.

Aloe is believed to kill certain types of bacteria and fungi making it a traditional component in household cleaning products.

Aloe is traditionally used as a poultice for wound care because it is believed to have antibacterial, antifungal, and antiviral compounds that help to prevent wound infections.

The Food and Drug Administration (FDA) has approved aloe vera as a natural food flavoring.

**Part Used:**  Gel, Juice, Leaf

**Side Effects:**  Aloe bitters and aloe juice should not be taken internally during pregnancy, during menstruation, or in cases of rectal bleeding.

The laxative compounds in aloe are passed into mother's milk, so nursing mothers should avoid internal use of aloe.

Aloe can cause intense intestinal cramps if overused.

Overuse of aloe juice can cause diarrhea.

The FDA banned the use of aloe as a laxative ingredient in over-the-counter drug products in 2002, but it is widely used is commercial pharmaceuticals outside the United States.

The oral consumption of aloe leaf may cause cancer.

Consumption of aloe may cause lowered glucose levels.

Additional uses and side effects may exist but further research is necessary to determine the exact properties and effects of use.

**General:** Aloe is succulent native to Africa but can be grown as a garden plant in other warm climates to zone 10 and is cultivated as an indoor plant worldwide. Aloe prefers moderately fertile, sandy soil with good drainage and full sunlight. Aloe is related to the cactus and each part of the plant contains substances that are used in supplement treatments.

The green part of the leaf that surrounds the gel is used to produce aloe juice or dried latex.

**Alum, Alumroot, Coral Bell, Rock Geranium**
**Botanical Name:** Heuchera americana

**Properties:** Analgesic, Antibacterial, Anti-inflammatory, Antiseptic, Astringent, Cancer Mordant, Styptic

**Traditional Use:** Alum root has antiseptic, analgesic, and styptic properties that make it a traditional powder for the topical treatment of the pain, inflammation and bleeding associated with skin sores, ulcers, and wounds while acting to prevent infection.

Alum root powder is traditionally added to sprays or used as a gargle for relief from mouth and throat pain or inflammation and as an infection control agent.

**Part Used:** Leaf, Root - Powdered

**Side Effects:** Alum Root is not recommended for use by women who are pregnant or nursing.

Internal use of alum root may interfere with the absorption of other supplements.

Internal use of alum root may cause stomach irritation.

Internal use of alum root may cause kidney and liver damage.

Alum root is not recommended for internal use.

Additional uses and side effects may exist but further research is necessary to determine the exact properties and effects of use.

**General:**  Alum Root is an evergreen perennial ground cover with a mounding habit that grows to approximately 1 foot by 1 foot.  Native to eastern North America, it is hardy to zone 4.  Alum Root flowers during the summer and the seeds ripen in the early fall.  Alum Root grows easily in sandy or loamy soil and requires good drainage and full to partial shade.  Alum is easily propagated by direct seeding in the late spring or division in the early fall.  Transplants must be deeply planted with only the crown of the plant showing to ensure it thrives in its new environment.

Alum Root has been used as an alum substitute mordant in traditional dying and is harvested at the end of the flowering season for use in salads.  The mature root is also harvested, dried, and powdered for use in traditional supplement infusions and topical treatments.

## American Agave
**Botanical Name:**  Agave americana

**Properties:**  Antiseptic, Diaphoretic, Diuretic, Laxative

**Traditional Use:**  Agave stem sap has been used as a traditional topical or supplement preparation to treat bacterial infections.

Agave stem sap has traditionally been used as a gargle to treat bacterial infections in the throat, gums, and mouth.

Agave stem sap has been used as a traditional poultice component to help reduce infection and speed healing of skin sores and wounds.

**Part Used:**  Juice

**Side Effects:**  American Agave is not recommended for use by women who are pregnant or nursing.

American Agave may cause blood sugar changes.

American Agave sap may cause skin irritation in some people.

Additional uses and side effects may exist but further research is necessary to determine the exact properties and effects of use.

**General:**  American Agave is a succulent native to the Southern United States and South America but is cultivated in other regions.  Hardy to zone 9, it is not particular regarding soil or moisture composition but does require full sun.  American Agave can be propagated by seed sown out in the spring or by division of offsets any time.

Agave leaf and root extracts are used in soap making and the leaves are used to make rope or pulped to make paper. Agave hearts are eaten as a baked vegetable and the seeds are harvested and ground for use as a thickening agent or flour. The stem sap is used as a syrup substitute or the whole stem is eaten as a cooked vegetable.

## Andrographis, Indian Echinacea, Sambiloto
**Botanical Name:** Andrographis paniculata

**Properties:** Analgesic, Antibacterial, Antifungal, Anti-inflammatory, Antimicrobial, Antispasmodic, Antiviral, Astringent, Cholesterol, Febrifuge, Laxative, Immunostimulant, Sedative, Vermifuge

**Traditional Use:** Recent studies indicate that Andrographis may help to stimulate the immune system and it has traditionally been used to lessen the frequency & severity of infections when ingested regularly as a tea or juice and immediately upon noticing the symptoms of an infection.

Andrographis has strong antibacterial and antiviral properties making it a traditional component in natural cleaning products.

Andrographis is traditionally used in skin washes & topical ointments to prevent infection and speed healing of wounds, ulcers, and sores.

**Part Used:** Leaf, Juice

**Side Effects:** Andrographis is not recommended for us by women who are pregnant or nursing.

Andrographis is not recommended for use by women or men who are attempting to conceive.

Andrographis is not recommended for use by people who have an autoimmune disease like Multiple Sclerosis or Lupus.

Overuse of Andrographis may cause serious allergic reactions.

Additional uses and side effects may exist but further research is necessary to determine the exact properties and effects of use.

**General:** Andrographis is an herbaceous perennial native to Asia where it grows wild in the forests and wastelands. It can be cultivated elsewhere by direct or greenhouse sown seeds but needs 3-4 months of hot, humid weather to reach maturity.

The flower, leaf, and underground stem are harvested and juiced or dried for use in traditional supplement infusions sipped on an empty stomach.

## Anise
**Botanical Name:** Pimpinella anisum

**Properties:** Abortifacient, Antibacterial, Antiseptic, Antispasmodic, Aphrodisiac, Cancer, Carminative, Diaphoretic, Digestive, Diuretic, Expectorant, Galactogogue, Insect Repellant, Insecticide, Laxative, Phyto-estrogen, Stimulant, Tonic, Vermifuge

**Traditional Use:** Anise is traditionally used as a tea infusion, cough drop, or syrup made as 1 part anise seed essence to 4 parts base. It is given to break up mucus, ease congestion, and stop coughs associated with respiratory infections while having a secondary benefit of aiding in the elimination of germs.

Anise is traditionally given as an herbal tea to aid digestion, relieve upset stomach, and reduce flatulence while combating associated gastrointestinal bacteria.

**Part Used:** Seeds, Essential Oils

**Side Effects:** Anise is not recommended for use by women who are pregnant or nursing without the guidance of a qualified herbalist or physician.

Anise seed can be narcotic in large doses.

Anise seeds contain anethole, a plant hormone similar to human estrogen, and are not recommended for use by women who are pregnant, nursing, or for use by young babies.

Anise essential oil is for topical use only.

Anise may cause skin irritation, gastrointestinal upset or allergic reactions in some people.

Additional uses and side effects may exist but further research is necessary to determine the exact properties and effects of use.

**General:** Anise is an annual native to Africa and Southern Europe. It is cultivated worldwide as a garden or kitchen herb. Hardy to zone 8, Anise prefers a rich, well-drained soil in full sun. Anise should be planted after all danger of frost has passed and propagates easily from seeds. Anise does not care for transplanting but can be left to self-seed year after year.

Essential oils gathered from the seed have been used in perfumery, medicinal and dental care. Anise is used as an insect repellant, especially growing in the garden where it can repel vermin like slugs and act to protect nearby plants. Anise oils are sometimes diluted and sprayed on plants to protect against insects like spider mites and aphids.

Anise oil is often rubbed on traps to bait mice and other vermin. Gather the seeds when they begin to brown for the highest oil potency.

Young anise leaves and seeds are used as a raw or cooked vegetable and as a seasoning for a variety of dishes. Overcooking anise leaves can diminish the flavor. Anise seed oils are often added to sweets like ice cream and drinks.

Harvest Anise by cutting the ripe aerial parts along the length of the stalk and hang them to dry. The seeds can be harvested directly from the drying plant. Seed oil is extracted through steam distillation for liquid preparations.

**Traditional Delivery:**

1 teaspoon crushed anise seeds steeped 30 minutes in 1-cup boiling water.

1 to 2 drops of anise essential oil in an air diffuser.

2-3 drops of anise oil in 1 tablespoon massage base.

Anise seeds are used as a food seasoning.

Chewing anise seeds is sometimes used as an alternative to the tea.

**Annatto, Achiote, Bixin, Roucou, Lipstick Tree**
**Botanical Name**: Bixa orellana

**Properties:** Antibacterial, Antifungal, Antimicrobial, Antioxidant, Aphrodisiac, Astringent, Colorant - Culinary, Digestion, Febrifuge, Insect Repellant, Vermifuge

**Traditional Use:** Annatto leaf infusion has traditional been used to treat gram-positive bacterial infections.

Annatto leaf extract is traditionally used in creams and ointments to inhibit the growth of bacteria, speed healing and reduce blistering from burns, skin ulcers and wounds.

Annatto leaf and seeds are used as an infusion in cleaning agents designed to inhibit the growth of bacteria.

**Part Used:** Leaves, Seed, Pod

**Side Effects:** Annatto is not recommended for use by women who are pregnant or nursing.

Annatto may affect blood sugar levels.

Annatto may cause allergic reactions in some sensitive individuals.

Additional uses and side effects may exist but further research is necessary to determine the exact properties and effects of use.

**General:** Annatto is in actuality the extraction from the seeds of the Achoite tree. The tree is commonly called Annatto. Native to Central and South America, it has been naturalized to other tropical areas. Annatto is usually propagated by seed planted while still fresh. It is also possible to propagate Annatto by cuttings or air layering.

The entire plant is harvested, separated, and processed for use in a variety of preparations.

The seeds yield a yellow food colorant sometimes used for cosmetics and other items. The dye is water soluble and extracted by agitating the seeds in water.

The pulp remaining after the colorant has been extracted from the seeds has been used as a poultry feed or ground fine and used as a flour substitute.

The waxy residue left after the colorant has been removed from the seed coat is used as an insect repellant and has been used as a traditional treatment for treating intestinal parasites in animals.

Traditional supplement are made by simmering Annatto seeds in water for 5 – 10 minutes before grinding for use as an additive in traditional supplements.

The oils are extracted for flavoring or coloring by covering a layer of seeds with oil and heating on high until the seeds pop. The seeds are removed and the resulting oil is used as a colorant additive in foods and cosmetics.

## Apple
**Botanical Name:** Malus domestica

**Properties:** Amaphoretic, Antibacterial, Antifungal, Anti-inflammatory, Antioxidant, Astringent, Cancer, Cardio-Tonic, Cholesterol, Laxative, Vermifuge

**Traditional Uses:** Apple leaves have traditionally been used to treat gram-positive and gram-negative bacterial infections.

**Parts Used:** Fruit

**Side Effects:** Apple is not recommended beyond dietary uses for women who are pregnant or nursing.

Apple seeds contain cyanide and are poisonous.

Some people may have an allergic reaction to apple.

Additional uses and side effects may exist but further research is necessary to determine the exact properties and effects of use.

**General:** Most people are familiar with apples and eat them as part of their diet but the apple is also harvested for use as a traditional medicinal or as a dietary supplement. Studies indicate that the wild crab apple tree is now considered more beneficial than modernly cultivated apple trees.

Apple is used as a thickening agent in jams and other sweet culinary and the seed oil has been used in lamps. The wood is durable and hard making it desirable for use in small woodcraft.

Apple trees are not particular regarding soil composition but do prefer full to partial sun and consistent moisture. They can be propagated by seed with some care but are more commonly propagated by division of the suckers or by cuttings taken at the end of the growing season.

## Aquatic Apple Moss, Philonotis Moss
**Botanical Name:** Philonotis fontana

**Properties:** Analgesic, Antibacterial, Anti-inflammatory

**Traditional Use:**  Aquatic Apple Moss has traditionally been crushed and incorporated into a topical preparation to sooth and heal burns, cuts, and wounds while acting to inhibit bacterial infections.

**Part Used:**  Whole

**Side Effects:**  Aquatic Apple Moss is not recommended beyond dietary uses for women who are pregnant or nursing.

Additional uses and side effects may exist but further research is necessary to determine the exact properties and effects of use.

**General:**  Aquatic Apple Moss is a nonvascular moss plant native to most areas in the United States where it can be found growing wild in wet areas.  It is not particular regarding soil but prefers high moisture levels.  Aquatic Apple Moss's use as a topical treatment for skin wounds, ulcers and burns dates back to the Native Americans where the moss was crushed and incorporated into a honey poultice for wound healing and used as padding for broken bones.

## Arborvitae, American Cedar, Emerald Green, Thuja, Tree of Life, White Cedar, Yellow Cedar

**Botanical Name:**  Thuja occidentalis

**Properties:**  Abortifacient, Antibacterial, Antifungal, Anti-inflammatory, Antiseptic, Antiviral, Arthritis, Astringent, Coagulant, Depurative, Diaphoretic, Diuretic, Emmenagogue, Expectorant, Immunostimulant, Nervine, Rubefacient, Sedative, Styptic, Vermifuge

**Traditional Use:**  Arborvitae leaves and twigs are used as a traditional supplement tea or extract for their stimulating, expectorant, and astringent properties in treatments for respiratory problems like asthma, bronchitis, colds, congestion, influenza, and pneumonia.  Arborvitae is traditionally used to help stimulate antibodies and shorten the intensity and duration of bacterial and viral conditions.

**Part Used:**  Green Branches / Twigs, Leaf - Oil

**Side Effects:**  Arborvitae is a known abortifacient and should not be used by women who are pregnant or nursing.

Arborvitae has been used as an abortifacient in some cultures.

Arborvitae oil is toxic and should not be taken internally for extended periods.

Arborvitae oil should only be used under the care of a qualified herbalist or physician.

Arborvitae oil is a neurotoxin and use may cause convulsions, diarrhea, gastro-enteritis, increased heart rate, and spasms in high doses.

Arborvitae has immunostimulant properties and should not be used by individuals who have an immunoreactive illness like Multiple Sclerosis and Lupus.

Additional uses and side effects may exist but further research is necessary to determine the exact properties and effects of use.

**General:**
Arborvitae is an evergreen shrub native to North America and Asia that grows easily and is adapted to a variety of soil, sun, and water conditions though it prefers humid weather and regular watering.  Arborvitae is propagated by seeds sown out as soon as they are ripe or by cuttings taken in the late summer.

Arborvitae wood is used in crafts, fence posts, and shingle making,  The oils of the Arborvitae have been used as cleaners and insecticides.  The foliage is used as a source of vitamin C.  The shoot pith is eaten as a cooked vegetable or added to stews.  The inner bark is cooked and eaten or dried and ground to flour.

Arborvitae is typically harvested in the spring when the oil is extracted by steam distillation and the leaves & twigs are dried, powdered, and incorporated into traditional supplement infusions. 1 teaspoon of the leaves and tops were boiled in 2 cups of water by the Native Americans who then administered 1 tablespoon at a time to alleviate most internal symptoms or the oils were incorporated into recipes for topical preparations.

**Arrowleaf, Balsamroot, Oregon Sunflower**
**Botanical Name:**  Balsamorhiza sagittata

**Properties:**  Antibacterial, Antiseptic, Cathartic, Diaphoretic, Diuretic, Expectorant, Febrifuge, Immunostimulant, Sedative, Stimulant, Vulnerary

**Traditional Use:**  Arrowleaf root is believed to strengthen the immune system in a manner similar to Echinacea and is used in traditional preparations at a rate of 1-teaspoon tincture 2 times a day.

Arrowleaf sap and leaves have traditionally been used as a wound cleanser and balm to help speed healing and prevent infection in burns, ulcers, and wounds.

Arrowleaf root has traditionally been chewed or incorporated into sprays to alleviate throat pain, infection, & inflammation.

Arrowleaf root, stem, and leaf infusions have traditionally been used to reduce fever, expel excess mucus and increase immunity in common infections like bronchitis, colds, and influenza while acting to reduce the severity and duration of the underlying infection.

**Part Used:**  Root

**Side Effects:**  Arrowleaf is not recommended for use by women who are pregnant or nursing.

Arrowleaf may cause an allergic reaction in some people.

Additional uses and side effects may exist but further research is necessary to determine the exact properties and effects of use.

**General:** Arrowleaf is native to much of Western North America and is able to adapt to a variety of environmental conditions from desert to grassland to forest. A member of the sunflower family, it prefers moist soil and full sun and is propagated by seed but does not transplant well.

Arrowleaf roots, young shoots, and seeds have been eaten as a raw or cooked vegetable. The seeds are ground for a highly nutritious flour product and the leaves are boiled and eaten. The seeds yield a rich oil and the root has been roasted and ground as a coffee substitute.

Arrowleaf roots have been harvested for use as a traditional supplement for hundreds of years. The most common use for Arrowleaf is as an immunostimulant traditionally given as 1 teaspoon of the root tincture twice daily.

## Astragalus, Bei Qu, Huang Qi, Milk Vetch, Mongolian Milk, Ogi
**Botanical Name:** Astragalus membranaceus

**Properties:** Adaptogen, Antibacterial, Antihistamine, Anti-inflammatory, Antiviral, Cancer, Cardiotonic, Diuretic, Febrifuge, Hypoglycemic, Hypotensive, Immunostimulant, Nervine, Stimulant, Vasodilator

**Traditional Use:** Astragalus contains bioflavonoid, choline, and polysaccharide that have traditionally been used to strengthen the immune system and act as a preventative against bacterial & viral infections.

Astragalus capsules or teas are traditionally taken as an immunostimulant and preventative.

Astragalus has traditionally been used as part of a regimen geared toward helping to restore immune function in compromised individuals.

**Part Used:** Root

**Side Effects:** Astragalus is not recommended for use by women who are pregnant or nursing.

Astragalus may increase bleeding.

Astragalus may interfere with the effectiveness of a class of high blood pressure medications known as beta-blockers and with drugs that suppress the immune system.

Astragalus may affect blood sugar levels and blood pressure.

Caution should be used if you are on an immunosuppressive therapy as Astragalus may have immunostimulant properties.

Additional uses and side effects may exist but further research is necessary to determine the exact properties and effects of use.

**General:** Astragalus is native to China but can be cultivated in full sun, sandy and well-drained soil in other regions. Growing up to 6 feet tall, Astragalus is hardy to zone 6. It flowers in the late summer with the seeds ripening as the blooms pass their peak. Astragalus is difficult to propagate, as seed germination tends to be erratic. The seeds should be harvested when they are fresh, soaked, and then planted out immediately.

The roots of mature plants are harvested and incorporated into soups and teas or ingested as a tincture or powder capsule traditionally given at a rate of up to 5 tablespoons of the dried herb daily.

**Autumn Olive, Autumn Berry, Japanese Silverberry**
**Botanical Name:** Elaeagnus umbellata

**Properties:** Antibacterial, Astringent, Cancer, Cardiotonic, Stimulant

**Traditional Use:** The flowers of the Autumn Olive are traditionally used to treat bacterial infections such as aga e. coli, p. aeruginosa, s. aureus, and b. subtilis while the leaves have illustrated some abilities against both gram positive and gram-negative bacteria.

The leaves and flowers have been used in traditional supplements to help strengthen the immune system and shorten the length of common infections.

The antibacterial and astringent effects of the Autumn Olive have made it a traditional supplement for the treatment of urinary tract infections.

**Part Used:** Flower, Leaf, Seed, Oil

**Side Effects:** Autumn Olive is not recommended for use by women who are pregnant or nursing.

Autumn Olive flowers are believed to be a cardiac stimulant and should not be used without the advice of a physician or qualified herbalist.

Additional uses and side effects may exist but further research is necessary to determine the exact properties and effects of use.

**General:** Autumn Olive is deciduous shrub common in thin woods and lowland areas of Asia. It has been naturalized in other regions of the world where it is easily propagated by seed. Autumn Olive is hardy to zone 3 and is considered an invasive species in some parts of the Eastern United States. The Autumn Olive is often propagated by seed but may take two years to germinate. It can also be propagated by air layering or cuttings of branches taken in mid-summer. Autumn Olive is cultivated for its ability to fix nitrogen into poor quality or exhausted soils.

The fruit is eaten raw or cooked and is a source of essential fatty acids. The flowers, leaves, and seed are harvested for use in traditional supplements

**Babchi, Bu Gu Zhi**
**Botanical Name:** Psoralea corylifolia

**Properties:** Antibacterial, Antidepressant, Anti-inflammatory, Antioxidant, Antiviral, Astringent, Cancer, Cardiotonic, Diaphoretic, Diuretic, Laxative, Stimulant, Tonic

**Traditional Use:**  Bachi fruit extracts have traditionally been used to inhibit the growth of drug resistant bacteria.

**Part Used:**  Fruit, Leaf, Seed, Stem

**Side Effects:**  Babchi is not recommended for use by women who are pregnant or nursing.

Babchi may cause photosensitivity.

Babchi may cause excessive pigmentation.

Overuse of Babchi may be toxic.

Babchi seeds may interfere with treatments for depression.

Additional uses and side effects may exist but further research is necessary to determine the exact properties and effects of use.

**General:**  Babchi is an annual native to Asia.  It is not particular regarding soil composition but does prefer full sun and consistent moisture.  Babchi can be propagated by seeds soaked and sown out in the spring.

**Bachelor's Buttons, Blue Bottle, Bluebonnet, Bluebow, Blue Cap, Blue Centaury, Cornflowers, Cyani Flowers, Hurtsickle**
**Botanical Name:**  Centaurea cyanus

**Properties:**  Antibacterial, Antifungal, Anti-inflammatory, Antiseptic, Antitussive, Astringent, Diuretic, Emmenagogue, Febrifuge, Laxative, Purgative, Sedative, Tonic

**Traditional Use:**  Bachelor's Button or cornflower tea is traditionally used as a mild antiseptic and astringent eyewash for conjunctivitis and inflammation of the eyes.

Bachelor Button tea is traditionally used as an anti-inflammatory and antiseptic skin wash for cleansing of skin sores, ulcers, and wounds.

Bachelor Button flower tea has been used in traditional gargles to help sooth and promote healing of mouth ulcers & bleeding gums while minimizing related infections.

Bachelor Button tea has been used as a traditional treatment to alleviate urinary tract infections.

**Part Used:**  Flowers

**Side Effects:**  Bachelor Button is not recommended for use by women who are pregnant or nursing.

Bachelor Button may cause an allergic reaction in some people.

Additional uses and side effects may exist but further research is necessary to determine the exact properties and effects of use.

**General:** Bachelor Buttons are an annual, flowering plant native to Europe but have naturalized over much of North America growing wild in woodlands, fields, and along roadways. They can thrive in nearly any soil but prefer good drainage and full sun. Bachelor Buttons are propagated by seed and will self-seed readily once a bed has been established.

The young shoots and flowers are eaten as a raw or cooked vegetable. The flowers yield a blue toned dye product that is often used to color confectionaries and other foods. The colorant is mixed with alum to make a blue ink or dye.

The flowers are harvested during the summer months and used fresh or dried in traditional supplement infusions applied directly to the skin.

### Bael, Bilva, Bengal Quince, Stone Apple, Wood Apple
**Botanical Name:** Aegle marmelos

**Properties:** Antibacterial, Antimicrobial, Astringent, Demulcent, Digestive, Laxative

**Traditional Use:** The essential oil extracted from the Bael tree has traditionally been used to treat or prevent bacterial infections including infections of the gastrointestinal tract.

**Part Used:** Leaf, Fruit

**Side Effects:** Bael is not recommended for use by women who are pregnant or nursing.

Additional uses and side effects may exist but further research is necessary to determine the exact properties and effects of use.

**General:** Bael is a tree native to India and cultivated elsewhere as an ornamental and for its fruit. The fruit is eaten raw, cooked or sun dried. It is also used in drink making. The leaves and small shoots are eaten as a raw vegetable. The fruits & leaves are also harvested for use as traditional supplements.

### Bai Tou Weng
**Botanical Name:** Pulsatilla chinensis

**Properties:** Analgesic, Antibacterial, Anti-inflammatory, Antispasmodic, Cardiotonic, Detoxificant, Hepatic, Sedative

**Traditional Use:** Fresh Bai Tou Weng root has traditionally been used in topical preparations to ease the pain, inflammation, and bleeding associated with wounds while minimizing the likelihood of infection.

**Part Used:** Root

**Side Effects:** Bai Tou Weng is not recommended for use by women who are pregnant or nursing.

Fresh Bai Tou Weng may cause sedation, cardiac changes, paralysis, or even death.

Additional uses and side effects may exist but further research is necessary to determine the exact properties and effects of use.

**General:** Bai Tou Weng is native to Asia. Hardy to zone 6, it prefers sandy to loamy soil and requires full sun and consistent moisture. Bai Tou Weng can be propagated by seeds sown out as soon as they are ripe or by root cuttings taken in the fall after active growth has stopped.

Bai Tou Weng roots are harvested in the early spring or fall while the plant is not actively growing and used fresh or dried and powdered in traditional preparations.

## Balm of Gilead, Balsam Fir, Balsam Poplar, Canadian Balsam, Poplar
**Botanical Name:** Pinus balsamea

**Properties:** Analgesic, Anodyne, Anti-inflammatory, Antibacterial, Antimicrobial, Antiseptic, Astringent, Depurative, Diuretic, Stimulant

**Traditional Use:** Creams containing Balm of Gilead are traditionally used to ease pain, speed healing, and reduce infection in abrasions, burns, cuts, sunburn, and external hemorrhoids.

Balm of Gilead has been used as a traditional gargle to ease pain and inflammation, counter infection, and speed healing of a sore throat.

**Part Used:** Leaf Buds – Resin

**Side Effects:** Balm of Gilead is not recommended for use by women who are pregnant or nursing.

Balm of Gilead contains aspirin like substances and is not recommended for use in children's treatments or by those with sensitivity to aspirin.

Additional uses and side effects may exist but further research is necessary to determine the exact properties and effects of use.

**General:** Balm of Gilead is derived from the Poplar. The Poplar is a large tree up to 100 feet in height and 6 ½ feet in diameter. It can be found in many regions of the world and the American Poplar most commonly found in the United States contains the same supplement properties as those from other regions. It is hardy to zone 2 and is accepting of a variety of soil and shade conditions but requires protection from the wind and consistent moisture. It can be propagated by seed planted outdoors in the very early spring but germination is often poor so over-planting or indoor starts are beneficial. Some success has been had with propagation through air layering.

The inner bark is harvested, cooked, and ground into a fine flower for use as a thickening agent or mixed with other flour products for cereal and bread making. The bark is sometimes chewed raw and the resin is used as a gum or flavoring in sweet drinks and foods. The young shoots are sometimes used as a tea.

The buds are harvested in the late winter, boiled to separate the resin that is then dissolved in alcohol for use in traditional topical preparations.

**Balsam of Peru, Tolu, Quina**
**Botanical Name:** Myroxylon pereirae

**Properties:** Antibacterial, Anti-inflammatory, Antifungal, Antiseptic, Antiviral, Aromatic, Stimulant

**Traditional Use:** Balsam of Peru is an antiseptic that is traditionally used in washes & ointments to combat infection and help stimulate the repair of damaged tissues.

Balsam of Peru is an antiseptic that is traditionally used to help stimulate the repair of damaged tissues in washes & ointments to reduce infection and speed healing in skin sores, ulcers, and wounds.

**Part Used:** Bark Resin

**Side Effects:** Balsam of Peru is not recommended for use by women who are pregnant or nursing.

Balsam of Peru may be absorbed through the skin and prolonged or extensive use may cause kidney damage.

Balsam of Peru may cause allergic reactions in some people.

Balsam of Peru may cause sensitivity to sunlight.

Additional uses and side effects may exist but further research is necessary to determine the exact properties and effects of use.

**General:** Balsam of Peru is indigenous to the tropical forests of South America but is cultivated elsewhere for its wood and perfumery uses. It is mainly propagated by suckering but can also be propagated by seed and will self-propagate easily in a variety of soil, sun, and moisture conditions. It is considered an invasive species in some tropical regions.

The wood is sometimes used in woodcraft and the resin is frequently used in perfumery or as a flavoring. The oily resin is harvested for use in traditional topical preparations at a rate of 10% total volume, personal care products, and as a fragrance in perfumes, feminine care products, and household cleaners.

**Barberry, Agracejo, Berberry, Epine Vinette, Espino Cambron, Holly Leaved Barberry, Jaundice Berry, Mountain Grape, Oregon Grape, Pipperidge, Piprage, Sauderdorn, Sow Berry**
**Botanical Name:** Berberis vulgaris

**Properties:** Antibacterial, Anti-inflammatory, Antimicrobial, Antioxidant, Antiseptic, Antispasmodic, Cancer, Cholagogue, Colorant, Detoxification, Diuretic, Expectorant, Hepatic, Laxative, Immunostimulant, Laxative, Ophthalmic, Tonic

**Traditional Use:** An extract of Barberry bark is used in traditional preparations to treat conjunctivitis, sensitive eyes, and eyelid inflammation.

Barberry root & leaf tea is used as a traditional immunostimulant.

Barberry tea is traditionally given for its sedative effect that slows the passage of stool through the intestinal tract while inhibiting the ability of bacteria to implant in the intestine.

Barberry has been proven to help protect against various bacteria, fungus, and viruses making it a traditional component in a variety of washes, ointments, and supplements.

Barberry barks has traditionally been used as an antiseptic mouthwash to help speed the healing of mouth ulcers, kill mouth & throat infections, and alleviate inflamed throat and gum conditions.

Barberry contains berberine, a known anti-inflammatory and antimicrobial that is traditionally used to treat infections including salmonella, shingella staphylococci, streptococci, and yeast.

Studies show that barberry activates the macrophages, white blood cells that devour harmful microorganisms.

**Part Used:** Fruit, Root Bark, Stem Bark

**Side Effects:** Barberry should NOT be used by women who are pregnant or nursing.

Barberry should NOT be used in children's treatments.

Barberry is a Cox 2 Inhibitor and a qualified herbalist or physician should be consulted prior to use

Overdose may cause diarrhea, nosebleeds, stupor, or vomiting.

Barberry is not recommended for long-term use.

Additional uses and side effects may exist but further research is necessary to determine the exact properties and effects of use.

**General:** Barberry is indigenous to the United Kingdom and other parts of Europe but has naturalized throughout the eastern United States.  Often cultivated as an ornamental plant growing 1-3 feet in height and width, Barberry is hardy to zone 3.  It is not particular regarding soil composition or sunlight accepting semi or no shade.  Barberry seeds should be sown as soon as they are ripe, cuttings of this years growth can be taken in the early fall and suckers can be removed in the spring.

Barberry roots, bark, and stem produce a yellow toned dye product and the unripe berries have been used as beads.

Barberry fruits are eaten raw or cooked and are rich in vitamin C.  The fruits are used to make lemonade like beverage and as a culinary flavoring.  The leaves and shoot tips are used to make a hot or cold tea.

Barberry is harvested for either internal and external treatments where the fruit or root is traditionally made into a tea with 1 teaspoon used up to 2 times daily or a topical preparation at a rate of 10% barberry extract applied up to 3 times daily. The bark and leaf can be harvested, dried, and powdered for storage.

**Barberry - American**
**Botanical Name:** Berberis canadensis

**Properties:** Antibacterial, Cancer, Colorant

**Traditional Use:** American Barberry root is traditionally given to treat bacterial infection.

**Part Used:** Fruit, Root Bark, Stem Bark

**Side Effects:** American Barberry is not recommended for use by women who are pregnant or nursing.

Additional uses and side effects may exist but further research is necessary to determine the exact properties and effects of use.

**General:** American Barberry is native to eastern North America. Hardy to zone 5, it is not particular regarding soil composition but does prefer full to partial sun and dry to slightly moist conditions. It can be propagated by seeds sown out as soon as they are ripe or by cuttings taken in the mid-summer.

American Barberry root yields a yellow toned colorant used as a textile dye. The fruit is eaten raw or cooked and the leaves are eaten as a raw vegetable. The root is harvested for use in traditional supplemental preparations.

**Bay, Bay Laurel, Daphne, Grecian Laurel, Mediterranean Bay, Roman Laurel, Sweet Bay, True Bay**
**Botanical Name:** Laurus nobilis

**Properties:** Abortifacient, Analgesic, Antibacterial, Antifungal, Antimicrobial, Antiseptic, Aromatic, Astringent, Cancer, Carminative, Diaphoretic, Diuretic, Emmenagogue, Insect Repellant, Narcotic, Nervine, Rubefacient, Sedative, Stimulant, Vermifuge

**Traditional Use:** Bay leaves and leaf oils are antibacterial, antifungal, and antiseptic making them a common inclusion in household cleaning powder and spray preparations.

**Part Used:** Fruit, Leaves, Oil

**Side Effects:** Bay is not recommended for use beyond dietary by women who are pregnant or nursing.

Bay fruits have been used in some cultures as an abortifacient.

Bay may cause an allergic reaction in some people.

Bay may irritate the skin and mucus membranes of some individuals and should be used with caution

Bay oil should not be taken internally. Oil is for external use only.

Additional uses and side effects may exist but further research is necessary to determine the exact properties and effects of use.

**General:** Bay is native to Southern Europe and has been cultivated in other regions. Hardy to zone 8, Bay Laurel is not a winter hardy plant and should be brought indoors in much of the northern parts of the country. Bay is not particular regarding soil composition but prefers full sun light and good drainage. Bay is cultivated by seeds or cuttings taken during mid-summer.

Bay fruits yield an oil used in soap making and the leaves are used in insect repelling preparations. The leaves are used fresh or dried as a flavoring, tea, or harvested for use in traditional supplement preparations.

**Bergamot, Beebalm, Fragrant Balm, High Balm, Indian Plume, Mountain Balm**
**Botanical Name:** Monarda didyma

**Properties:** Analgesic, Antibacterial, Antifungal, Antiviral, Antispasmodic, Digestive, Nervine, Sedative

**Traditional Use:** Bergamot is an antibacterial, antiviral, analgesic and has been used in traditional treatments.

Bergamot essential oil is traditionally used against a variety of microorganisms and is often included as part of natural antibacterial and antiviral cleaning agents.

Bergamot leaf tea is traditionally used as an antibacterial wash to help speed healing in skin wounds and reduce the likelihood of infection.

Bergamot has been used in traditional gargle treatments to ease a sore throat and combat infection in the throat and mouth by blending 3 drops of bergamot oil in ½-cup warm water with ¼-teaspoon salt.

**Part Used:** Fruit, Leaf, Peel Oil

**Side Effects:** Bergamot is not recommended for use by women who are pregnant or nursing.

Bergamot is not recommended for use in children's treatments.

Bergamot increases sun sensitivity. Do not use on the skin when sun exposure is likely.

Additional uses and side effects may exist but further research is necessary to determine the exact properties and effects of use.

**General:** Bergamot is native to Asia and Eastern North America. Hardy to zone 4, it is not particular regarding soil composition but does prefer steady moisture and full to partial sun. Bergamot is propagated by seed planted in the late spring or by division in the spring or fall.

Bergamot leaves and young shoots are eaten as a raw or cooked vegetable. Bergamot fruit and leaves are harvested for use in topical & internal preparations as well as in fragrances, inhalant therapy, and natural care products.

## Bilberry, Arielle, Black Whortles, Beaberry, Brimbelle, Burnet Myrtle, Dyeberry, Huckleberry, Hurtleberry, Trackleberry, Whortleberry, Wineberry
**Botanical Name:** Vaccinium myrtillus

**Properties:** Antibacterial, Anti-inflammatory, Antioxidant, Antiseptic, Antiviral, Astringent, Cardiac, Colorant, Diuretic, Hypoglycemic, Hypotensive, Laxative, Vasodilator

**Traditional Use:** Bilberry fruit and leaves are used as a traditional supplement to help alleviate intestinal inflammation and decrease harmful bacteria in the digestive tract.

Bilberry leaf is used in traditional sprays, gargles, or teas to help reduce mouth pain & inflammation while combating related infection.

Bilberry leaf tea is traditionally used to reduce urinary inflammation, irritation, and infection.

**Part Used:** Leaf, Fruit

**Side Effects:** Bilberry is not recommended for use beyond dietary by women who are pregnant or nursing.

Bilberry may thin the blood and is not recommended for use by people who are on blood thinning medications.

Bilberry may lower blood sugar

High doses of bilberry leaf may be toxic and should be used with caution.

Additional uses and side effects may exist but further research is necessary to determine the exact properties and effects of use.

**General:** Bilberry is a relative of the blueberry and grows well in Asia, Europe, and North America where it is a seasonally blooming shrub with interesting blue berries. Bilberry prefers damp, acidic soil and moderate sunlight. It can be propagated by seed planted after all chance of frost has passed, by cuttings taken mid-summer, sucker division in the spring, or through air layering.

Bilberry leaf and fruits yield a green toned colorant used as a textile dye product. Bilberry fruits yield a blue or black toned colorant used in ink making. Bilberry fruit is often added as a dietary supplement or made into an extract. The green leaves are harvested in the fall for use in traditional supplement teas. The most common delivery method in traditional supplements is 80 milligrams extract up to 3 times daily.

**Birch Bark, Cherry Birch, White Birch**
**Botanical Name:** Betula pubescens

**Properties:** Analgesic, Antibacterial, Antifungal, Anti-inflammatory, Antiparasitic, Antiseptic, Astringent, Colorant, Depurative, Diaphoretic, Disinfectant, Diuretic, Febrifuge, Insect Repellant, Insecticide, Tonic

**Traditional Use:** Birch Bark has been used as a traditional gargle or topical preparation to help alleviate mouth ulcers, canker sores, or mouth & throat inflammation and related infection.

Birch bark has been used as a traditional treatment for urinary tract infections, inflammation, and irritable bladder.

Birch has been used in skin washes to help disinfect wounds and promote healing.

**Part Used:** Bark, Leaf, Root

**Side Effects:** Birch may have a blood thinning effect and is not for use by people on blood thinning medication, anticoagulants, or who have a disorder related to blood.

Birch is not recommended for use by women who are pregnant or nursing.

Birch is not recommended for use in children's treatments.

Birch is not recommended for use by individuals who are allergic to aspirin.

Birch oil is for external use only.

Birch is not recommended for use without the advice of a qualified herbalist or physician.

Additional uses and side effects may exist but further research is necessary to determine the exact properties and effects of use.

**General:** Birch is native to cold, northern climates and is a deciduous tree that grows well in many types of soil and sun conditions. Hardy in all zones, it flowers in the early spring with the seeds ripening in mid summer. Birch tolerates wind well and is sometimes grown as a windbreak. It can be propagated by seed sown indoors in the spring.

Birch wood is waterproof and resinous making it useful for a variety of light woodcraft like canoe skins and roofing tiles. The tar oil obtained from the tree is used as an insect repellant and shoe polish. Birch bark is powdered and used to repel insects from home perimeters and stored goods while the tar is used in liquid insect repelling applications. The inner bark yields a brown toned colorant used as a textile dye. Birch bark and roots yield natural dye products ranging in tone from red to purple-black. The inner bark has been used to make rope and as a paper making component. Birch sap is used as an adhesive and the inner bark is used to make cord and paper.

The young leaves are eaten as a raw or cooked vegetable and the inner bark of the Birch is eaten cooked or dried and ground into flour. The sap is used as a sweet flavoring or concentrated into a sugar by boiling it in water until the water evaporates. The sap has also been fermented into Birch Beer. Birch bark is harvested in the late spring and is peeled from the living tree rather than felling the entire tree for the harvest.

The bark and leaves are harvested, dried, and powdered for use in traditional supplement preparations and the oil is extracted from the leaf buds through steam distillation.

The bark and leaves are harvested, dried, and powdered for use in traditional supplement preparations and the oil is extracted from the leaf buds through steam distillation.

Betula lenta – Cherry Birch, Silver Birch - Betula pendula and Sweet Birch - Betula lenta have been used in much the same way as the White Birch.

## Birthwort, Guang Fang Ji, Pelican Flower, Pipevines, Red River Snakeroot, Sangree Root, Sangrel, Snakeroot, Snakeweed, Virginia Serpentary
**Botanical Name:** Aristolochia clematitis

**Properties:** Abortifacient, Antibacterial, Anti-inflammatory, Antispasmodic, Antiviral, Cancer, Depurative, Diaphoretic, Emmenagogue, Febrifuge, Immunostimulant, Nervine

**Traditional Use:** Birthwort has shown some ability to stimulate the immune system and is used in traditional immunity building regimen.

Birthwort has shown some ability to promote antibacterial and antiviral effects in the body and has traditionally been used to treat a wide array of infections.

Birthwort has been used in traditional topical preparations to cleanse, prevent infection, and speed healing in skin sores, ulcers, and wounds.

**Part Used:** Blooming Flower, Root

**Side Effects:** Birthwort is not recommended for use by women who are pregnant or nursing.

Birthwort has been used as an abortifacient in some cultures.

Birthwort contains aristolochic acid that is considered toxic and has been banned for use in many parts of the world.

Birthwort can cause nausea, abdominal pain, and vomiting.

Overuse of birthwort is toxic and can cause gastrointestinal upset, kidney damage, respiratory paralysis, spasms, vomiting, and even death.

Do not use birthwort until you have consulted a qualified herbalist or physician to determine if there is a less dangerous and more effective treatment available for your particular needs.

Additional uses and side effects may exist but further research is necessary to determine the exact properties and effects of use.

**General:** Birthwort is native to Europe, North America, and Mexico but has been naturalized to other parts of the world and is considered an invasive weed by some. Hardy to zone 6, it prefers rich, shady woods for growth but will grow in any soil composition or sun situation. Birthwort can be propagated by seed sown as soon as they are ripe in the fall, division in the fall, or by root cuttings taken in the late winter.

Birthwort was once a commonly used supplement treatment for a variety of body systems but has fallen out of preference due to the potential for toxicity. If Birthwort is indicated for a particular disorder, the advice of a qualified herbalist or physician should be sought.

### Biscuit Root, Fernleaf Biscuit Root
**Botanical Name:** Lomatium dissectum

**Properties:** Antibacterial, Antiviral, Antimicrobial, Expectorant, Immunostimulant, Ophthalmic, Stimulant

**Traditional Use:** Biscuit Root has both antibacterial and antiviral properties making it a common traditional supplement or topical preparation to help treat bacterial and viral infections.

Biscuit Root is commonly used in traditional disinfectant cleansers and as a steam air purifier.

Biscuit Root has traditionally been used in eye rinses to treat infections and inflammation of the eye.

Biscuit Root is used as a traditional preparation to stimulate the immune system helping to prevent or shorten the duration and severity of infections.

Biscuit Root is traditionally used as a wash to prevent or treat infections in skin sores, ulcers, and wounds.

Biscuit Root has been used as a traditional gargle to alleviate mouth & throat infections.

**Part Used:** Rosin, Root

**Side Effects:** Biscuit Root is not recommended for use by women who are pregnant or nursing.

Biscuit Root is not recommended for use by people with an immunoreactive disorder like Multiple Sclerosis or Lupus.

Biscuit Root may cause an allergic reaction or a full body skin rash in some people.

Additional uses and side effects may exist but further research is necessary to determine the exact properties and effects of use.

**General:** Biscuit Root is a flowering plant native to western North America and adaptable to a wide range of soil and water conditions. It does require full sun. Biscuit Root is propagated by seed sown as soon as it is ripe and self-seeds readily.

The root is eaten as a cooked vegetable or dried and ground for use as a thickening agent or flour additive. The root and resin have been harvested for hundreds of years for use in supplement preparations to alleviate a variety of infectious conditions.

**Bistort, Adderwort, Dragonwort, Easter Giant, Knotweed, Odorwort, Poor Man's Cabbage, Red Legs, Snakeweed, Sweet Dock**
**Botanical Name:** Persicaria bistorta

**Properties:** Antibacterial, Anti-inflammatory, Astringent, Demulcent, Diuretic, Febrifuge, Laxative, Styptic

**Traditional Use:** Bistort has been used as a traditional mouthwash or dental care ingredient to alleviate bleeding gums, mouth ulcers, mouth inflammation, and infection.

Bistort has been incorporated into a traditional gargle to treat throat inflammation, pain, and infection.

Bistort root has strong astringent effects and has shown an ability to stop bleeding, inhibit infections, and stimulate healing making it a traditional component in wound care preparations.

Bistort has been used as a traditional topical and supplement preparation to help treat ulcers caused by bacterial infection and as part of a treatment for peptic ulcers and ulcerative colitis.

**Part Used:** Leaf, Root

**Side Effects:** Bistort is not recommended for use by women who are pregnant or nursing.

Additional uses and side effects may exist but further research is necessary to determine the exact properties and effects of use.

**General:** Bistort is perennial native to Europe and adapted to North America where it can be found growing wild in damp meadows and near water. Hardy to zone 4, it is not particular regarding soil composition but prefers full or partial sun and consistently moist or wet soil. Bistort grows well in bog gardens and can be propagated by seed, self-sowing readily. The clumps can also be divided in the fall.

The young leaves are harvested for use as a salad or cooked vegetable and the leaves have been a traditional ingredient for an Easter pudding eaten during Lent. The seeds are boiled to remove the tannins and then salted and eaten plain or cooked in soups. The seeds have also been ground for use as flour.

The mature roots and young leaves are harvested in the spring when the plant begins to bud and dried in the sun for use in infusions at a rate of 2 teaspoons of the dried root in 2 cups of water steeped overnight delivered at a rate of 1 cup up to 3 times daily. Powdered bistort is typically included in external wound care preparations.

**Bitter Apple**
**Botanical Name:** Citrullus colocynthis

**Properties:**  Antibacterial, Anti-inflammatory, Antimicrobial, Cathartic, Purgative

**Traditional Use:**  Bitter Apple fruit, leaf, and root extract has been used as a traditional treatment against a variety of gram-positive bacterial infections.

**Part Used:**  Fruit, Leaf

**Side Effects:**  Bitter Apple is not recommended for use by women who are pregnant or nursing.

Bitter Apple is a strong purgative and is not recommended for internal use without the advice of a qualified herbalist or physician.

Additional uses and side effects may exist but further research is necessary to determine the exact properties and effects of use.

**General:**  Bitter Apple is a hardy perennial native to India and cultivated elsewhere.  It can be propagated by seed but is more often grown through division or cuttings taken in the spring.  It prefers sandy, well-drained soil, is drought tolerant, and is not particular regarding sun conditions.

The oils are extracted from the seed for use as a lamp fuel or culinary oil and the seeds are sometimes eaten fresh or cooked.  The fruits are harvested for use in dietary and supplemental treatments.

**Bitter Damson, Dysentery Bark, Mountain Damson, Simarouba, Slave Wood, Stave Wood**
**Botanical Name:**
Simarouba amara

**Properties:**
Abortifacient, Analgesic, Antibacterial, Antiviral, Astringent, Cancer, Diuretic, Febrifuge, Immunostimulant, Tonic, Vermifuge

**Traditional Uses:**
Bitter Damson leaf and bark tea contains high levels of tannins and are used in traditional supplement to alleviate severe diarrhea dysentery and malarial conditions.  Research indicates that Bitter Damson is effective at killing the salmonella and shingella bacteria.

Bitter Damson has been used as a traditional supplement to stimulate the immune system acting to prevent infection or shorten the duration of infection when taken as soon as systems appear.

Bitter Damson is traditionally used to treat both bacterial and viral infections.

**Parts Used:**
Bark

**Side Effects:**
Bitter Damson is not recommended for use by women who are pregnant or nursing.

Bitter Damson has been used as an abortifacient.

Overuse of Bitter Damson may cause gastrointestinal upset.

Additional uses and side effects may exist but further research is necessary to determine the exact properties and effects of use.

**General:**
Bitter Damson is a tree native to the Caribbean and South America but has been cultivated in other regions. It is not particular regarding soil composition but requires full sun and high moisture. \

Bitter Damson is used in woodcraft and papermaking but is most valued as a veneer product. The wood requires pest protection treatment. The bark is harvested, dried, and powdered for use in traditional supplements. Bitter Damson has recently gained interest by researches for its potential in treating viral infections, stimulating the immune system, and preventing or treating cancer.

**Bitter Wintergreen, Ground Holly, King's Cure, Love In Winter, Pipisissewa, Prince's Pine, Rheumatism Weed, Spotted Wintergreen**
**Botanical Name:** Chimaphila umbellata

**Properties:** Anodyne, Antibacterial, Antiviral, Anti-inflammatory, Astringent, Diuretic, Glycemic, Rubefacient, Stimulant

**Traditional Uses:** Bitter Wintergreen is traditionally used to treat urinary system disorders like bladder or kidney stones and urinary tract infections.

Bitter Wintergreen is included in traditional ointments and washes to treat skin and wound infections.

**Parts Used:** Leaf, Stem

**Side Effects:** Bitter Wintergreen is not recommended for use by women who are pregnant or nursing.

Bitter Wintergreen may affect blood sugar.

Additional uses and side effects may exist but further research is necessary to determine the exact properties and effects of use.

**General:** Bitter Wintergreen is an evergreen shrub native to Europe and Western North America but it has been naturalized in other regions. Hardy to zone 4, it is not particular regarding soil composition but does prefer full or semi-shade and moist soil. Bitter Wintergreen can be propagated by seed but is somewhat difficult to germinate. It does better when propagated by spring division or softwood cuttings taken in the early summer.

Bitter Wintergreen leaf and stem are harvested for use as a food, flavoring in root beer, or tea. The sprouted seeds have been brewed into an alcoholic beverage. Bitter Wintergreen has been used in traditional supplements for hundreds of years.

**Black Alder, Alder, Smooth Alder, Tag Alder**

**Botanical Name:** Alnus glutinosa

**Properties:** Antiparasitic, Antiviral, Astringent, Cathartic, Colorant, Dental, Emetic, Febrifuge, Galacogogue, Insecticide, Purgative, Styptic, Tonic, Vermifuge

**Traditional Use:** Black Alder bark decoctions have been used as a traditional topical preparation to reduce inflammation, treat infection, and speed healing in skin condtions like contact dermatitis, persistent sores, ulcers, and wounds.

Black Alder leaves and dried bark are traditionally powdered for use as a gargle to treat throat pain and inflammation and has shown some ability to clear staph and strep infections.

**Part Used:** Bark, Leaves

**Side Effects:** Black Alder is not recommended for use by women who are pregnant or nursing.

Black Alder bark is purgative when fresh. Only dried and powdered bark is used in supplement preparations.

Additional uses and side effects may exist but further research is necessary to determine the exact properties and effects of use.

**General:**
Black Alder is native to Asia, Europe, and North America. Hardy to zone 3, it prefers loamy or clay soil, full or partial sun, and moist to wet conditions. Black Alder grows quickly and has a reputation for fixing nitrogen into poor quality soil. Black Alder is cultivated by seeds sown as soon as they are ripe or by cuttings taken in the late fall and planted in sandy soil throughout the winter.

Black Alder is prized for yielding a wide range of dye products. The bark of the Black Alder yields a red toned dye used as a textile colorant and to make ink. The buds yield a green toned dye. Fresh, green Black Alder wood yields a fawn colored dye product. The bark and young shoots yield a yellow toned dye. Shoots harvested as soon as they appear yield a dusky brown toned colorant. The fruits yield a dark red toned dye.

Black Alder wood is water durable and has been used in a variety of maritime woodcraft.

Black Alder bark and leaves are harvested in the spring, dried and powdered for use in traditional supplements made with 1 teaspoon powder in 1 cup liquid. Fresh bark is purgative so only the dried bark is traditionally used for most treatments.

**Black Cherry, Black Choke, Chokecherry, Rum Cherry, Virginian Prune, Wild Cherry**
**Botanical Name:** Prunus serotina

**Properties:** Anodyne, Antibacterial, Anti-inflammatory, Antitussive, Antiviral, Astringent, Colorant, Expectorant, Sedative, Tonic

**Traditional Use:** Black Cherry bark and fruits are a traditional tincture cough remedy and is a primary component in many commercial cough treatments. Black cherry contains compounds that are excreted through the lungs increasing respiration and sedating the nerves that provoke a cough reflex that combines well with the antibacterial and antiviral effect to make it a treatment in asthma, bronchitis, colds, congestion, non-productive coughs, influenza, pneumonia, and whooping cough.

Black Cherry is antiviral & antibacterial and is traditionally used to minimize the length and severity of infections including upper respiratory infections like the common cold, bacterial pneumonia, and influenza.

An infusion of the Black Cherry bark has traditionally been used to reduce infection and inflammation of the eyes.

Black Cherry root bark infusions are used as a traditional topical wash to alleviate pain, speed healing, and combat infection in skin sores, ulcers, and wounds.

**Part Used:** Bark, Fruit

**Side Effects:** Black Cherry is not recommended for use by women who are pregnant or nursing.

Black Cherry is not for long-term use.

Black Cherry bark contains a highly poisonous substance called prussic acid and overuse can be toxic.

Additional uses and side effects may exist but further research is necessary to determine the exact properties and effects of use.

**General:** Black Cherry is deciduous tree native to North America and cultivated in Europe. Hardy to zone 3, it is not particular regarding soil composition but requires full sun and consistent moisture. It can be propagated by seed sown out as soon as it is ripe, by air layering in the spring, or by cuttings taken between spring and mid summer.

Black Cherry leaves yield a green toned dye product and the fruit yields a grayish green colorant. The wood is valued in woodcraft and the fruit is eaten raw or cooked in jams, preserves, and pastry. The juices of the fruit have also been used as a food, beverage, or medicinal flavoring. A decoction of the bark is used as a flavoring in baked goods, beverages, and medicinals while the young twigs are used as a hot or cold beverage.

Black Cherry bark and fruits are harvested for use in commercial and traditional supplement syrups. The bark separates from the tree easily making it easy to harvest, dry and power for use in traditional supplement tinctures, syrups, or infusions. It should not be boiled since this may destroy some of the active components so it is traditionally administered at a rate of 1-teaspoon bark steeped in 1-cup warm water given in 2 teaspoonful doses up to 3 times a day.

**Black Currant, Cassis**

**Botanical Name:** Ribes nigrum

**Properties:** Antiinflammatory, Antimicrobial, Astringent, Cholesterol, Colorant, Diaphoretic, Diuretic, Febrifuge, Immuno-Stimulant

**Traditional Uses:** Black Currents contain high levels of GLA and is used as a traditional supplement to help stimulate the immune system and ward off or shorten the duration and severity of infections.

Black Current leaf has traditionally been used as a gargle to help speed the healing of mouth ulcers and to alleviate the associated infection, pain & inflammation in both the sores and in sore throats.

Black Current has been used as a traditional wash to help prevent infection and speed the healing of wounds and skin ulcers.

**Parts Used:** Fruit, Leaf, Seed – Oil

**Side Effects:** Black Currant is not recommended for use by women who are pregnant or nursing.

Black current may slow blood clotting.

Additional uses and side effects may exist but further research is necessary to determine the exact properties and effects of use.

**General:**
Black Current is a berry native to Asia and Europe but cultivated in many other regions. Hardy to zone 5, it is not particular regarding soil composition but does prefer good drainage, consistent moisture, and full or partial sun. It is propagated by seed planted out in the fall as soon as they are ripe or by cuttings taken in the late summer or early winter with a heel of old growth.

The fruits yield a blue or light purple dye product and are eaten raw or cooked as a food or drink component. The leaves are used as a soup seasoning or tea substutite and the seed oil is valued for natural skin care preparations. The leaves are harvested for use fresh or dried in traditional topical and tea supplements.


**Black Jujube, Azufaifo, Badar, Ber, Black Date, Chinese Date, Da Zao, Jujube Plum, Red Date**
**Botanical Name:** Ziziphus jujuba

**Properties:** Anodyne, Antibacterial, Antifungal, Anti-inflammatory, Astringent, Cancer, Contraceptive, Diuretic, Emollient, Expectorant, Hepatic, Hypnotic, Hypotensive, Immunostimulant, Laxative, Narcotic, Sedative

**Traditional Uses:** Jujube fruit has traditionally been used to stimulate the immune system.

Powdered Jujube root has been used as a traditional topical preparation component to help heal skin sores, ulcers, and wounds while acting to prevent infection.

**Parts Used:** Fruit, Leaf, Root

**Side Effects:** Jujube is not recommended for use by women who are pregnant or nursing.

Jujube is not recommended for use by people who are trying to conceive.

Jujube may lower the blood pressure.

Additional uses and side effects may exist but further research is necessary to determine the exact properties and effects of use.

**General:** Black Jujube is a tree like shrub native to Eastern Asia and parts of Europe. Hardy to zone 6, it is not particular regarding soil composition but does prefer good drainage and dry or moist conditions. It requires full sun and is propagated by seed planted out as soon as it is ripe. Root cuttings can be taken while the plant is dormant or mature cuttings can be taken in early winter. The suckers can also be removed from the mother plant during dormancy. All winter propagation requires a greenhouse for growth.

Black Jujube fruit is eaten raw or cooked but can also be dried and eaten as a nutritive trail food or powdered for incorporation into recipes. The leaves are eaten as a cooked vegetable. The dried fruits are used whole or powdered for bread and cake making.

Black Jujube yields a hard wood used in tool making and other small woodcraft.

The fruit is harvested for use fresh or dried and powdered for incorporation in traditional supplements.

**Bladderwrack, Atlantic Kelp, Black Tang, Bladder Fucus, Cutweed, Fucus, Kelp, Kelpware, Knotted Wrack, Marine Oak, Norwegian Seaweed, Marina Rockweed, Rockweed, Rockwrack, Sea Kelp, Seaweed, Seawrack, Tang, Varech**
**Botanical Name:** Fucus vesiculosus

**Properties:** Analgesic, Antibacterial, Antiviral, Anti-inflammatory, Appetite Suppressant, Contraceptive, Laxative, Hyperthyroid, Hypoglycemic, Laxative

**Traditional Use:** Bladderwrack has shown some level of antiviral and antibacterial ability and has traditionally been used to inhibit bacterial infections and viruses.

**Part Used:** Whole

**Side Effects:** Bladderwrack is not recommended for use by women who are pregnant or nursing.

Bladderwrack is not recommended for use by individuals attempting to conceive as it may lower fertility.

Bladderwrack is a thyroid stimulant and is not recommended for use by people who have a thyroid condition or are on medication affecting the thyroid without the guidance of a qualified physician or herbalist.

Bladderwrack contains high amounts of iodine and may affect the thyroid in individuals who do not have a previous thyroid disorder and may raise the risk of thyroid cancer.

Bladderwrack may cause an allergic reaction in some people.

Additional uses and side effects may exist but further research is necessary to determine the exact properties and effects of use.

**General:** Bladderwrack is seaweed found growing on the coasts of the northern water bodies including the Atlantic Ocean, Baltic Sea, Pacific Ocean, and the North Sea. It is harvested year round along both the east and west coastline of North America and other countries and used at a 1:1 dilution in extracts for supplement use with the traditional dosage being 1 teaspoon administered 3 times daily.

**Blanket Flower**
**Botanical Name:** Gaillardia pinnatifida

**Properties:** Analgesic, Antibacterial, Antispasmodic, Colorant, Diuretic

**Traditional Use:** The leaves of the Blanket Flower have been used in traditional supplement teas to help alleviate the symptoms of an irritable bladder and painful urination or to treat a urinary tract infection.

**Part Used:** Leaves

**Side Effects:** Blanket Flower is not recommended for use by women who are pregnant or nursing.

Blanket Flower may cause an allergic reaction in some people.

Additional uses and side effects may exist but further research is necessary to determine the exact properties and effects of use.

**General:** Blanket Flower is a perennial that can be found growing wild in open fields. It is cultivated by seed in southern North America. Hardy to zone 8, it is not particular regarding soil composition but does prefer some sun and consistent moisture. Blanket Flower is sometimes propagated by root cuttings taken during the cold season months.

The seeds are traditionally harvested, dried, and powdered for use as a food and the leaves are harvested for use in traditional supplements.

**Blood Grass, Buchid, Cogon Grass, Gacon, Spear Grass, Wooly Grass**
**Botanical Name:** Imperata cylindrica

**Properties:** Antibacterial, Astringent, Cancer, Diuretic, Emollient, Febrifuge, Styptic

**Traditional Use:** Blood Grass has traditionally been used to treat bacterial infections like bacillus dysenteriae and staphylococcus.

Blood Grass flowers are used in traditional decoction washes to treat bacterial infections of the skin and urinary tract.

Blood Grass is strongly astringent, styptic, and antibacterial making it a traditional topical preparation to speed healing of skin sores, ulcers, and wounds while acting to prevent infection.

**Part Used:** Flower, Root

**Side Effects:** Blood Grass is not recommended for use by women who are pregnant or nursing.

Additional uses and side effects may exist but further research is necessary to determine the exact properties and effects of use.

**General:** Blood Grass is native to eastern Asia but has been cultivated as an ornamental grass in other parts of the world including North America. Hardy to zone 6, it is not particular regarding soil composition or water but does require full sun. Blood Grass can be propagated by seeds sown in the spring or division of the clumps.

Blood Grass fronds are used in basketry and as a filling for pillows and other soft products. The leaves yield a fiber used in papermaking. The young shoots are eaten as a cooked vegetable and the roots are chewed for their flavor. Burnt Blood Grass ashes are used as a salt substitute. The flower and roots are harvested for use in traditional topical and medicinal preparations.

**Bloodroot, Bloodwort, Coon Root, Indian Paint, Red Root, Sanguinaria, Sweet Slumber, Tetterwort**
**Botanical Name:** Sanguinaria canadensis

**Properties:** Antibacterial, Antifungal, Anti-inflammatory, Cancer, Cathartic, Colorant, Diuretic, Emetic, Emmenagogue, Expectorant, Febrifuge, Narcotic, Sedative, Stimulant

**Traditional Use:** Bloodroot is traditionally used to encourage the expulsion of excess mucus in conditions like asthma, bronchitis, and bacterial pneumonia while combating related infection.

Bloodroot is used in commercial and traditional mouth & tooth care preparations to prevent the formation of plaque, reduce gingivitis, and inhibit bacteria growth in the mouth. Bloodroot should not be ingested and is commonly used only in preparations that will be spit out of the mouth.

**Part Used:** Root

**Side Effects:** Bloodroot should not be used without the advice of a qualified herbalist or physician.

Bloodroot is not recommended for use by women who are pregnant or nursing.

Bloodroot is not recommended for use by people who have an inflammatory disease.

Bloodroot is for external use only.

Ingesting Bloodroot may cause drowsiness, nausea, and vomiting.

Overuse of Bloodroot may cause coma, low blood pressure, shock, and vision disorders.

Bloodroot may cause an allergic reaction in some people.

The FDA has ruled Bloodroot to be unsafe for use in foods, drugs, herbals, and beverages.

Additional uses and side effects may exist but further research is necessary to determine the exact properties and effects of use.

**General:** Bloodroot is a hardy perennial that grows to a height of 6-12 inches with white flowers that bloom in the spring. The root contains a natural red juice that looks like blood when the root is bruised or broken. It can be found in much of the United States and prefers low hillsides and forest borders. Hardy to zone 3, it is not particular regarding soil composition but does require full to partial sun and consistent moisture. Bloodroot is often propagated by seed sown in the spring, division in the early spring or late fall, or by cuttings of shoots taken in the late spring.

Bloodroot roots have a distinctive reddish-orange color and were used by Early Americans as a dye product. Orange colors are achieved without a mordant, alum yields a rust tone, and tin gives a reddish pink colorant.

The root has also been crushed for use as an insecticide or harvested in the fall, dried, and powdered for use in traditional treatments.

**Blueberry, Highbush Blueberry, Hillside Blueberry, Lowbush Blueberry, Rabbiteye**
**Botanical Name:** Vaccinium angustifolium

**Properties:** Antibacterial, Antioxidant, Astringent, Colorant, Hypoglycemic

**Traditional Uses:** Blueberry leaves are traditionally made into a tea or gargle for relief from the pain and inflammation of the throat and mouth and related bacterial infection.

Blueberry is a traditional treatment for bacterial urinary tract infections.

**Parts Used:** Fruit, Leaf

**Side Effects:** Blueberry is not recommended for use beyond dietetic by women who are pregnant or nursing.

Blueberry may lower blood sugar.

Additional uses and side effects may exist but further research is necessary to determine the exact properties and effects of use.

**General:** Blueberries are found in many regions of the world where they are consumed as a food and harvested for use in traditional supplements. Hardy to zone 2, blueberry is not particular regarding soil composition but it does prefer full to partial sun and dry to moist soil. Blueberries can be propagated by seed sown out as soon as they are ripe or by air layering.

Blueberry fruits are eaten as a dried, raw, or cooked food and the leaves and berries have been used as a tea. The antioxidant properties of the blueberry are being studied to determine the potential benefits blueberries may provide as supplements.

**Buckhorn Plantain, Chimney-Sweeps, Headsman, Hoary Plantain, Lamb's Tongue, Ribgrass, Ribleaf, Ribwort Plantain, Ripplegrass, Soldier's Herb**
**Botanical Name:** Plantago lanceolata

**Properties:** Antibacterial, Anti-inflammatory, Astringent, Colorant, Demulcent, Diuretic, Expectorant, Haemostatic, Laxative, Vermifuge

**Traditional Uses:** Buckhorn Plantain leaf is traditionally used in gargles and sprays for relief of mouth and throat inflammation and infection

Buckhorn Plantain leaves are traditionally used as part of a supplement to treat or prevent peptic ulcers.

Buckhorn Plantain leaf has been used in traditional topical washes and hot poultices to prevent infection and speed healing in wounds, ulcers, and other skin disorders.

**Parts Used:** Leaf, Seed

**Side Effects:** Buckhorn Plantain is not recommended for use by women who are pregnant or nursing.

Additional uses and side effects may exist but further research is necessary to determine the exact properties and effects of use.

**General:** Buckhorn Plantain is one of about 200 species of plantain found worldwide. Buckhorn is native to Asia and Europe. Hardy to zone 6, it is not particular regarding soil composition but does prefer full sun and consistent moisture. Buckhorn is propagated by seeds sown in the spring.

The whole plant yields a golden brown toned colorant used as a culinary, cosmetic or textile dyeing. The leaves are used in papermaking or eaten as a raw or cooked vegetable. The seeds have been eaten cooked or ground for flour. The leaves and seeds have been harvested for hundreds of years for use as a traditional supplement component.

**Buffalo Gourd**
**Botanical Name:** Cucurbita foetidissima

**Properties:** Analgesic, Antibacterial, Anti-inflammatory, Detergent, Insecticide, Laxative, Solvent, Vermifuge

**Traditional Use:** Buffalo Gourd fruits have been used as a natural cleaning product to remove grease spots from wood, the root as a lathering soap ingredient, and the root juices as a natural disinfectant.

Buffalo Gourd fruits have traditionally been mashed and incorporated into a topical salve or poultice to speed healing and prevent infection in skin sores, ulcers, and wounds.

**Part Used:** Fruit, Root, Seed

**Side Effects:** Buffalo Gourd is not recommended for use by women who are pregnant or nursing.

Buffalo Gourd may cause gastrointestinal irritation.

Additional uses and side effects may exist but further research is necessary to determine the exact properties and effects of use.

**General:** Buffalo Gourd is a climbing vine native to the Southwestern United States. Hardy to zone 10, it is not particular regarding soil composition but does prefer full to partial sun and dry to moist conditions. Buffalo Gourd can be propagated by seed sown out in the spring.

Buffalo Gourd has been used for hundreds of years as a food, the oils in cosmetics, the fruit as a soap product and the whole gourd as a ritual item. It is also used as a traditional supplement.

## Bupleurum, Bei Chai Hu, Hare's Ear, Sickle Leaf, Thoroughwax
**Botanical Name:** Bupleurum falcatum

**Properties:** Analgesic, Antibacterial, Anti-inflammatory, Antitussive, Antiviral, Carminative, Diaphoretic, Emmenagogue, Febrifuge, Hepatic, Immunostimulant, Sedative

**Traditional Use:** Bupleurum has been used in traditional supplements to help reduce the fever and cough associated with conditions like bronchitis, colds, influenza, and pneumonia and to help reduce the length and severity of the infection.

Buplerum has been used in traditional paste or poultice preparations to alleviate pain, prevent infection, and speed healing in skin boils, sores, ulcers, and wounds.

**Part Used:** Root

**Side Effects:** Bupleurum is not recommended for use by women who are pregnant or nursing.

Bupleurum is not recommended for use by people with an autoimmune disorder like Multiple Sclerosis or Lupus.

Bupleurum is not recommended for use by people who are undergoing treatment for hepatitis or are taking antibiotics.

Additional uses and side effects may exist but further research is necessary to determine the exact properties and effects of use.

**General:** Bupleurum is native to Asia and Europe but is cultivated in other regions. Hardy to zone 3, it is not particular regarding soil composition but does prefer full to partial sun and dry to moist soil. Bupleurum can be propagated by seed sown out in the spring or by division of the clumps.

The root, leaves, and young shoots are eaten as a cooked vegetable and the root has been harvested, dried, and powdered for thousands of years for use in traditional supplements.

**Burdock, Arctium, Bardana, Bardane, Begger's Buttons, Bur Oil, Burr Seed, Clotbur, Cocklebur, Gobo, Happy Major, Hardock, Harebur, Lappa, Love Leaves, Thorny Bur**
**Botanical Name:** Arctium lappa

**Properties:** Antibacterial, Antifungal, Anti-inflammatory, Antioxidant, Cancer, Carminative, Cholagogue, Depurative, Detoxification, Diaphoretic, Digestive, Demulcent, Detoxification, Diaphoretic, Diuretic, Hypoglycemic, Liver Function, Stimulant

**Traditional Use:** Burdock leaves, roots, and seeds are traditionally used to help to destroy bacteria, reduce inflammation, increase blood flow, and detoxify the blood.

Burdock roots & seeds are antibacterial and antifungal making them a traditional supplement and topical preparation ingredient to treat bacterial and fungal infections.

Burdock leaves are used in antibacterial and antifungal household cleaning preparations.

Burdock leaves have been used in traditional topical ointments and poultices to reduce inflammation, minimize infection and speed healing in skin sores, ulcers, and wounds.

**Part Used:** Leaf, Root, Seed

**Side Effects:** Burdock is not recommended for use by women who are pregnant or nursing.

Burdock may cause an allergic reaction in some people.

Burdock may lower blood sugar.

Consumption of Burdock root may cause flatulence in some people.

Additional uses and side effects may exist but further research is necessary to determine the exact properties and effects of use.

**General:** Burdock is a biennial native to Asia and Europe but has been introduced to North America and can often be found growing wild along ditches and roads. Hardy to zone 3, Burdock is not particular regarding soil composition but does prefer full or part sun and consistent moisture. It is propagated by seeds sown directly in the garden in the fall.

The roots are eaten as a raw or cooked vegetable or dried for later use. The roots have been dried and powdered for use as a sugar substitute in diabetic care recipes. The young leaves and stalks are harvested for use as a raw or cooked vegetable and the seeds are sprouted and eaten in a manner similar to bean sprouts.

The leaves, roots, and seeds are harvested in the first year during the peak growth for use as a food or made into traditional and commercial pharmaceuticals that are usually boiled at a rate of ½ - 1 teaspoon in 1 cup of water, allowed to steep for 30 minutes. Up to 3 x's daily.

## Burning Bush, Dittany, Gas Plant
**Botanical Name:** Dictamnus albus

**Properties:** Abortifacient, Antibacterial, Antifungal, Antispasmodic, Contraceptive, Digestive, Diuretic, Emmenagogue, Expectorant, Febrifuge, Galactogogue, Sedative, Stimulant, Tonic, Vermifuge

**Traditional Uses:** Burning Bush root bark infusions are traditionally used to treat bacterial infections.

**Parts Used:** Root Bark

**Side Effects:** Burning Bush is not recommended for use by women who are pregnant or nursing.

Burning Bush may have a contraceptive affect and is not recommended for use by women who are trying to conceive.

Burning Bush may cause photosensitivity in some people.

Additional uses and side effects may exist but further research is necessary to determine the exact properties and effects of use.

**General:** The Burning Bush is native to Asia & Europe and is cultivated in the United States. Hardy to zone 3, it prefers sandy to loamy soil, full sun, and consistent moisture. It can be propagated by seeds sown out as soon as they are ripe, spring division or winter root cuttings.

Burning Bush yields an essential oils used in cosmetics and the root bark is harvested in the fall, dried, and powdered for use in traditional preparations.

## Cajeput, Paperbark Tree, Swamp Tea Tree, White Tea Tree
**Botanical Name:** Melaleuca leucadendron

**Properties:** Analgesic, Antibacterial, Antimicrobial, Antiviral, Astringent, Carminative, Emollient, Estrogenic, Expectorant, Febrifuge, Immunostimulant, Insect Repellant, Insecticide, Rubefacient

**Traditional Use:** Cajeput has been added to household cleansing preparations to help reduce bacteria and viruses on solid and soft surfaces.

Cajeput is traditionally used in a hot vapor air purification treatments to cleanse the air of bacteria and viruses.

Cajuput is used as part of a traditional aromatic treatment for the relief of sinus and chest congestion associated with conditions like bronchitis, colds, allergies, and pneumonia and to help shorten the duration or lessen the severity of common infections.

**Part Used:**  Leaves, Twigs

**Side Effects:**  Cajeput is not recommended for use by women who are pregnant or nursing.

Cajeput is not recommended in children's treatments.

Cajeput is not recommended for use by people with kidney problems.

Cajeput may worsen asthma symptoms in some people.

Cajeput may cause skin irritation.  You should dilute it before applying Cajeput to the skin and it is not recommended for use in the facial area.

Additional uses and side effects may exist but further research is necessary to determine the exact properties and effects of use.

**General:**  Cajeput is native to Australia and Asia preferring extremely wet conditions for optimal growth.

Cajeput oil is extracted from the leaves and twigs of the tree and blended with other oils for use as a traditional supplement diluted at 5 drops Cajeput to 1-tablespoon carrier oil.

**Calafate, Chitra, Magellan Barberry**
**Botanical Name:**  Berberis microphylla

**Properties:**  Antibacterial, Astringent, Cancer, Colorant, Diaphoretic, Febrifuge, Laxative, Tonic

**Traditional Use:**  Calafate root infusions are traditionally used to treat bacterial infections in the gastrointestinal system.

Calafate root has been used as a traditional soak wash for the treatment of conjunctivitis, sun damage to the eyes, and to reduce swollen eyes.

**Part Used:**  Root, Stem

**Side Effects:**  Calafate is not recommended for use by women who are pregnant or nursing.

Additional uses and side effects may exist but further research is necessary to determine the exact properties and effects of use.

**General:**  Calafate is an evergreen shrub native to South America.  Hardy to zone 5, it is not particular regarding soil composition, but does prefer full to partial sun and dry to moist soil.  Calafate can be propagated by seed sown out as soon as it is ripe or by cuttings taken in mid summer.

Calafate fruit is eaten raw or cooked and has been dried in a manner similar to the raisin.  The stem and root are harvested, dried, and powdered for use in traditional preparations.

**Calendula, Bull Flower, Gold Bloom, Holligold, Marigold, Mercadela, Pot Marigold, Zergul**
**Botanical Name:** Calendula officinalis

**Properties:** Analgesic, Antibacterial, Antifungal, Anti-inflammatory, Antioxidant, Antispasmodic, Astringent, Cancer, Colorant, Contraceptive, Detoxification, Estrogenic, Febrifuge, Hepatic, Immunostimulant

**Traditional Use:** Calendula blossoms are anti-inflammatory, astringent, and antibacterial making them a traditional component in topical washes and ointments for the treatment of wounds and injuries including acne, burns, bruises, skin sores, skin ulcers, and minor wounds. Simmer with preferred ingredients, like milk or a lotion base and apply directly to the skin.

Calendula tea is a gentle antibacterial and anti-inflammatory that has been used as part of traditional eyewash for inflammation and in treatments for conditions like pink eye and other infections.

Calendula is traditionally used to help enhance the immune system by neutralizing the free radicals that suppress the body's immune function.

Calendula infusions have been used as a traditional gargle to reduce pain, infection, & inflammation in the throat & mouth and to speed the healing of mouth ulcers.

Calendula is traditionally used to minimize infection and accelerate healing in skin sores, ulcers, and wounds.

Calendula has been used as a traditional supplement to prevent and treat the bacteria that causes some peptic ulcers.

**Part Used:** Flowers, Oil

**Side Effects:** Calendula is not recommended for use by women who are pregnant or nursing.

Calendula has been used as a male contraceptive and should not be used by men and women who are trying to conceive.

Calendula may cause an allergic reaction in some people.

Additional uses and side effects may exist but further research is necessary to determine the exact properties and effects of use.

**General:** Calendula is an annual native to the Mediterranean but is cultivated as an annual garden plant in much of the world. Hardy to zone 6, it is not particular regarding soil composition but does prefer good drainage, full or part sun, and consistent moisture. Calendula is easy to grow from seed and will self-seed readily if given its own place in the garden.

The leaves are eaten raw and the flowers are eaten raw or dried for use as a seasoning and as a saffron substitute. The seeds are nutritive and have been ground for use as a nutritional supplement.

Calendula is grown as an insect repellant in the garden, helping to protect nearby plants from infestation. Calendula flowers yield a dye product in tones of yellow, gold, and orange and calendula oils from the plant are used in perfumery.

The deep orange flowers should be harvested while in bloom and dried in the shade. Calendula is traditionally dried and powdered for use as a tea up to 3 times daily but has also been used as a tincture or topical salve additive.

## Camu Camu, Cacari, Camo Camo, Rumberry
**Botanical Name:** Myrciaria dubia

**Properties:** Antibacterial, Antioxidant, Antiviral, Balancing, Immunostimulant, Neuroprotective

**Traditional Uses:** Camu Camu is traditionally used in supplements to protect against and treat common bacterial and viral infections.

Camu Camu contains large amounts of vitamin C and is used as a traditional preparation to help strengthen the immune system.

**Parts Used:** Fruit, Leaf

**Side Effects:** Camu Camu is not recommended for use by women who are pregnant or nursing.

Additional uses and side effects may exist but further research is necessary to determine the exact properties and effects of use.

**General:** Camu Camu is native to the rainforests of South America and has been cultivated indoors in other regions. Camu Camu requires damp, warm surroundings in order to thrive and it can be propagated by seeds or division of the suckers in the spring.

The fruit is used as a food and the fruit and leaves are harvested for use in traditional supplements.

## Cancer Bush, Copperleaf, Field Copperleaf
**Botanical Name:** Acalypha arvensis

**Properties:** Antibacterial, Antifungal, Diuretic, Insecticide

**Traditional Use:** Cancer Bush is traditionally used to prevent bacterial infections like staphylococcus, fungal infections like athlete's foot, or parasitic infestations like scabies.

Cancer Bush has been used as a traditional powder application or strong tea wash to speed healing in skin sores, ulcers, and wounds while acting to prevent infection.

Cancer Bush has traditionally been used in supplements to increase urination and alleviate the bacteria associated with a urinary tract infection.

**Part Used:** Whole

**Side Effects:**  Cancer Bush is not recommended for use by women who are pregnant or nursing.

Additional uses and side effects may exist but further research is necessary to determine the exact properties and effects of use.

**General:**  Cancer Bush is native to Central America, North America, and South America where the whole plant has been harvested and dried for use as a powder topical application or as a traditional tea based internal or external treatment.  Do not confuse cancer bush Acalypha arvensis with Sutherlandia frutescens that is called by the same common name.

### Cannabis, Anashca, Banji, Bhang, Blunt, Bud, Charas, Ganga, Grass, Hash, Hemp, Marijuana, Mary Jane, Sawi, Sinsemilla
**Botanical Name:**  Cannabis sativa

**Properties:**  Analgesic, Anodyne, Antibacterial, Antispasmodic, Cancer, Cholagogue, Demulcent, Diuretic, Emmenagogue, Emollient, Febrifuge, Hypnotic, Narcotic, Nervine, Psychedelic, Sedative, Tonic

**Traditional Use:**  Cannabis has traditionally been used in treatment plans against gram-positive bacteria and may be a natural antibiotic.

**Part Used:**  Flower, Leaf, Seed

**Side Effects:**  Cannabis is not recommended for use by women who are pregnant or nursing.

Cannabis is not recommended for use by people who have heart disease, lung disease, a weakened immune system, or seizure disorders.

Cannabis is a psychotropic plant and use or overuse can be hazardous.

Cannabis is an illegal substance in the United States.

Additional uses and side effects may exist but further research is necessary to determine the exact properties and effects of use.

**General:**  Cannabis is native to Asia but has been naturalized in many parts of the world.  Hardy to zone 9, it is not particular regarding soil composition but does require full sun and consistent moisture.  Cannabis can be propagated by seeds sown in the spring after all danger of frost has passed.

Female Cannabis seeds yield oil used in lighting, soap making, and paints while the male yields a fiber used in paper, clothing, and rope making.  Cannabis seeds are eaten raw or cooked and the male plant leaves are harvested for use in traditional preparations.

### Carlina, Carline Thistle, Dwarf Carline, Ground Thistle, Stemless Carline
**Botanical Name:**  Carlina acaulis

**Properties:**  Antibacterial, Antibiotic, Antifungal, Antiseptic, Antispasmodic, Antiviral, Carminative, Diaphoretic, Diuretic, Emetic, Febrifuge, Vermifuge

**Traditional Use:** The essential oil of the Carline Thistle root have been incorporated into steam based air purification recipes to eliminate bacteria and viruses in the home.

The essential oil of the Carline Thistle root has antibacterial and antiviral properties and has been incorporated into household cleaners.

Carline Thistle is traditionally included in topical washes and ointments to prevent infection and speed healing of skin sores, ulcers, and wounds.

Carline Thistle has been used as a traditional gargle component for throat & mouth inflammation, sores, and infections.

**Part Used:** Root - Oil

**Side Effects:** Carline Thistle is not recommended for use by women who are pregnant or nursing.

Carline Thistle may cause an allergic reaction in some people.

Overuse of Carline Thistle is purgative.

Additional uses and side effects may exist but further research is necessary to determine the exact properties and effects of use.

**General:** Carline Thistle is native to Europe and naturalized to North America. Hardy to zone 4, it is not particular regarding soil composition but does prefer full sun and consistent moisture. It is propagated by seed surface sown in the spring.

Carline Thistle flowering heads are eaten as a cooked vegetable and the root and stems are peeled and steamed. The root is harvested in the fall and dried for use in tea traditionally given at a rate of 2 teaspoons root powder to 1 cup of water 3 times daily. The root is also steam distilled to extract the essential oils.

**Cashew, Cajueiro, Jambu**
**Botanical Name:** Anacardium occidentale

**Properties:** Antibacterial, Antimicrobial, Antiviral, Astringent, Hypoglycemic, Insecticide, Stimulant, Vermifuge

**Traditional Use:** Cashew essential oil has illustrated antimicrobial effects and has traditionally been used in treatments against gram-positive bacteria such as bacillus subtilis, and staphylococcus aureus.

The bark of the Cashew tree has astringent properties as well as infection fighting elements and is used in traditional gargles for the relief from gum inflammation, toothaches, and throat infections including strep throat.

**Part Used:** Bark, Nut, Resin - Oil

**Side Effects:** Cashew shell oils can cause skin irritation. Always heat the oils before use to minimize the caustic effect and dilute them when possible.

Use only roasted nuts.

Additional uses and side effects may exist but further research is necessary to determine the exact properties and effects of use.

**General:** The cashew is an evergreen native to Central & South America and cultivated in other tropical zones.

The nut is used as a food and the fruits are eaten or fermented into alcohol. The bark, hulls, and hull oil are often harvested for use in supplement poultices, rinses, and ointments.

## Century Plant, Mescal Agave, Parry's Agave
**Botanical Name:** Agave parryi

**Properties:** Antiseptic, Diaphoretic, Diuretic, Laxative

**Traditional Use:** Century Plant stem sap has been used as a traditional topical or supplement preparation to treat bacterial infections.

Century Plant stem sap has traditionally been used as a gargle to treat bacterial infections in the throat, gums, and mouth.

Century Plant stem sap has been used as a traditional poultice component to help reduce infection and speed healing of skin sores and wounds.

**Part Used:** Juice

**Side Effects:** Century Plant is not recommended for use by women who are pregnant or nursing.

Century Plant may cause blood sugar changes.

Century Plant sap may cause skin irritation in some people.

Additional uses and side effects may exist but further research is necessary to determine the exact properties and effects of use.

**General:** Century Plant is native to the Southwestern United States and Mexico and naturalized to other regions. Hardy to zone 8, it prefers sandy or loamy soil, full sun, and consistent moisture. Century Plant is easily propagated by seed or by division of the suckers growing around the mother plant.

Century Plant leaf and root extracts are used in soap making and the leaves are used to make rope or pulped to make paper. Century Plant hearts are eaten as a baked vegetable and the seeds are harvested and ground for use as a thickening agent or flour. The stem sap is used as a syrup substitute or the whole stem is eaten as a cooked vegetable.

**Chanca Piedra, Amli, Bhonya, Cane Peas, Cane Senna, Creole Senna, Hurricane Weed, Jar Amla, Mapatan, Quebrapedera, Quinine Weed, Rami Buah, Sasha Foster, Shatter Stone, Stone Breaker, Tamalaka**
**Botanical Name:** Phyllanthus niruri

**Properties:** Antibacterial, Anti-inflammatory, Antispasmodic, Antiviral, Diuretic, Emmenagogue, Febrifuge, Hypoglycemic, Immunostimulant

**Traditional Use:** Chanca Piedra has been used in traditional preparations to alleviate infection, pain, and spasms of the urinary tract.

**Part Used:** Flower, Leaf

**Side Effects:** Chanca Piedra is not recommended for use by women who are pregnant or nursing.

Chanca Piedra may affect blood sugar.

Additional uses and side effects may exist but further research is necessary to determine the exact properties and effects of use.

**General:** Chanca Piedra is a common tropical plant and is considered an invasive species in some regions. Hardy to zone 6, It is not particular regarding soil or sun conditions but does prefer consistent moisture. It can be propagated by seeds soaked and sown in the spring and will self-sow readily if given its own place in the garden.

The supplement benefits of the plant are usually extracted using a water bath method and taken as a tincture. Chanca Piedra has been used for thousands of years as a traditional supplement and is being researched for inclusion in commercial pharmaceuticals.

**Chaparral, Creosote Bush, Greasewood, Hedionilla, Jarilla**
**Botanical Name:** Larrea tridentata

**Properties:** Analgesic, Antibacterial, Antifungal, Antioxidant, Expectorant, Laxative

**Traditional Use:** Chaparral tincture is used as a traditional ingredient in alcohol based topical treatments to reduce pain and deter infection in skin sores, ulcers, and wounds.

A decoction of Chaparral twigs and leaves is traditionally used as a gargle to alleviate tooth, throat, and mouth pain while helping to fight bacterial infection in the throat or mouth.

**Part Used:** Flower, Leaf, Fruit

**Side Effects:** Chaparral is not recommended for use by women who are pregnant or nursing.

Chaparral is for external use only – prolonged ingestion of chaparral can cause liver damage.

Chaparral is not recommended for long-term use.

Chaparral may cause diarrhea, fever, headache, kidney damage, liver damage, nausea, stomach pain, weight loss, and allergic skin reactions.

Additional uses and side effects may exist but further research is necessary to determine the exact properties and effects of use.

**General:** Chaparral is an evergreen shrub native to the southwestern regions of the United States and Mexico. Hardy to zone 8, it is not particular regarding soil composition but does prefer full or part shade and consistent moisture. It is typically propagated by seed but can also be grown from cuttings of new growth taken in the late spring.

The flower bulbs are eaten as a pickled vegetable. The stems and leaves are used as a tea alternative. The leaves and twigs are juiced and the resulting resin is used as a preservative to keep oils from becoming rancid.

The flower, leaf, and fruit of the Chaparral are harvested for use as a tincture or traditional supplement up to 3 times daily.

### Chaulmoogra, De Feng Zi, Hydnocarp, Gynocardia Oil
**Botanical Name:** Hydnocarpus wightiana

**Properties:** Antibacterial, Antimicrobial, Febrifuge, Nervine, Sedative, Tonic

**Traditional Uses:** Chaulmoogra has traditionally been used as part of a topical preparation to prevent infection and speed healing of skin sores, ulcers, and wounds.

**Parts Used:** Seed - Oil

**Side Effects:** Chaulmoogra is not recommended for use by women who are pregnant or nursing.

Chaulmoogra should NOT be taken internally. Chaulmoogra contains Cyanide.

Additional uses and side effects may exist but further research is necessary to determine the exact properties and effects of use.

**General:** Chaulmoogra is native to India and cultivated in other regions where the seed is harvested for use in traditional topical preparations.

### Cherokee Rose, Brier Rose, Dog Rose, Hip Rose
**Botanical Name:** Rosa laevigata

**Properties:** Antibacterial, Antioxidant, Astringent, Cancer, Carminative, Depurative, Diuretic, Emmenagogue, Vulnerary

**Traditional Use:** Cherokee Rose hips, leaves, and roots have traditionally been used as a supplement infusion to alleviate bacterial infections of the urinary tract.

**Part Used:** Hip, Leaf, Root

**Side Effects:**  Cherokee Rose is not recommended for use by women who are pregnant or nursing.

Cherokee Rose may cause an allergic reaction in some people.

Additional uses and side effects may exist but further research is necessary to determine the exact properties and effects of use.

**General:**  Cherokee Rose is native to Asia and North America.  Hardy to zone 7, it is not particular regarding soil composition but does prefer full sun and consistent moisture.  Cherokee Rose can be propagated by seeds but is often slow to germinate.  It can also be propagated by cuttings taken in mid summer, division of suckers during the dormant season or layering.

Cherokee Rose fruits are eaten raw or cooked and the hips have been harvested as a sugar substitute, wine ingredient, and food product.  The hip, leaf, and root have also been harvested for use as a tea option and as a traditional supplement.

**Chicory, Achicoria, Succory, Wild Endive**
**Botanical Name:**  Cichorium intybus

**Properties:**  Abortifacient, Antibacterial, Anti-inflammatory, Cardio-Tonic, Depurative, Diuretic, Immunostimulant, Laxative

**Traditional Use:**  Chicory contains a photochemical that supports the immune system as well as compounds that help to fight inflammation and bacterial infections making it a traditional addition to immunity building and infection control treatments.

Bruised Chicory leaves have traditionally been used in fresh poultice preparations and soaks to fight infection and reduce inflammation in skin sores, ulcers, and wounds.

Chicory has been used in traditional supplements to reduce irritation of the urinary tract and as part of a treatment for urinary tract infections.

**Part Used:**  Leaf, Root

**Side Effects:**  Chicory is not recommended for use by women who are pregnant or nursing.

Chicory is known to have an abortifacient effect and is used in commercial treatments for abortion in some countries.

Chicory may affect the heart and should not be used without the advice of a qualified herbalist or physician.

Chicory may cause an allergic reaction in some people.

Additional uses and side effects may exist but further research is necessary to determine the exact properties and effects of use.

**General:** Chicory is native to eastern North America and can be found growing wild in fields and along the sides of roads. Hardy to zone 3, it is not particular regarding soil composition but does require full sun and consistent moisture. It can be propagated by seed sown out in the late spring.

The leaves are eaten as a raw or cooked vegetable and the root is harvested in the fall for use as a coffee substitute or supplement with the traditional dosage being 1-teaspoon root to 1-cup boiling water. Steep for 15-30 minutes. Strain before consumption.

## Chitra, Barberry, Tree Turmeric
**Botanical Name:** Berberis aristata

**Properties:** Antibacterial, Astringent, Cancer, Colorant, Diaphoretic, Febrifuge, Laxative, Tonic

**Traditional Use:** Chitra root infusions are traditionally used to treat bacterial infections in the gastrointestinal system.

Chitra root has been used as a traditional soak wash for the treatment of conjunctivitis, sun damage to the eyes, and to reduce swollen eyes.

**Part Used:** Root, Stem

**Side Effects:** Chitra is not recommended for use by women who are pregnant or nursing.

Additional uses and side effects may exist but further research is necessary to determine the exact properties and effects of use.

**General:** Chitra is an evergreen shrub native to Asia. Hardy to zone 6, it is not particular regarding soil composition but does prefer full to partial sun and dry to moist soil. Chitra can be propagated by seed sown out as soon as it is ripe or by cuttings taken in the mid summer.

Chitra fruit is eaten raw or cooked and has been dried in a manner similar to the raisin. The stem and root are harvested, dried, and powdered for use in traditional preparations.

## Chrysanthemum, Mum
**Botanical Name:** Dendranthema x grandiflorum

**Properties:** Antibacterial, Antifungal, Anti-inflammatory, Antimicrobial, Carminative, Demulcent, Depurative, Diaphoretic, Febrifuge, Hypotensive, Sedative

**Traditional Use:** Chrysanthemum has traditionally been used in topical and internal preparations to alleviate bacterial infections and has shown an ability to treat staphylococcus and streptococcus infections.

Chrysanthemum has been used as a traditional topical soak to alleviate sore, tired eyes and as part of an eye infection treatment.

Chrysanthemum has traditionally been used as part of a topical preparation to reduce inflammation, inhibit infection and speed healing in skin sores, ulcers, and wounds.

**Part Used:** Flower

**Side Effects:** Chrysanthemum is not recommended for use by women who are pregnant or nursing.

Chrysanthemum may cause an allergic reaction in some people.

Chrysanthemum flowers may have an affect on the heart and are not recommended for use without the guidance of a qualified herbalist or physician.

Additional uses and side effects may exist but further research is necessary to determine the exact properties and effects of use.

**General:** Chrysanthemum is a perennial aromatic cultivated as a flowering herb in most regions of the world. Hardy to zone 4, it is not particular regarding soil composition but prefers full sun and moist soil. It is easily propagated by seed.

Chrysanthemum has been cultivated as an indoor plant to remove toxins from the environment and purify the air. The flower heads and petals have been parboiled and eaten as a cold vegetable or pickled. The leaves are eaten as a cooked vegetable and the flower petals are used to brew a sweet tea.

The essential oils are extracted or the flowers are dried, powdered, and used as a traditional supplement tea or capsule supplement up to 3 times daily.

### Cilantro, Chinese Parsley, Coriander, Dhanyaka, Kustumburi
**Botanical Name:** Coriandrum sativum

**Properties:** Analgesic, Antibacterial, Antifungal, Anti-inflammatory, Antiseptic, Carminative, Depurative, Digestive, Expectorant, Hypoglycemic, Immunostimulant, Narcotic, Vermifuge

**Traditional Use:** Cilantro seed oil has traditionally been used to treat bacterial infections.

Cilantro infusions have been used in traditional preparations for the treatment of conjunctivitis.

Cilantro is traditionally added to a specialized immunity building diet to help eliminate chronic infections.

Cilantro oil is added to traditional mouthwashes or skin ointments to help reduce infection and speed the healing of mouth & skin ulcers.

**Part Used:** Leaf, Oil, Seed

**Side Effects:** Cilantro is not recommended for use beyond dietary by women who are pregnant or nursing.

Cilantro may cause photosensitivity.

Cilantro may cause an allergic reaction in some people.

Cilantro may cause severe reactions in those suffering from asthma or bronchial congestion.

Overuse of Cilantro seed may have a narcotic like effect.

Additional uses and side effects may exist but further research is necessary to determine the exact properties and effects of use.

**General:** Cilantro is native to Asia and Europe but has been cultivated as a kitchen herb in much of the world. Hardy to zone 5, it prefers sandy to loamy soil, full to partial sun and dry to moist conditions. Cilantro can be propagated by seed sown out in the spring.

Cilantro seed yields an essential oil used as a flavoring, in perfumery or in soap making. The root is harvested, dried, and powdered for use as a flavoring and the leaves are eaten as a raw or cooked food flavoring or for supplement use as an infusion of 1-cup fresh cilantro or 1 teaspoon dried and powdered cilantro daily. The seeds are commonly called coriander while the leaves are called cilantro but both come from the same plant.

**Cinnamon, Cannelle de Ceylan, Cassia Bark**
**Botanical Name:** Cinnamomum zeylanicum

**Properties:** Analgesic, Anti-inflammatory, Antibacterial, Antifungal, Antimicrobial, Antioxidant, Antiperspirant, Antispasmodic, Antiviral, Aphrodisiac, Astringent, Cancer, Deodorant, Digestive, Estrogenic, Hypotensive, Insect Repellant, Stimulant

**Traditional Use:** Cinnamon oil is used in cleaning products to reduce fungus and bacteria. A recent study indicates that cinnamon oil has antimicrobial properties that make it effective against certain infections like streptococcus, staphylococcus, & drug resistant infections like MRSA. Cinnamon is traditionally blended with other oils like thyme, lemon, and lemon grass to make an effective disinfectant.

Cinnamon is used as a traditional infusion to ease symptoms of IBS by relaxing muscles and relieving gas while its antibacterial properties are used as an aid in countering bacterial infections.

**Part Used:** Bark, Leaf, Oil

**Side Effects:** Cinnamon is not recommended for use beyond dietary by women who are pregnant or nursing.

Cinnamon oil may be irritating to the skin and should be handled with care and diluted in any remedy.

Cinnamon may lower blood sugar.

Additional uses and side effects may exist but further research is necessary to determine the exact properties and effects of use.

**General:** Cinnamon is a common culinary additive grown in hot, tropical climates and used worldwide. Cinnamon bark is also harvested, dried, and used as a traditional supplement tea.

**Clove, Ding Xiang, Girofle, Kreteks, Lavanga**
**Botanical Name:** Syzygium aromaticum

**Properties:** Anodyne, Antibacterial, Antifungal, Antioxidant, Antiperspirant, Antiseptic, Antispasmodic, Antiviral, Aphrodisiac, Carminative, Digestive, Headache, Hypoglycemic, Insect Repellant, Stimulant, Tonic

**Traditional Use:** Clove oil is added to aromatherapy lamps, room cleaners, and vaporizers as a disinfecting agent.

Clove has traditionally been used as a wash or topical ointment to relieve dental pain and reduce mouth & tooth infections.

Clove is almost pure eugenol that is a photochemical that numbs pain while acting to kill bacteria, viruses, and fungus making it a traditional choice for household cleaners and for treatments for bacterial, fungal, and viral infections.

Clove has traditionally been used in topical preparations to inhibit infection and reduce the pain and inflammation of skin sores, ulcers, and wounds.

**Part Used:** Flower, Leaf, Stem - Oil

**Side Effects:** Clove is not recommended for use beyond dietary by women who are pregnant or nursing.

Clove is not recommended for use beyond dietary by people who are taking blood-thinning medication or who have a bleeding disorder.

Clove oil is highly irritating to the skin and should be handled with caution.

Clove may cause an allergic reaction in some people.

Clove may increase the allergic reactions to other irritants in some people.

Clove may lower blood sugar.

Additional uses and side effects may exist but further research is necessary to determine the exact properties and effects of use.

**General:** Clove is the flower from Syzygium aromaticum native to Indonesia but cultivated in many areas of the world. Clove is not particular regarding soil composition but does prefer high moisture and plentiful sun.

Cloves are used as a spice worldwide and have been smoked as a tobacco alternative. Clove is a common ingredient in insect repelling preparations and is especially effective against ants.

The flowers are harvested before blooming and dried or the oils are extracted from the flowers for use in traditional aromatherapy or topical preparations.

## Coca, Cocaine, Go Ko Yi, Inca Health Tea, Java Coca, Spadic
**Botanical Name:** Erythroxylum coca

**Properties:** Anesthetic, Antibacterial, Depurative, Local Anesthetic, Psychedelic, Stimulant

**Traditional Use:** Coca has been used in traditional preparations to alleviate bacterial infections and has been shown to be effective against gram-negative bacteria.

**Part Used:** Leaves

**Side Effects:** Coca is not recommended for use by anyone without the guidance of a qualified herbalist or physician.

Coca may cause heart attack, high blood pressure, kidney failure, liver failure, migraine headache, seizures, or stroke.

Additional uses and side effects may exist but further research is necessary to determine the exact properties and effects of use.

**General:** Coca is native to the Columbia, Peru, and the Andes. Coca has been used as a traditional supplement for thousands of years and is still used as a supplement in some cultures but is considered an illegal substance in the United States.

## Cocklebur, Clotbur, Woolgarie
**Botanical Name:** Xanthium strumarium

**Properties:** Anodyne, Antibacterial, Antifungal, Antiseptic, Antispasmodic, Antitussive, Astringent, Cancer, Colorant, Diaphoretic, Diuretic, Emollient, Febrifuge, Hypoglycemic, Laxative, Sedative, Tonic

**Traditional Use:** Cocklebur seeds have traditionally been used in topical preparations to help speed healing and prevent infection in skin sores, ulcers, and wounds.

Cocklebur leaves have been used as a traditional supplement treatment for chronic or resistant bacterial urinary tract infections.

**Part Used:** Fruit, Root, Seed

**Side Effects:** Cocklebur is not recommended for use by women who are pregnant or nursing.

Cocklebur is not recommended for use in children's treatments.

Cocklebur may affect blood sugar.

Cocklebur seeds and roots are avoided by foraging animals and may be toxic if used internally.

Additional uses and side effects may exist but further research is necessary to determine the exact properties and effects of use.

**General:**  Cocklebur is a hardy, self-seeding annual that can be found growing along wetlands in many parts of the world.  Hardy to zone 7, it is not particular regarding soil composition but does prefer full sun and wet conditions.

Cocklebur leaves yield a self-mordanting yellow toned colorant used in culinary, cosmetic and textile dyes.  Cocklebur seeds yield a blue dye product that is self-mordanting.

Cocklebur leaves have been harvested for use as a cooked vegetable and the seeds have been harvested and ground into a flour product.  The fruits, root, and seeds are harvested, dried, and powdered for use in traditional topical and supplement infusions.

**Cockscomb**
**Botanical Names:**  Celosia argantea

**Properties:**  Antibacterial, Astringent, Hypotensive, Parasiticide, Styptic

**Traditional Use:**  Cockscomb flowers and seeds have traditionally been used to stop internal and external bleeding and to help reduce infection while speeding healing in skin sores, ulcers, and wounds.

Cockscomb seed and flower infusions have been used as a traditional treatment for bacterial urinary tract infections.

**Part Used:**  Flower, Seed

**Side Effects:**  Cockscomb is not recommended for use by women who are pregnant or nursing.

Cockscomb may affect the blood pressure.

Cockscomb is not recommended for use by people with glaucoma or similar eye conditions because it is known to dilate the pupils.

Additional uses and side effects may exist but further research is necessary to determine the exact properties and effects of use.

**General:**  Cockscomb is native to the tropical regions and cultivated as an interesting ornamental.  Hardy to zone 9, it is not particular regarding soil composition but does require full sun and consistent moisture.  It can be propagated by seed sown out in the spring.

The leaves and young shoots are eaten as a cooked vegetable and the flower and seed are harvested for use in traditional preparations.

**Columbine, Culverwort, European Columbine, Granny's Nightcap**
**Botanical Name:**  Aquilegia vulgaris

**Properties:** Anodyne, Antibacterial, Antifungal, Antiviral, Astringent, Diuretic, Diaphoretic, Insecticide, Nervine, Sedative

**Traditional Use:** Columbine has been used in traditional supplements to treat bacterial, fungal, and viral infections including staphylococcus aureus, micrococcus luteus, bacillus subtilus, and candida albicans, and all strains of influenza.

**Part Used:** Leaf, Flower, Stem

**Side Effects:** Columbine is not recommended for use by women who are pregnant or nursing.

Overuse of Columbine may be toxic.

Additional uses and side effects may exist but further research is necessary to determine the exact properties and effects of use.

**General:** Columbine is native to Asia and Europe and has been naturalized to the United States. Hardy to zone 3, it prefers sandy to loamy soil with full to partial sun and consistent moisture. Columbine is propagated by seeds sown out as soon as they are ripe.

The aerial parts of the plant are harvested while in bloom and dried and powdered for use in a traditional teas or topical preparations.

### Corncockle, Cockle, Corn Campion, Corn Cockle, Corn Rose, Crown of the Field
**Botanical Name:** Agrostemma githago

**Properties:** Antibacterial, Antiviral, Diuretic, Expectorant, Vermifuge

**Traditional Uses:** Corncockle is traditionally used in topical ointments to help kill bacteria, viruses, and parasites.

**Parts Used:** Root, Seed

**Side Effects:** Corncockle is not recommended for use by women who are pregnant or nursing.

The leaves and seeds of the Corncockle are toxic and are not recommended for internal use. The sapopins may be absorbed through the skin and should be used only under the guidance of a qualified herbalist or physician.

Corn Cockle is for external use only. Internal use may cause breathing difficulty, diarrhea, dizziness, paralysis, vomiting, coma, and even death.

Additional uses and side effects may exist but further research is necessary to determine the exact properties and effects of use.

**General:** Corncockle is an annual plant native to Asia & Europe but naturalized in other areas where it is considered an invasive weed by some. It is not particular regarding soil composition but prefers full to partial sun and dry to moist conditions. Corncockle can be found growing wild in cornfields or propagated by seeds sown out as soon as they are ripe.

The leaves have been cooked as a vegetable and the root & seed have been harvested for use in traditional supplements.

## Couch Grass, Twitch Grass, Witch Grass
**Botanical Name:** Agropyron repens

**Properties:** Antibacterial, Antibiotic, Antifungal, Anti-inflammatory, Antibacterial, Antimicrobial, Colorant, Demulcent, Diuretic, Expectorant, Vermifuge

**Traditional Use:** Couch Grass has been used in traditional gargles or tea treatments to coat the throat and reduce inflammation, infection, & pain in the throat and mouth.

A tea made of couch grass roots contains both antibiotic and diuretic properties and has traditionally been used to treat painful urination and urinary tract infections.

**Part Used:** Rhizome

**Side Effects:** Couch Grass is not recommended for use by women who are pregnant or nursing.

Couch Grass is not recommended for use by people with edema.

Couch Grass may lower blood sugar in some people.

Additional uses and side effects may exist but further research is necessary to determine the exact properties and effects of use.

**General:** Couch Grass is native to North & South America, Asia, Australia, and Europe. It is considered an invasive weed by some and grows readily in open grasslands, gardens, and other sunny locations. It is not particular regarding growing conditions and will self-sow readily if given its own place in the garden.

Couch Grass roots yield a grey toned colorant used as a traditional dye product. The roots have also been roasted and ground for use in baking. The rhizome is harvested in the spring or fall, dried, and powdered for use in traditional supplement teas.

## Crab Claw
**Botanical Name:** Peperomia pellucida

**Properties:** Analgesic, Antibacterial, Antifungal, Anti-inflammatory, Antimicrobial, Astringent, Diuretic

**Traditional Use:** Crab Claw has traditionally been used in topical and internal preparations to alleviate bacterial infections and studies illustrate that it has broad-spectrum antimicrobial properties against infections like bacillus subtilis, e coli, pseudomonas aeruginosa, and staphylococcus aureus.

Crab Claw has been used in traditional eyewash preparations to reduce eye inflammation and combat common eye infections.

Crab Claw has traditionally been used as a gargle or spray to alleviate pain, infection, & inflammation in the mouth or throat.

**Part Used:** Leaf, Juice, Stem

**Side Effects:** Crab Claw is not recommended for use by women who are pregnant or nursing.

Crab Claw may cause an allergic reaction or asthma like symptoms in some people.

Additional uses and side effects may exist but further research is necessary to determine the exact properties and effects of use.

**General:** Crab Claw is a clumping herb native to Asia and South America but is cultivated in other regions. It prefers loamy soils, partial or full shade and moist conditions. It is easily propagated by seed or by division of clumps in the fall.

Crab Claw leaves and stems are eaten as a raw or cooked vegetable, dietary supplement, or in traditional topical and supplement preparations.

**Dandelion, Blowball, Cankerwort, Clock Flower, Cochet, Dudhal, Endive, Fairy Clock, Fortune Teller, Irish Daisy, Lion's Tooth, Priest's Crown, Puff Ball, Swine Snout, Wild Endive**
**Botanical Name:** Taraxacum officinale

**Properties:** Antibacterial, Antifungal, Anti-inflammatory, Antioxidant, Astringent, Colorant, Cholagogue, Digestive, Depurative, Detoxification, Diuretic, Hepatic, Hypoglycemic, Laxative, Stimulant

**Traditional Use:** Dandelion has been used as a traditional treatment and cleaning component against bacterial infections including bacillus dysenteriae, meningococci, pneumococci, and staphylococcus aureus.

Dandelion has been used as a traditional infusion to irrigate urinary tract infections while acting against related bacteria.

**Part Used:** Leaf, Flower, Root

**Side Effects:** Dandelion is not recommended for use by women who are pregnant or nursing.

Dandelion is not recommended for use by people with gall bladder disease without the guidance of a qualified herbalist or physician.

Dandelion is not recommended for use by people with stomach ulcers or gastritis.

Dandelion may cause stomach upset and diarrhea in some people.

Dandelion may cause an allergic reaction in some people.

Additional uses and side effects may exist but further research is necessary to determine the exact properties and effects of use.

**General:** Dandelion is native to Asia, Europe, and North America where it is considered an invasive weed growing easily in a variety of sun, soil, and moisture conditions.

Dandelion root and leaf extract is used to make a liquid plant food that is said to help stimulate growth in other plants. The roots juices are used to create latex and they yield an orangish-brown colorant used as a textile dye. The dandelion flower yields a natural yellow colorant used as a textile, culinary or cosmetic dye. Mordant – Alum.

Dandelions leaves, roots, and flowers are eaten as a raw or cooked vegetable or to flavor beer or soft drinks and the roots are roasted for use as a coffee substitute. The flowers are used to make tea or wine.

Dandelion has been used by a variety of societies, including the Native Americans, as a supplement treatment. Dandelion is root is harvested from mature plants, preferably in their second season of growth and the leaves, stems, and flowers are harvested anytime for use in traditional teas, washes, and supplements up to 3 times daily.

**Day Flower**
**Botanical Name:** Commelina communis

**Properties:** Antibacterial, Astringent, Colorant, Depurative, Diuretic, Febrifuge

**Traditional Use:** Day Flower is traditionally included as part of a topical preparation to reduce bleeding, inflammation, and infection in skin sores, ulcers, and wounds.

Day Flower has been used as a traditional gargle or spray to relieve infection of the throat & mouth.

**Part Used:** Leaf

**Side Effects:** Day Flower is not recommended for use by women who are pregnant or nursing.

Additional uses and side effects may exist but further research is necessary to determine the exact properties and effects of use.

**General:** Day Flower is a perennial native to Asia but cultivated in other areas as an ornamental. Hardy to zone 7, it prefers sandy to loamy soil, full to partial sun and consistent moisture. Day Flower can be propagated by seeds sown out in the spring after all danger of frost has passed, cuttings or by division.

The flowers, leaves, and shoots are harvested for use as a cold vegetable or as a flavoring. The petals yield a bright blue colorant used as a dye product and the leaves are harvested, dried, and powdered for use as a traditional supplement.

**Devil's Claw, Grapple, Wood Spider**
**Botanical Name:** Harpagophytum procumbens

**Properties:** Analgesic, Antibacterial, Anti-inflammatory, Antispasmodic, Cancer, Cardio-Tonic, Digestive, Hepatic

**Traditional Use:** Doses of 50 mg to 100 mg of devils claw are available in commercial preparations.

Devils Claw has been used as a part of a traditional topical preparation to reduce pain, treat infection, reduce inflammation and speed healing of mouth ulcers, skin ulcers, skin sores, and wounds.

**Part Used:** Root

**Side Effects:** Devils Claw is not recommended for use by women who are pregnant or nursing.

Devils Claw is not recommended for use by people who have an ulcer or other stomach condition.

Devils Claw may cause gastrointestinal upset, headaches, loss of appetite, tinnitus or other side effects.

High doses of Devils Claw could interfere with blood pressure, heart, and diabetes medications.

Research is being conducted to determine if Devil's Claw may be beneficial at stabilizing heart rhythms in certain conditions.

Additional uses and side effects may exist but further research is necessary to determine the exact properties and effects of use.

**General:** Devils Claw is native to the deserts of Africa and has been cultivated in other regions where the tubers and roots are harvested at the end of the rainy season, chopped, dried in the sun, and powdered for use in traditional supplement teas given up to 3 times daily.

### Devil's Club, Cukilanarpak, Devil's Root, Fatsia
**Botanical Name:** Echinopanax horridum

**Properties:** Antibacterial, Antifungal, Antiviral, Expectorant, Stimulant

**Traditional Uses:** Devil's Club is traditionally included in liquid preparations to kill bacteria, fungus, and viruses on the skin and in surface cleaners.

**Parts Used:** Inner Root Bark

**Side Effects:** Devil's Club is not recommended for use by women who are pregnant or nursing.

Devil's Club may affect blood sugar.

Additional uses and side effects may exist but further research is necessary to determine the exact properties and effects of use.

**General:** The root of the Devil's Claw is harvested and peeled so that the inner root can be dried, powdered, and incorporated into topical preparations or for supplement uses. The essential oils are extracted for use in liquid preparations.

### Dill, Aneth, Dillweed, Dilly, Eneldo, Madhura, Sotapa, Sowa
**Botanical Name:** Anethum graveoleus

**Properties:** Abortifacient, Antibacterial, Antifungal, Antispasmodic, Cancer, Carminative, Digestive, Disinfectant, Diuretic, Galactogogue, Insect, Muscle Relaxant, Sedative

**Traditional Use:** Dill tea or oil is traditionally used to kill bacteria in the intestine, ease flatulence, and to calm the symptoms of colic, IBS, and uneasy digestion.

Dill has been used as a traditional supplement to alleviate bacteria in the intestinal tract.

**Part Used:** Leaf, Oil, Seed, Stem, Whole

**Side Effects:** Dill is not recommended for use beyond dietetic by women who are pregnant or nursing. Dill seeds are an abortifacient.

Dill oil may irritate the skin.

Dill may cause an allergic reaction in some people.

Dill may cause photosensitivity.

Overuse of Dill may cause disorientation, dizziness, or hallucinations.

Additional uses and side effects may exist but further research is necessary to determine the exact properties and effects of use.

**General:** Dill is native to Asia but is cultivated worldwide as an annual kitchen herb. Hardy to zone 8, Dill grows easily from seed in well-drained, acidic soil with full sun.

Dill leaves are eaten raw or cooked or dried for culinary use while the seed is harvested, dried, and powdered or the oils are extracted for use in traditional supplement preparations.

### Dong Quai, Chinese Angelica, Dang Gui
**Botanical Name:** Angelica sinensis

**Properties:** Adaptogen, Analgesic, Antibacterial, Antibiotic, Anti-inflammatory, Antispasmodic, Antiviral, Aphrodisiac, Emollient, Hepatic, Laxative, Phytoestrogen, Sedative, Stimulant, Vasodilator

**Traditional Use:** Dong Quai is used as a traditional agent to prevent bacterial infections like bacillus dysenteriae, bacillus typhi, and streptococci.

**Part Used:** Root

**Side Effects:**  Dong Quai is not recommended for use by women who are pregnant or nursing.

Dong Quai is not recommended for use by people with a hormone sensitive condition like endometriosis, fibroids, or certain types of cancer.

Dong Quai has been shown to have anticoagulant effects and may stimulate bleeding – do not use if you have a bleeding disorder and discontinue use during the monthly menstrual cycle.

Dong Quai may cause photosensitivity in come people.

Additional uses and side effects may exist but further research is necessary to determine the exact properties and effects of use.

**General:**  Dong Quai is native to the mountainous regions of Asia but is cultivated in other parts of the world as an ornamental and medicinal plant.  Hardy to zone 7, it is not particular regarding soil composition but does prefer full to partial sunlight and consistent moisture.

The mature roots are harvested for use in a traditional supplement of 2 tbsp. of fresh root or 1 tbsp. of dried root daily.

**Drumstick**
**Botanical Name:**  Moringa oleifera

**Properties:**  Abortifacient, Antibacterial, Antifungal, Anti-inflammatory, Antioxidant, Antiseptic, Antispasmodic, Cancer, Cardio-Tonic, Cholesterol, Diuretic, Emmenagogue, Expectorant, Hypoglycemic, Hypotensive, Rubefacient

**Traditional Use:**  Drumstick root has been used to reduce congestion in conditions like asthma, bronchitis, colds, influenza, and pneumonia and to help shorten the duration and severity of infections.

Drumstick has been used as part of a gargle to alleviate pain & inflammation while fighting infection in the mouth, teeth, or throat.

Drumstick has traditionally been used to purify bacteria laden drinking water.

**Part Used:**  Whole

**Side Effects:**  Drumstick is not recommended for use by women who are pregnant or nursing.

Drumstick has been used as an abortifacient in some cultures.

Drumstick is not recommended for use by women who are trying to conceive as it may affect fertility.

Drumstick may affect blood sugar.

Additional uses and side effects may exist but further research is necessary to determine the exact properties and effects of use.

**General:** Drumstick is a tree native to Africa and Asia where the leaves and seed are harvested for use as a highly nutritional food product and the bark, leaves, and roots are harvested for use in traditional supplements.

Drumstick has been used in traditional supplements to treat over 200 diseases and research has been conducted to verify some of the many uses of this highly nutritive tree. Additional research is being conducted to determine other potential uses and benefits.

**Echinacea, Black Samson, Purple Coneflower**
**Botanical Name:** Echinacea angustifolia, Echinacea purpurea

**Properties:** Adaptogen, Antibacterial, Anti-inflammatory, Antiseptic, Antibacterial, Antiviral, Depurative, Digestive, Immunostimulant

**Traditional Use:** Echinacea is used in traditional supplements to alleviate chronic bacterial infections.

All types of Echinacea contain compounds that support disease resistance and are traditionally used to help to shorten the length of common infections when taken as soon as symptoms appears.

Extracts of Echinacea root have shown immunostimulatory effects in clinical trails and Echinacea has been used as a traditional supplement to inhibit viruses and increase antibacterial and microphage activity.

Echinacea has traditionally been used to help to alleviate inflammation of the mucus membranes of the digestive and respiratory system and to alleviate the pain of a sore throat or tonsils while combating infection.

**Part Used:** Flower, Leaf, Root, Stem

**Side Effects:** Echinacea is not recommended for use by women who are pregnant or nursing.

Echinacea may cause an allergic reaction, skin rash, or gastrointestinal upset in some people.

Echinacea is not recommended for use by people who have an autoimmune disease like Multiple Sclerosis or Lupus.

Overuse of Echinacea may cause fever, nausea, and vomiting.

Extended use of Echinacea may cause immunosuppression.

Additional uses and side effects may exist but further research is necessary to determine the exact properties and effects of use.

**General:** There are nine known species of Echinacea native to the United States & Canada. The most potent species are Echinacea angustifolia (white flower) and Echinacea purpurea (purple flower). Hardy to zone 3, Echinacea is drought resistant once established but requires full sun for optimal growth. It can be propagated by seed sown out in the spring, spring division, or root cuttings in the late fall.

The entire plant including flower, leaf, root, and stem are used to make teas, juice, extracts or in preparations for external use. The root contains the highest concentration of beneficial compounds. Therapeutic levels of Echinacea are delivered in tincture form at a rate of 50 drops up to 5 times daily.

### Edelweiss, Lion's Paw, Queen's Flower
**Botanical Name:** Leontopodium alpinum

**Properties:** Antibacterial, Anti-inflammatory, Antiviral, Antimicrobial, Antioxidant

**Traditional Use:** Edelweiss has traditionally been used as part of natural cleaning products to kill bacteria and viruses in the air and on hard surfaces.

Edelweiss has illustrated ability against e. coli, enterococcus faecium, pseudomonas aeruginosa, staphylococcus aureus, streptococcus pneumoniae, and streptococcus pyogenes in European research studies.

Edelweiss has traditionally been used in topical ointments to promote cell regeneration, alleviate infection, and speed wound healing.

**Side Effects:** Edelweiss is not recommended for use by women who are pregnant or nursing.

Additional uses and side effects may exist but further research is necessary to determine the exact properties and effects of use.

**General:** Edelweiss can be found growing in higher altitudes and is cultivated as an ornamental or for disinfectant and supplement uses.

### Elecampane, Alant, Aster, Elfdock, Elfwort, Horse Elder, Horseheal, Indian Elecampane, Scabwort, Velvet Dock, Wild Sunflower, Yellow Starwort
**Botanical Name:** Inula helenium

**Properties:** Analgesic, Antibacterial, Antifungal, Anti-inflammatory, Antimicrobial, Antiseptic, Astringent, Cholagogue, Colorant, Demulcent, Detoxification, Diaphoretic, Diuretic, Expectorant, Vermifuge

**Traditional Use:** The ooze of the Elecampane root has traditionally been used in steam treatments to cleanse the air of common bacteria, fungus, and viruses.

Elecampane tea has been used as a traditional component in treatments for common bacterial and fungal infections.

Elecampane is traditionally used in surface, air, and wound cleaning products to kill bacteria, fungus, and viruses.

**Part Used:** Flower, Rhizome, Root

**Side Effects:** Elecampane is not recommended for use by women who are pregnant or nursing.

Elecampane may cause allergies to people sensitive to plants in the sunflower family.

Elecampane may irritate the mucus membranes.

Elecampane may affect blood sugar.

Additional uses and side effects may exist but further research is necessary to determine the exact properties and effects of use.

**General:** Elecampane is a perennial native to Europe and naturalized in many other areas of the world. It is not particular regarding soil composition but does prefer full or partial sun and consistent moisture. Elecampane grows easily from root cuttings or seed.

Elecampane leaves are eaten as a raw or cooked vegetable or bitter seasoning and the roots are candied and eaten as a sweet vegetable. The root is harvested in the fall from mature plants, air dried, and ground or made in an alcohol extract for inclusion in traditional supplement preparations.

**Elephant Tree**
**Botanical Name:** Bursera microphylla

**Properties:** Antibacterial, Antiviral, Astringent, Expectorant, Immunostimulant

**Traditional Use:** Elephant Tree bark, leaves, and resin have traditionally been used in alcohol tinctures to alleviate pain and inflammation while reducing infection and speeding healing in cold sores, mouth sores, and tooth abscesses.

Elephant Tree leaves have been used as a traditional supplement tea to help build the immune system and ward off common infections.

**Part Used:** Bark, Leaf, Resin

**Side Effects:** Elephant Tree is not recommended for use by women who are pregnant or nursing.

Additional uses and side effects may exist but further research is necessary to determine the exact properties and effects of use.

**General:** Elephant Tree is a small shrub native to Central America and the southern United States. The resin is harvested for use in varnish products and the bark, leaf and resin are harvested, dried, and powdered for use as a traditional supplement.

**Embauba, Snakewood Tree, Trumpet Tree**

**Botanical Name:** Cecropia peltata

**Properties:** Abortifacient, Analgesic, Antibacterial, Antifungal, Anti-inflammatory, Antioxidant, Antispasmodic, Astringent, Cardio-Tonic, Diuretic, Emollient, Hypoglycemic, Stimulant, Vasodilatation

**Traditional Use:** Embauba leaf extract has traditionally been used as part of a preparation to alleviate bacterial infections like e. coli, salmonella, shingella, and staphylococcus.

**Part Used:** Leaf, Resin

**Side Effects:** Embauba is not recommended for use by women who are pregnant or nursing.

Embauba has been used as an abortifacient in some cultures.

Embauba is believed to affect the heart and is not recommended for use without the advice of a qualified herbalist or physician.

Embauba may affect blood sugar.

Additional uses and side effects may exist but further research is necessary to determine the exact properties and effects of use.

**General:** Embauba is a small, fast growing tree native to tropical and sub-tropical regions of Central and South America and cultivated as an ornamental in frost-free zones. Embauba is considered an invasive species in some regions of the world.

The wood is used as a lightweight craft product, the inner bark is used as a fiber product, and the leaves are harvested for use as natural sandpaper. The young buds are harvested for use as a cooked vegetable and the leaves are harvested, dried, and powdered for use in traditional supplements.

### Eucalyptus, Blue Gum Blue Mallee, Gully Gum, Gum Tree, Red Gum, Stringy Bark Tree, Sagandhapara
**Botanical Name:** Eucalyptus globulus

**Properties:** Analgesic, Antibacterial, Antifungal, Anti-inflammatory, Antiperspirant, Antiseptic, Antispasmodic, Antiviral, Astringent, Cancer, Colorant, Depurative, Diuretic, Expectorant, Febrifuge, Hypoglycemic, Insect Repellant, Rubefacient, Vermifuge

**Traditional Use:** Eucalyptus is traditionally added to vapor inhalants for relief from bronchial congestion while acting to shorten the duration of common infections.

Eucalyptus oils have been used in natural cleaning products as an agent to kill airborne or surface bacteria, viruses, and fungus.

Eucalyptus has been used at a rate of 2% in traditional topical lotions to reduce infection and speed healing in burns and other types of wounds.

**Part Used:** Leaf, Oil

**Side Effects:** Eucalyptus is not recommended for use by women who are pregnant or nursing.

Eucalyptus is not recommended for use in children's treatments.

Eucalyptus is not recommended for use by people with a history of seizure disorders.

Eucalyptus may lower blood sugar.

Undiluted Eucalyptus oil is toxic both internally and externally. Always dilute Eucalyptus Oil before use. The leaf is generally considered safe in teas.

Overuse of Eucalyptus oil may cause difficulty breathing, dizziness, gastrointestinal irritation, hallucinations, nausea, vomiting, paralysis, convulsions, and even death.

Additional uses and side effects may exist but further research is necessary to determine the exact properties and effects of use.

**General:** Eucalyptus is native to Australia but is cultivated in many other parts of the world. Hardy to zone 9, it is not particular regarding soil composition but does prefer full sun and moist to wet conditions. Eucalyptus can be propagated by seeds sown after all danger of frost has passed. If sown indoors, seedlings should be transplanted to their permanent location as soon as the second set of leaves appear.

Eucalyptus leaf oil is used in insect repelling preparations. According to the CDC, Lemon Eucalyptus has proven to be as effective as DEET at repelling insects like mosquitoes. The oils are also used as a cleanser effective against grease, bacteria, and a variety of fungal growths. The wood is valued for indoor and outdoor woodcraft or pulped for making paper. The young leaves yield a self-mordanting yellow to tan colorant, the young shoots yield tones of grey to green and the young bark yields a darker green. Eucalyptus is one of the most commonly used treatments for cough, congestion, and household disinfecting cleaners. The oil is extracted from fresh or partially dried leaves for use in aromatherapy and traditional supplements.

**Evodia, Gosyuyu, San Cha Ku, Wu Chu Yu**
**Botanical Name:** Evodia officinalis

**Properties:** Analgesic, Antibacterial, Anti-inflammatory, Astringent, Hypotensive, Vermifuge

**Traditional Uses:** Evodia has been used as a traditional supplement to help alleviate the symptoms of diarrhea and has illustrated an ability to combat heliobacter pylori bacteria.

Evodia has been a traditional supplement in the treatment of stomach ulcers and appears to be especially effective in treating bacterially related ulcers.

**Parts Used:** Fruit, Root

**Side Effects:** Evodia is not recommended for use by women who are pregnant or nursing.

Evodia may affect the heart.

Evodia may decrease clotting ability.

Additional uses and side effects may exist but further research is necessary to determine the exact properties and effects of use.

**General:** Evodia is a deciduous tree native to Asia where the fruit & root have been used as a traditional supplement for thousands of years. The fruits are used fresh or dried and the roots are dried and powdered.

**Fennel, Biri Sanuf, Bitter Fennel, Carosella, Hinojo, Sweet Fennel, Wild Fennel, Xiao Hui Xiang**

**Botanical Name:** Foeniculum vulgare

**Properties:** Adaptogenic, Analgesic, Anodyne, Antidepressant, Antifungal, Antiinflammatory, Antimicrobial, Antiseptic, Antispasmodic, Antiviral, Appetite Depressant, Carminative, Colorant, Depurative, Detoxification, Diaphoretic, Diuretic, Emmenagogue, Estrogenic, Expectorant, Galactagogue, Hallucinogenic, Insect Repellant, Laxative, Vulnerary

**Traditional Use:** Fennel tea or syrup contains more creosol and alpha-pinene than anise making it a traditional supplement for helping the body expel excess mucus and in calming dry coughs in conditions like asthma, bronchitis, colds, influenza and sinusitis while acting to treat the underlying infection.

Fennel has been included in traditional sprays & gargles to alleviate throat & mouth inflammation and infection.

Fennel has traditionally been used to treat urinary tract infections.

Fennel oil has antiviral properties and is used in air purifiers to clear the air of viral infections.

**Part Used:** Leaf, Oil, Root, Seed, Whole

**Side Effects:** Fennel is not recommended for use by women who are pregnant or nursing.

Fennel is a uterine stimulant.

Fennel may cause photosensitivity, indigestion, pulmonary edema, and vomiting.

Fennel is not recommended for use by women who have an estrogen sensitive disorder like endometriosis, fibroids or certain types of cancer.

Fennel can affect blood sugar.

Fennel oil may affect liver function.

Additional uses and side effects may exist but further research is necessary to determine the exact properties and effects of use.

**General:**
Fennel is an annual plant native to the Mediterranean but is cultivated worldwide as it is easily grown from seed in rich soil with plenty of sun and moderate moisture. It grows to a height of 3-6 feet and has yellow flowers that bloom in the summer months. Fennel should be grown away from other plants since it may inhibit their growth.

Fennel leaves, stalks, and flower heads are eaten as a raw or cooked vegetable and the seeds are used as an anise-like flavoring. Dried fennel leaves have been used as part of insect repellant powders especially to protect pets against fleas.

The leaf and root are harvested for use fresh or dried and powdered for use in traditional supplements. The oils are extracted from the crushed seed for use in topical and aromatherapy treatments.

## Fiddlewood
**Botanical Name:** Vitex gaumeri

**Properties:** Antibacterial, Antifungal, Antiseptic, Vermifuge

**Traditional Use:** Fiddlewood bark tea has been used as a traditional skin wash to disinfect and speed healing in skin sores, ulcers and wounds.

**Part Used:** Bark

**Side Effects:** Fiddlewood is not recommended for use by women who are pregnant or nursing.

Fiddlewood is for external use only.

Additional uses and side effects may exist but further research is necessary to determine the exact properties and effects of use.

**General:** Fiddlewood is native to Central & South America where the bark has been harvested, dried, and powdered for generations as a traditional topical supplement.

## Fishwort, Chameleon Plant, Heartleaf, Lizard tail
**Botanical Name:** Houttuynia cordata

**Properties:** Antibacterial, Antibiotic, Anti-inflammatory, Antiviral, Astringent, Depurative, Diuretic, Emmenagogue, Febrifuge, Hypoglycemic, Laxative, Tonic

**Traditional Uses:** Fishwort roots have traditionally been used to treat bacterial infections, especially gram-positive infection.

**Parts Used:** Whole

**Side Effects:** Fishwort is not recommended for use by women who are pregnant or nursing.

Additional uses and side effects may exist but further research is necessary to determine the exact properties and effects of use.

**General:** Fishwort is native to Asia. Hardy to zone 8, it is not particular regarding soil composition but does prefer full to partial shade and moist to wet conditions. Fishwort can be propagated by seed sown in the spring or division of the clumps.

Fishwort shoots and leaves are harvested early in the growing season and eaten raw or cooked and the root is eaten cooked. The whole plant is harvested and juiced or made into an extract or strong decoction for use in traditional preparations.

**Fleabane**
**Botanical Name:** Pulicaria dysenterica

**Properties:** Antibacterial, Antimicrobial, Astringent

**Common Uses:** Bacterial Infections, Wound Care

**Traditional Use:** Fleabane has been used as a traditional supplement to treat bacterial infections and to kill bacteria on hard and soft surfaces.

Fleabane has traditionally been used in topical washes and ointments to prevent infection and speed healing in wounds.

**Side Effects:** Fleabane is not recommended for use by women who are pregnant or nursing.

Additional uses and side effects may exist but further research is necessary to determine the exact properties and effects of use.

**General:** Fleabane is a member of the daisy family native to Europe and cultivated in other regions as an ornamental. Hardy to zone 7, It is not particular regarding soil composition but does require full sun and moist to wet soil. Fleabane can be propagated by seeds sown in the spring after all danger of frost has passed and will self sow readily if given its own place in the garden.

Fleabane leaves are harvested for use fresh or dried and powdered for use as a traditional supplement primarily for its antibacterial and antimicrobial effects.

**Fo-Ti, Chinese Cornbind, Chinese Knotweed, Climbing Knotweed, Flowery Knotweed, He-Shou-Wu, Tuber Fleeceflower**
**Botanical Name:** Polygonum multiflorum

**Properties:** Adaptogen, Analgesic, Antibacterial, Antioxidant, Antispasmodic, Astringent, Cancer, Cardiotonic, Detoxification, Hypoglycemic, Hypotensive, Laxative, Phytoestrogen, Sedative, Skin Care, Tonic

**Traditional Use:** Fo Ti has traditionally been used to stimulate the immune system and to ward off viruses or bacterial infections.

**Part Used:** Root, Stem

**Side Effects:** Fo Ti is not recommended for use by women who are pregnant or nursing.

Fo Ti is not recommended for use in children's treatments.

Fo-Ti may increase blood sugar.

Fo Ti is not recommended for use by people liver or kidney disease without the guidance of a qualified herbalist or physician.

Overdose or overuse of Fo Ti may cause numbness, tingling in the extremities, abdominal pain, diarrhea, and nausea.

Additional uses and side effects may exist but further research is necessary to determine the exact properties and effects of use.

**General:** Fo-Ti is native to China and Japan and can be found growing along forest edges and open fields. Hardy to zone 7, it is not particular regarding soil composition but does prefer full to partial sun and consistent moisture. Fo-Ti can be propagated by seed sown out in the spring or through division of the clumps.

Fo-Ti leaves and seeds are eaten raw or cooked and the root is soaked to remove the bitterness and then eaten as a cooked vegetable. Fo-Ti is a very popular traditional supplement in China where the roots are harvested in the fall, dried, and powdered or steam processed for use as a traditional supplement with the most mature roots holding the most supplement value. The stems are harvested in the fall and used fresh or dried and powdered for use in traditional infusions. Extracts of the entire plant have been used in traditional cancer treatment plans.

**Forsythia, Forsitia, Golden Bell, Lian Qiao, Lien Chiao, Rengyo, Yellow Bell, Weeping Golden Bell**
**Botanical Name:** Forsythia suspensa

**Properties:** Antibacterial, Anti-inflammatory, Antitussive, Antiviral, Antiseptic, Astringent, Cancer, Diuretic, Emmenagogue, Febrifuge, Natural Skin Care, Vermifuge

**Traditional Use:** Forsythia flowers have been used as a traditional treatment to treat common infections like bacillus typhi, mycobacterium tuberculi, pneumococcus, shigella dysenteriae, staphococcus aureus, and streptococcus.

Forsythia leaves have been used as part of a traditional topical poultice to combat infection, alleviate pain & inflammation, and speed healing associated with hemorrhoids, skin ulcers, and wounds.

Forsythia is traditionally added to gargles or sprays to alleviate throat & mouth inflammation and infection.

**Part Used:** Flower, Leaf, Twig

**Side Effects:** Forsythia is not recommended for use by women who are pregnant or nursing.

Additional uses and side effects may exist but further research is necessary to determine the exact properties and effects of use.

**General:** Forsythia is native to Asia but is now found in many regions of the world. Hardy to zone 5, it is not particular regarding soil composition or sun conditions but does prefer consistent moisture.  Forsythia can be propagated by seeds sown in the spring, cutting, air layering, or division.

Forsythia has been used as a traditional supplement for thousands of years and the twigs, fruit, and leaves have been harvested, dried, and powdered for use internally and externally.

## Garden Cress, Cress, Pepper Grass
**Botanical Name:**
Lepidium sativum

**Properties:**
Abortifacient, Antibacterial, Antiviral, Diuretic, Expectorant, Galactogogue, Immunostimulant

**Traditional Use:**
Garden Cress has traditionally been used to calm coughs and congestion associated with asthma, bronchitis, colds, and influenza and as a component in traditional supplements to shorten the length of common bacterial and viral infections.

Garden Cress is rich in Vitamin C and is traditionally used in conditions arising from a Vitamin C deficiency and has shown high levels of antibacterial and antiviral effects in laboratory testing leading to its inclusion in immunity related therapy.

**Part Used:**
Flower, Leaf, Stem

**Side Effects:**
Garden Cress was traditionally used as an abortifacient and should never be used by a pregnant or nursing woman.

The oil of the plant may cause skin irritation, blisters, and even necrosis.

Additional uses and side effects may exist but further research is necessary to determine the exact proportios and effects of use.

**General:**
Garden Cress is an annual grown in many parts of the world as a food.  Hardy to zone 7, it is not particular regarding soil composition but does prefer full to partial sun and consistent moisture. Garden Cress can be propagated by seed sown in the spring.

Garden Cress seeds yield an edible oil used in candle making and lighting.  The leaf is eaten as a raw or cooked vegetable, the root is used as a condiment, and the seeds are used as a seasoning.  The flower, leaf, and stem are harvested during the flowering season for use fresh or as a traditional tea supplement.

## Garlic, Allium, Lasuna, Poor Man's Treacle, Rason, Rust Treacle, Stinking Rose
**Botanical Name:** Allium sativum

**Properties:** Antibacterial, Antifungal, Antimicrobial, Antioxidant, Antiseptic, Antispasmodic, Astringent, Chalagogue, Cholesterol, Depurative, Diaphoretic, Diuretic, Emmenagogue,

Expectorant, Febrifuge, Hypotensive, Immunostimulant, Stimulant, Insect Repellant, Rubefacient, Vermifuge

**Traditional Use:**  The juices of Garlic have been used as a disinfecting agent in household cleansing products.

Garlic contains antibacterial and antifungal compounds that make it a traditional ingredient in topical treatments for bacterial and fungal infections.

Garlic contains a broad spectrum antimicrobial and has traditionally been used in supplements to shorten the length of infections.

Garlic has been used in traditional dietary plans to boost the body's immune response helping to ward off common infections.

Garlic juice is traditionally used as a topical poultice or wash to disinfect wounds.

**Part Used:**  Bulb, Whole

**Side Effects:**  Garlic is not recommended for use beyond dietary for women who are pregnant or nursing.

Garlic is not recommended for use beyond dietary in children's treatments.

Overuse of Garlic may cause heartburn in some people.

Overuse of Garlic may burn the skin in some people.

Garlic may cause bad breath, body odor, upset stomach, and rarely allergic reactions.

Garlic may reduce blood clotting ability.  Do not use garlic supplements if you are planning to have surgery, dental work, or have a bleeding disorder.

Additional uses and side effects may exist but further research is necessary to determine the exact properties and effects of use.

**General:**  Garlic is the edible bulb from a plant in the lily family and has been used as a spice and supplement for thousands of years.  Garlic bulbs are traditionally given in high quantities to obtain the supplement value.  Two cloves daily is a baseline for supplement use.  Garlic can be consumed raw, juiced, or dried into a powder supplement.

The juices of the Garlic have been used as an insect repellant primarily against insects like moths.  The bulbs, leaves, and flowers are eaten as a raw or cooked vegetable and the aroma increases as the plant ripens.

Wild Garlic is similar in composition and uses to cultivated Garlic but has a milder aroma and weaker action making it more common for use in traditional treatments given over a longer period.  Other types of Garlic including Allium canadense – Canadian Garlic and Allium vineale – Crow Garlic have similar properties with milder aroma and weaker action.

## Garlic Mustard
**Botanical Name:** Alliaria petiolata

**Properties:** Antibacterial, Antiseptic, Colorant, Detoxification, Diaphoretic, Vermifuge, Vulnerary

**Traditional Use:** Garlic Mustard juices have shown effectiveness against certain types of gram-negative bacteria like typhoid and have been used in traditional treatments to alleviate infections.

Garlic Mustard has been used as a traditional topical poultice or ointment to prevent infection and speed healing in skin sores, ulcers, and wounds.

**Part Used:** Leaf, Seed

**Side Effects:** Garlic Mustard is not recommended for use beyond dietary for women who are pregnant or nursing.

Additional uses and side effects may exist but further research is necessary to determine the exact properties and effects of use.

**General:** Garlic Mustard is native to Africa and Asia but has been naturalized to Europe and North America where it is considered an invasive species by some. It is not particular regarding soil composition but does prefer full shade and consistently moist or wet soil. It is propagated by seed and will self-seed readily if given its own place in the garden.

Garlic Mustard yields a yellow toned colorant used as a traditional dye product. The young leaves are harvested for use as a raw or cooked vegetable or dried for use as a seasoning. The flowers and young seedpods are eaten raw in salads.

The leaf and seed are harvested before flowering for use fresh or dried and powdered in traditional supplements.

## Glossy Privet, Aligustre, Linguster, Joteishi, Ligustro, Tree Privet, Tureno, White Waxtree, Yojungja
**Botanical Name:** Ligustrum lucidum

**Properties:** Antibacterial, Anodyne, Antiseptic, Cancer, Cardio-Tonic, Diuretic, Immunostimulant, Tonic

**Traditional Uses:** Glossy Privet has been used as a traditional supplement to combat bacterial respiratory and digestive tract infections.

**Parts Used:** Fruit

**Side Effects:** Glossy Privet is not recommended for use by women who are pregnant or nursing.

Glossy Privet may cause an allergic reaction in some people.

Additional uses and side effects may exist but further research is necessary to determine the exact properties and effects of use.

**General:**  Glossy Privet is native to China but is cultivated in other regions as an ornamental tree. It is considered invasive in some areas.  The fruit is harvested when ripe and used fresh or dried while the leaves are harvested year round and dried & powdered for use in traditional supplements.

## Goldenrod, Aaron's Rod, Woundwort
**Botanical Name:**  Solidago virgaurea

**Properties:**  Analgesic, Antibacterial, Antifungal, Anti-inflammatory, Antioxidant, Antiseptic, Antispasmodic, Astringent, Carminative, Colorant, Diaphoretic, Diuretic, Expectorant, Febrifuge, Hypoglycemic, Stimulant

**Traditional Use:**  Goldenrod is traditionally used in topical washes and ointments to reduce infection and speed healing of skin sores, ulcers, and wounds.

Goldenrod tea is used as a traditional gargle or spray to ease mouth & throat pain & inflammation while helping to combat infection.

Goldenrod is an effective diuretic that provides antiseptic benefits making it a traditional treatment for urinary tract infections.

**Part Used:**  Flower, Leaf

**Side Effects:**  Goldenrod is not recommended for women who are pregnant or nursing.

Goldenrod may cause an allergic reaction in some people.

Goldenrod is not recommended for people who have edema, kidney disease, heart problems, or high blood pressure.

Additional uses and side effects may exist but further research is necessary to determine the exact properties and effects of use.

**General:**  Goldenrod is a perennial wildflower that grows up to 5 feet in height.  It is native to Asia, Europe, and North America where it can be found growing wild in fields and along roads. Hardy to zone 5, it is not particular regarding soil composition or moisture but does prefer full to partial sun.  Goldenrod can be propagated by seeds sown out in the spring and will self-sow readily if given its own place in the garden.  Clumps can also be divided in the spring or fall.

Goldenrod flowers and stalks are used to create bright yellow and gold dye products.  Mordant – Alum.  The whole plant can provide a brown toned dye product.  Mordant – Chrome. Goldenrod leaves are used as a tea and the leaves and flowers are traditionally used as a cold extract or infusion.

**Goldenseal, Eye Balm, Eye Root, Goldenroot, Ground Raspberry, Indian Dye, Indian Plant, Indian Turmeric, Jaundice Root, Orange Root, Turmeric Root, Wild Curcuma, Yellow Indian Pain, Yellow Puccoon, Yellow Root**
**Botanical Name:** Hydrastis canadensis

**Properties:** Antibacterial, Antifungal, Anti-inflammatory, Antiseptic, Antispasmodic, Antiviral, Astringent, Cholagogue, Colorant, Detoxifier, Diuretic, Emmenagogue, Expectorant, Hypoglycemic, Hypotensive, Laxative, Immunostimulant

**Traditional Use:** Goldenseal is traditionally used in topical antiseptic and antibacterial ointments to speed healing and prevent infection in abrasions, cuts, and other wounds.

Goldenseal is a traditional ingredient in eliminating conjunctivitis and the astringent and antibacterial action helps to reduce redness and inflammation associated with other eye conditions.

Goldenseal contains active compounds that are used to in traditional preparations to stimulate white blood cells to seek out active infections including bacteria, fungi, viruses, and tumor cells.

Goldenseal is traditionally believed to be as effective if not more effective as prescription pharmaceuticals at treating gastrointestinal infections including those that cause diarrhea.

Goldenseal is included in traditional poultices, ointments, or gargles to treat mouth sores and throat or mouth infections.

**Part Used:** Leaf, Root, Underground Stem

**Side Effects:** Goldenseal is not recommended for use by women who are pregnant or nursing.

Goldenseal is not recommended for use in children's treatments.

Goldenseal is not intended for long-term use.

Goldenseal contains alkaloids that are toxic in large doses.

Overdose of goldenseal can cause vomiting, diarrhea, or stomach upset in some people.

Goldenseal may lower blood sugar levels, raise blood pressure, or cause gastrointestinal upset.

Goldenseal may change the way your body reacts to other prescription drugs.

Additional uses and side effects may exist but further research is necessary to determine the exact properties and effects of use.

**General:** Goldenseal is a perennial native to Eastern North America. Hardy to zone 3, it can be found growing wild in part of the US or cultivated in many supplement gardens. It is not particular regarding soil composition but does prefer full to partial shade and consistent moisture. It can be propagated by seed planted out as soon as they are ripe or by divisions of larger clumps in the fall.

The roots and stalk of the goldenseal yield a yellow colorant used as a textile dye product. The juices pounded out of the roots are used as an insect repellant. The underground stem and root of the Goldenseal plant are harvested in the fall for use fresh or dried, and powdered for use in supplement teas or made into an extract.

## Graviola, Brazilian Cherimoya, Brazilian Paw Paw, Guanabana, Guanavana, Nangka Blanda, Soursop
**Botanical Name:** Corossol epineux

**Properties:** Antibacterial, Antiparasitic, Antiviral, Cancer, Purgative

**Traditional Uses:** Graviola infusions are traditionally used to treat internal and external bacterial and viral infections.

**Parts Used:** Leaf, Fruit, Seed

**Side Effects:** Graviola is not recommended for use by women who are pregnant or nursing.

Graviola may be cause nerve damage or death.

Graviola may worsen the symptoms of Parkinson's Disease or cause symptoms similar to Parkinson's Disease.

Additional uses and side effects may exist but further research is necessary to determine the exact properties and effects of use.

**General:** Graviola is a small evergreen tree native to Brazil where it is harvested and used a seasoning or in beverages. The fruits, leaves, and seeds are also harvested, dried, and powdered for use in traditional supplements.

## Grindelia, Gum plant, Gumweed, Tarweed
**Botanical Name:** Grindelia robusta

**Properties:** Antibacterial, Anti-inflammatory, Antispasmodic, Antitussive, Colorant, Demulcent, Depurative, Emollient, Expectorant, Sedative

**Traditional Use:** Grindelia has been used as a traditional supplement to treat urinary tract infections, spasms, and irritable bladder.

**Part Used:** Flower, Leaf, Stem

**Side Effects:** Grindelia is not recommended for use by women who are pregnant or nursing.

Overuse of Grindelia may cause gastrointestinal upset.

Grindelia may have an effect on the heart and should be used under the guidance of a physician or qualified herbalist.

Additional uses and side effects may exist but further research is necessary to determine the exact properties and effects of use.

**General:** Grindelia is native to Central and North America. Hardy to zone 7, it prefers sandy to loamy soil, full sun, and dry to moist conditions. Grindelia can be propagated by seed sown in the spring and will self sow readily if given its own place in the garden.

Grindelia flowers yield a yellow toned colorant and the seedpods yield a green toned colorant. The leaf and flowers are harvested before the buds open, dried in full sunlight, powdered, and incorporated into traditional supplement infusions up to 3 times daily.

### Guduchi, Ambervel, Amrita, Gilo, Glunchanb, Gurcha, Indian Tinospora, Jetwatika, Teluga, Tinospora
**Botanical Name:** Tinsospora cardiofolia

**Properties:** Adaptogenic, Antibacterial, Antimicrobial, Antiseptic, Astringent, Detoxificant, Hyperglycemic, Immunostimulant, Stimulant, Tonic

**Traditional Use:** Guduchi stem extracts have been used as a traditional treatment for bacterial infections like e. coli.

Guduchi has traditionally been given as a treatment component to stimulate the production of white blood cells helping to increase immunity and ward off common infections.

**Part Used:** Leaf, Root, Stem

**Side Effects:** Guduchi is not recommended for use by women who are pregnant or nursing.

Guduchi may lower blood sugar.

Additional uses and side effects may exist but further research is necessary to determine the exact properties and effects of use.

**General:** Guduchi is a semi-parasitic vine native to India and found growing other subtropical regions. It is not particular regarding soil composition but does prefer full to partial sun and dry soil.

The entire plant is harvested, dried, and powdered for use in traditional infusions or the compounds extracted through as a strong decoction.

### Gumbo Limbo
**Botanical Name:** Bursera simaruba

**Properties:** Antibacterial, Anti-inflammatory, Astringent, Diuretic

**Traditional Use:** Gumbo Limbo has traditionally been used in gargles and sprays to reduce inflammation and treat infection in the mouth and throat.

Gumbo Limbo has been used as a traditional supplement to treat urinary tract infection.

**Part Used:**  Leaf

**Side Effects:**  Gumbo Limbo is not recommended for use by women who are pregnant or nursing.

Additional uses and side effects may exist but further research is necessary to determine the exact properties and effects of use.

**General:**  Gumbo Limbo is native to Central America, southern North America, and South America.  It is easily grown from cuttings and cultivated as wind resistant hedge rows.  The wood is used for craftwork and the resin is used as a glue or varnish product.

## Gurmar, Gemnema, Gurmarbooti, Miracle Plant, Shardunika, Vishani
**Botanical Name:**  Gymnema sylvestre

**Properties:**  Antibacterial, Antiviral, Astringent, Cholesterol, Diuretic, Hypoglycemic

**Traditional Use:**  Gurmar has shown an ability to kill bacteria and viruses and is often included in household cleaning preparations.

**Part Used:**  Leaf, Root

**Side Effects:**  Gurmar is not recommended for use by women who are pregnant or nursing.

Gurmar affects blood sugar.

Additional uses and side effects may exist but further research is necessary to determine the exact properties and effects of use.

**General:**  Gumar is native to Asia, Africa, and India where the leaves are harvested for use in traditional treatments at a rate of 7-10 grams of powdered leaf per dose.

## Hairy Agrimony
**Botanical Name:**  Agrimonia pilosa

**Properties:**  Analgesic, Antibacterial, Anti-inflammatory, Astringent, Cardio-Tonic, Haemostatic, Hypoglycemic, Vasoconstrictor, Vermifuge

**Traditional Use:**  The juice from Hairy Agrimony has been used as a traditional supplement to treat and prevent peptic ulcers.

Hairy Agrimony is traditionally used as part of a gargle or spray to reduce mouth & throat inflammation, infection, and pain.

Hairy Agrimony is used in traditional topical preparations to reduce infection, relieve pain, stop bleeding and speed healing in wounds.

**Part Used:**  Whole

**Side Effects:** Hairy Agrimony is not recommended for use by women who are pregnant or nursing.

Hairy Agrimony may lower blood sugar.

Hairy Agrimony may cause heart palpitations when taken internally.

Additional uses and side effects may exist but further research is necessary to determine the exact properties and effects of use.

**General:** Hairy Agrimony is a perennial native to Asia and Europe but cultivated in many regions of the world as an ornamental. It is not particular regarding soil composition but does prefer full to partial sun and dry to moist soil. Hairy Agrimony can be propagated by seed sown out in the spring or allowed to self-sow in the fall. It can also be divided at the end of the growing season.

The leaves are harvested and eaten as a cooked vegetable while the seeds are harvested, dried and powdered for use as flour. The whole plant is harvested at the beginning of the flowering season, dried, and powdered for use in traditional supplements.

**Henna, Alcanna, Egyptian Privet, Mehndi, Mendee, Mignonette Tree, Reseda, Smooth Lawsonia**
**Botanical Name:** Lawsonia inermis

**Properties:** Analgesic, Antibacterial, Antifungal, Anti-inflammatory, Astringent, Cancer, Colorant, Diuretic, Emmenagogue

**Traditional Use:** Henna leaves have been used as a traditional preparation to treat both gram positive and gram-negative bacterial infections.

Henna leaves are traditionally used in an infusion to treat severe bacterially caused diarrhea and dysentery.

Henna leaf tea has been used as a traditional gargle or spray to alleviate bacteria infections of the throat or mouth and reduce related inflammation.

**Part Used:** Bark, Fruit, Leaf

**Side Effects:** Henna is not recommended for use by women who are pregnant or nursing.

Henna has been used as a uterine stimulant and may have abortifacient properties.

Henna is not recommended for use in children's treatments.

Henna is not recommended for internal treatments without the advice of a physician or qualified herbalist.

Henna may cause an allergic reaction or skin irritation.

Additional uses and side effects may exist but further research is necessary to determine the exact properties and effects of use.

**General:** Henna is a shrub or tree native to the Middle East and cultivated in other tropical and sub-tropical regions.

Henna powders can be colorless or finished in shades of red and are frequently used as colorants in natural care products. Henna is harvested, dried, and powdered for use in external applications or as a traditional supplement tea up to 3 times daily though the FDA has only approved Henna as a hair colorant.

### Herb Paris
**Botanical Name:** Paris polyphylla

**Properties:** Analgesic, Antibacterial, Antispasmodic, Expectorant, Febrifuge, Narcotic

**Traditional Use:** Herb Paris root decoctions have traditionally been used to treat bacterial infections like bacillus dysenteriae, bacillus typhi, e. coli, and staphylococcus aurus among others.

Herb Paris root decoctions have traditionally been used in topical preparations to alleviate pain, treat infection, and speed healing in skin sores, ulcers, and wounds.

**Part Used:** Root

**Side Effects:** Herb Paris is not recommended for use by women who are pregnant or nursing.

Additional uses and side effects may exist but further research is necessary to determine the exact properties and effects of use.

**General:** Herb Paris is native to Asia and cultivated in other parts of the world as an ornamental. Hardy to 8, It is not particular regarding soil composition but does prefer full to partial shade and consistent moisture. Herb Paris can be propagated by seeds sown as soon as they are ripe or division of mature plants.

The roots of mature Herb Paris plants are harvested for use in traditional decoctions.

Do not confuse Herb Paris, Paris polyphylla with Paris quadrifolia also commonly called Herb Paris.

### Herb Robert, Crow's Foot, Dove's Foot, Dragon's Blood, Mountain Geranium, Red Robin, Robert Geranium, Stinky Bob, Storksbill, Wild Crane's Bill
**Botanical Name:** Geranium robertianum

**Properties:** Antibacterial, Antimicrobial, Antiviral, Astringent, Colorant, Diuretic, Hypoglycemic, Vulnerary

**Traditional Use:** An extraction of Herb Robert mixed at a rate of 20/80 with ethyl alcohol has traditionally been used to treat infections and has shown an ability to inhibit or kill common bacteria and viruses including adeno, e. coli, and staphylococcus.

Herb Robert is used as a traditional topical preparation to prevent infection and speed healing of skin sores, ulcers, and wounds.

**Part Used:** Flower, Leaf, Root, Stem

**Side Effects:** Herb Robert is not recommended for use by women who are pregnant or nursing.

Herb Robert may affect blood sugar.

Additional uses and side effects may exist but further research is necessary to determine the exact properties and effects of use.

**General:** Herb Robert is native to Africa, Asia, and Europe and naturalized to North and South America. Hardy to zone 6, it is not particular regarding soil composition but does prefer full to partial sun and dry to moist soil. Herb Robert is propagated by seed sown in the spring and will self-sow readily if given its own place in the garden.

Herb Robert yields a brown colorant that has been used as a hair, skin, or textile dye. The colorant extracted as a dye product is used as a sunless tanning lotion that has a secondary benefit of repelling mosquitoes and other biting insects. Herb Robert is harvested during the flowering season and used fresh in traditional supplements or the oils are extracted for later use.

### Hibiscus, Gongura, Guinea Sorrel, Jamaica Sorrel, Karkade, Red Sorrel, Red Tea, Roselle, Sour Tea, Sudanease Tea
**Botanical Name:** Hibiscus sabdariffa

**Properties:** Antibacterial, Antispasmodic, Antiviral, Astringent, Colorant, Digestive, Diuretic, Emollient, Febrifuge, Hypotensive, Laxative, Sedative, Uterine Relaxant, Vermifuge

**Traditional Use:** Hibiscus leaves have traditionally been used in topical poultices to alleviate infection in skin sores, ulcers, and abscessed wounds.

**Part Used:** Flower, Leaf, Oil

**Side Effects:** Hibiscus flower is not recommended for use by women who are pregnant or nursing.

Hibiscus has been used as a uterine relaxant in some cultures.

Hibiscus may lower blood pressure.

Additional uses and side effects may exist but further research is necessary to determine the exact properties and effects of use.

**General:** Hibiscus is an annual cultivated in many warmer regions as an ornamental and as a container plant in other places. Hardy to zone 10, it is not particular regarding soil composition but does prefer full sun and consistent moisture. Hibiscus is propagated by bulbs planted out in the spring or by division and separation of the bulbs prior to winter storage.

Hibiscus stems are used to make a hemp like fiber. Yellow Hibiscus flowers yield a yellow toned dye. Red or purple Hibiscus flowers yield a dusky red toned colorant.

Hibiscus flowers are harvested for use in jams, drinks, and foods. The leaves and flowers are harvested and the oils extracted through steam distillation or dried and powdered for use in a traditional supplement tea.

### Holy Basil, Ajaka, Baranda, Brinda, Indian Basil, Kemangen, Sacred Basil, Tulsi
**Botanical Name:** Ocimum sanctum

**Properties:** Adaptogen, Antibacterial, Antifungal, Anti-inflammatory, Antioxidant, Antitussive, Cancer, Carminative, Cox-2 Inhibitor, Demulcent, Diuretic, Expectorant, Febrifuge, Hypoglycemic, Immunostimulant, Insect Repellant, Laxative

**Traditional Use:** Holy Basil has been used as a traditional treatment for staphylococcus infections and other types of bacterial infections.

Holy Basil has traditionally been used to stimulate the immune system helping to ward off common infections.

**Part Used:** Leaf, Seed, Stem

**Side Effects:** Holy Basil is not recommended for use by women who are pregnant or nursing.

Holy Basil may slow blood clotting.

Additional uses and side effects may exist but further research is necessary to determine the exact properties and effects of use.

**General:** Holy Basil is native to India and is cultivated elsewhere. It is considered an invasive weed in some areas. It is easily propagated by seed and will self-seed readily.

Holy Basil leaves have been used as an insect repellant. The leaves are used as a seasoning in a variety of dishes or as a tea. The leaves are harvested and the oils extracted or the leaf, seed, and stem are harvested, dried, and powdered for use in traditional supplements.

### Honey Locust
**Botanical Name:** Gleditsia sinensis

**Properties:** Antibacterial, Antifungal, Anti-inflammatory, Antiseptic, Antitussive, Astringent, Cancer, Diuretic, Emetic, Expectorant, Febrifuge, Haemostatic, Laxative, Stimulant, Vermifuge

**Traditional Use:** Honey Locust has traditionally been used as a gargle to help treat infection, reduce inflammation and speed healing in the mouth and throat.

A decoction of the Honey Locust thorn and leaf has been used in traditional topical washes or ointments to treat infection and speed healing of skin ulcers, sores, and wounds.

**Part Used:** Leaf, Seed, Thorn

**Side Effects:** Honey Locust may contain toxic compounds and it is not recommended for use without the advice of a qualified herbalist or physician.

Honey Locust is not recommended for use by women who are pregnant or nursing.

Additional uses and side effects may exist but further research is necessary to determine the exact properties and effects of use.

**General:** Honey Locust is a deciduous tree native to Asia, Europe, and North America. Hardy to zone 5, it is not particular regarding soil composition but does prefer full sun and consistent moisture. It is easily propagated by seeds soaked until they swell before planting.

The seedpod has been harvested for use as a soap product or as a source of tannin. The wood is used for construction. The seeds have been used as a sugar substitute or roasted, soaked and eaten as a sweet cooked vegetable.

The leaf, seed, and thorn are harvested for use fresh or dried in traditional topical and infusion preparations.

**Honeysuckle, Chevrefeuille, Goat's Leaf, Honey Suckle, Suikazura, Woodbine**
**Botanical Name:** Lonicera periclymenum

**Properties:** Antibacterial, Anti-inflammatory, Antispasmodic, Antiviral, Antiseptic, Cathartic, Diuretic, Emetic, Emollient, Expectorant, Febrifuge, Laxative, Sedative, Vulnerary

**Traditional Uses:** Honeysuckle has been used as a traditional gargle to reduce infection and speed the healing of mouth ulcers and reduce throat infections.

Honeysuckle is traditionally used in tropical preparations to speed healing in skin sores, ulcers, and wounds while preventing infections.

**Parts Used:** Flower, Leaf, Seed

**Side Effects:** Honeysuckle is not recommended for use by women who are pregnant or nursing.

Additional uses and side effects may exist but further research is necessary to determine the exact properties and effects of use.

**General:** Honeysuckle is a common bush or climbing vine cultivated in many regions of the world as a fragrant ornamental. Hardy to zone 5, it is not particular regarding soil composition or sun but does prefer consistent moisture. Honeysuckle can be propagated by seeds sown out as soon as they are ripe, cuttings taken in mid summer or layering.

Honeysuckle flowers yield a sweet, sugary nectar or the oils are extracted for use in perfumery. The fruits are eaten as a cooked food while the flowers have been used as an aromatic tea.

Honeysuckle leaf, seed, and flower are harvested, dried, and powdered for use in traditional supplement infusions.

## Honeysuckle – Japanese
**Botanical Name:** Lonicera japonica

**Properties:** Antibacterial, Anti-inflammatory, Antimicrobial, Antispasmodic, Antiviral, Astringent, Depurative, Diuretic, Febrifuge, Hypotensive

**Traditional Use:** Japanese Honeysuckle bark has traditionally been used to break up bladder and kidney stones and to alleviate urinary tract inflammation & infections.

Japanese Honeysuckle flowers & leaves are broad spectrum antimicrobials used in traditional supplements to treat a variety of bacterial and viral infectious agents including a numerous influenza strains, pseudomonas aeruginosa, salmonella typhi, staphylococcus aureus and streptococcus pneumoniae.

Japanese Honeysuckle flowers & leaves are used as a traditional gargle to reduce infection in the mouth and throat and to speed healing of mouth ulcers .

**Part Used:** Bark, Flower, Leaf

**Side Effects:** Japanese Honeysuckle is not recommended for use by women who are pregnant or nursing.

Additional uses and side effects may exist but further research is necessary to determine the exact properties and effects of use.

**General:** Japanese Honeysuckle is native to Asia and is commonly cultivated in many regions of the world as a fragrant and ornamental. Hardy to zone 4, it is not particular regarding soil composition but does prefer full or partial sun and consistent moisture. It can be propagated by seeds sown out as soon as they are ripe, cuttings taken in the mid summer or by layering in the fall.

Japanese Honeysuckle has been used in Chinese supplements for thousands of years. The leaves are harvested and eaten as a cooked vegetable while the flowers are used as a sweet syrup. The bark, flower, and leaves are harvested at the end of the growing season, dried, and powdered for use in traditional topical and infusion preparations.

## Hops, Houblon, Lupulin
**Botanical Name:** Humulus lupulus

**Properties:** Abortifacient, Anodyne, Antibacterial, Antifungal, Antimicrobial, Antiseptic, Cancer, Colorant, Diuretic, Emollient, Estrogenic, Febrifuge, Galactogogue, Hypnotic, Muscle Relaxant, Nervine, Sedative

**Traditional Use:** Hops have both antibacterial and antifungal properties making it a traditional treatment for common fungal infections like athlete's foot and bacterial infections like staphylococcus.

Hops have traditionally been used in topical preparations to reduce inflammation, pain, and infection while speeding healing in skin sores, ulcers, and wounds.

**Part Used:** Female Cone, Female Flower

**Side Effects:** Hops are not recommended for use by women who are pregnant or nursing.

Hops have been used as an abortifacient in some cultures.

Hops have a CNS depressant effect and should not be used in conjunction with CNS depressants, antipsychotic medications, or alcohol.

Hops can irritate the skin.

Overuse may cause confusion and dizziness.

Some people may react differently to hops and experience dizziness, menstrual disturbances, or nervousness.

Hops is not recommended for use by people who suffer from a psychotic disorder like bi-polar disorder, depression, or schizophrenia or for use by people taking prescription medications to treat these disorders.

Hops should not be used without the advice of a qualified herbalist or physician.

Additional uses and side effects may exist but further research is necessary to determine the exact properties and effects of use.

**General:** Hops are native to Asia & Europe but are cultivated in North America. Hardy to zone 5, it is not particular regarding soil composition but does prefer full or partial sun and moist soil though it can tolerate drought once established. Hops can be propagated by seed sown out in the spring or by cuttings taken early in the season.

Hops leaves and flower heads yield a brown toned colorant and the female fruits yield oil used in perfumery. The stems are used to make hemp like cording and are sometimes used to make cloth.

The whole female herb is harvested in the fall, dried at temperatures between 40 and 60 degrees, and powdered for use in traditional supplement teas or tincture preparations.

**Horehound**
**Botanical Name:** Marrubium vulgare

**Properties:** Analgesic, Antibacterial, Antiseptic, Antispasmodic, Appetite Stimulant, Cholagogue, Circulatory, Diaphoretic, Digestive, Diuretic, Emmenagogue, Expectorant, Hepatic, Hypoglycemic, Hypotensive, Insect Repellant

**Traditional Use:** Horehound has been used as a traditional preparation to treat bacterial infections especially against drug resistant bacteria.

**Part Used:** Flower, Leaf

**Side Effects:** Horehound is not recommended for use by women who are pregnant or nursing.

Horehound may affect blood sugar.

Additional uses and side effects may exist but further research is necessary to determine the exact properties and effects of use.

**General:** Horehound is a bitter herb that grows throughout the world and is considered an invasive weed in some areas. Hardy to zone 3, it is not particular regarding soil composition but does require full sun and consistent moisture. Horehound can be propagated by seed sown in the spring or division of the clumps.

Horehound yields an essential oil used as a flavoring in liquors or as an insect repellant. Horehound has been used as a respiratory supplement for hundreds of years and is traditionally harvested as it comes into flower and used fresh, dried, or as an extract.

**Horseradish, Great Raifort, Mountain Radish, Red Cole**
**Botanical Name:** Armoracia rusticana

**Properties:** Antibacterial, Antifungal, Anti-inflammatory, Antimicrobial, Antiseptic, Antispasmodic, Digestive, Diuretic, Expectorant, Rubefacient, Stimulant

**Traditional Use:** Horseradish has traditionally been used in topical and supplement preparations to treat both gram positive and gram-negative bacterial infections.

Horseradish has been used as a traditional supplement for urinary tract infections.

Horseradish has been used as an agent to purify drinking water and has proven effective against a variety of microbes.

**Part Used:** Root

**Side Effects:** Horseradish is not recommended for use beyond dietary by women who are pregnant or nursing.

Horseradish is not recommended for use by people with a history of kidney disease, an inflammatory bowel condition, an under active thyroid gland.

Children under 4 years of age should not consume horseradish supplement.

Horseradish may irritate the mucus membranes and should not be used when stomach or intestinal ulcers are present.

Additional uses and side effects may exist but further research is necessary to determine the exact properties and effects of use.

**General:** Horseradish is native to Europe but has naturalized in many regions of the world. Hardy to zone 5, it is not particular regarding soil composition but does prefer full to partial sun and consistent moisture. Horseradish can be propagated by division at almost any time during the growing season and even the smallest part of root will grow into a full plant.

Horseradish root is harvested and grated to make horseradish sauce. The young leaves are eaten as a raw or cooked component in dishes and the seeds are sprouted and eaten as a raw vegetable. The root is harvested for use in external preparations at a rate of 2% and internally as a traditional supplement tea up to 3 times daily.

**Hyssop, Curdukotu, Jufa, Ysop**
**Botanical Name:** Hyssopus officinalis

**Properties:** Abortifacient, Anti-inflammatory, Antimicrobial, Antiseptic, Antispasmodic, Antiviral, Astringent, Carminative, Diaphoretic, Diuretic, Emmenagogue, Expectorant, Hypertensive, Nervine, Sedative, Vermifuge, Vulnerary

**Traditional Use:** The leaves and oils of the hyssop have antimicrobial properties that are traditionally used to combat topical and internal bacterial and viral infections.

Hyssop is traditionally used in washes & topical ointments to help treat infection & speed healing in skin sores, ulcers, and wounds.

Hyssop has been used as a traditional gargle or spray to alleviate inflammation and infection in the throat & mouth.

Hyssop is traditionally used in supplements to treat urinary tract infections.

**Part Used:** Flower, Leaf, Oil

**Side Effects:** Hyssop is not recommended for use by women who are pregnant or nursing.

Hyssop has been used as an abortifacient in some cultures.

Hyssop is not recommended for use in children's treatments.

Hyssop is not recommended for use by people with a history of seizures.

Additional uses and side effects may exist but further research is necessary to determine the exact properties and effects of use.

**General:** Hyssop is native to the Mediterranean but is cultivated in the United States as an ornamental or for its oils. Hardy to zone 7, it prefers sandy to loamy soil, full sun, and consistent moisture. Hyssop can be propagated by seeds sown in the spring, cuttings taken in mid summer or division.

Hyssop oils are extracted through steam distillation for use in food, perfumery, aromatherapy, and traditional preparations. The flowers, leaves, and young shoots are eaten as a raw vegetable or flavoring additive. The whole plant, but especially the leaves are harvested during flowering, dried, and powdered for use in traditional supplemental infusions given throughout the day.

### Iceland Moss, Centaria, Liverwort, Iceland Lichen
**Botanical Name:** Cetraria islandica

**Properties:** Antibacterial, Antibiotic, Anti-inflammatory, Antimicrobial, Demulcent, Digestive, Galactogogue, Tonic

**Traditional Use:** Iceland Moss extracts have been used in commercial and traditional disinfecting products.

Iceland moss infusions have been used as a traditional gargle or spray to ease pain and inflammation in the throat and mouth while treating bacterial infections.

Iceland moss has traditionally been used in washes to treat skin inflammation, alleviate infections, and speed wound healing.

**Part Used:** Thallus - Moss

**Side Effects:** Iceland Moss is regulated in the United States. Iceland Moss is only approved for use as a flavoring agent.

Iceland Moss is not recommended for use by women who are pregnant or nursing.

Iceland Moss may irritate the mucus membranes and overuse may cause loose stools, nausea, and liver problems.

Additional uses and side effects may exist but further research is necessary to determine the exact properties and effects of use.

**General:** Iceland moss is a lichen that grows in the Alpine, Arctic, and Boreal biomes of the Northern Hemisphere. Hardy to zone 2, it is not particular regarding soil composition but does prefer full to partial sun and consistent moisture. Iceland Moss is propagated by division.

The moss is harvested, dried in the sun, and powdered for use as a flour product, food thickener, and in traditional supplement teas up to 4 times daily or as a wash prepared as an infusion and applied to the affected area 3-4 times daily.

### Ikhathazo, Lesoko
**Botanical Name:** Alepidea amatymbica

**Properties:** Antibacterial, Antifungal, Anti-inflammatory, Antimicrobial, Psychoactive, Sedative

**Traditional Use:** Ikhathazo has traditionally been used as a topical or supplement preparation to treat bacterial & fungal infections and has proven to have antimicrobial properties in laboratory studies.

Ikhathazo has been used as a traditional topical preparation to reduce inflammation, minimize the likelihood of infection, and speed healing in wounds.

**Part Used:** Rhizome

**Side Effects:** Ikhathazo is not recommended for use by women who are pregnant or nursing.

Ikathazo may cause intoxication, hallucinations or aggravate existing psychiatric disorders and is not recommended for use without the advice of a qualified herbalist or physician.

Additional uses and side effects may exist but further research is necessary to determine the exact properties and effects of use.

**General:** Ikhathazo is a perennial native to Africa where the plant has been used as a ceremonial psychoactive and as a traditional supplement.

## Immortelle, Shrubby Everlasting, Eternal Flower, Goldilocks, Sandy Everlasting, Strawflower, Yellow Chaste Weed
**Botanical Name:**
Helichrysum angustifolium

**Properties:**
Analgesic, Antibacterial, Anti-inflammatory, Antispasmodic, Antiviral, Cytophaylactic, Depurative, Diuretic, Expectorant, Hypoallergenic, Immunostimulant, Nervine

**Traditional Use:**
Immortelle has traditionally been used to alleviate constriction and excess congestion in conditions like asthma, bronchitis, colds, and influenza while acting to fight any bacteria or virus causing any related infection.

Immortelle has been used as a traditional supplement to help stimulate the immune system helping to prevent or shorten the duration of common infections.

**Part Used:**
Flower

**Side Effects:**
Immortelle is not recommended for use by women who are pregnant or nursing.

Immortelle is not recommended for use in children's treatments.

Immortelle is not recommended for use by people who have a blocked bile duct or gallstones.

Immortelle may cause an allergic reaction in some people.

Additional uses and side effects may exist but further research is necessary to determine the exact properties and effects of use.

**General:**
Immortelle is native to Europe and the United States. It prefers sandy or loamy soil, full or partial sunlight and consistent moisture. It is easily propagated by seeds direct sown as soon as they are ripe or by division of suckers in the spring.

The flowers are harvested as the buds begin to bloom. They are dried, powdered, and used in traditional supplement teas up to 3 times daily. Immortelle oil is steam distilled within 24 hours of harvesting the flower for use in topical and aromatherapy preparations.

**Indian Kamilla, Apuyot, Kamilla, Pikal, Rohini, Spoonwood, Tagusala**
**Botanical Name:** Mallotus philippensis

**Properties:** Antibacterial, Antifungal, Antihistamine, Antimicrobial, Colorant, Contraceptive, Purgative, Vermifuge

**Traditional Use:** Kamilla has been used as a traditional topical or supplement treatment to alleviate gram positive and gram-negative bacterial infections including e coli and pneumonia among others.

**Part Used:** Bark, Fruit Skin, Leaf, Seed – Oil

**Side Effects:** Kamilla is not recommended for use by women who are pregnant or nursing.

Kamala is not recommended for people who show symptoms of appendicitis.

Kamilla is not recommended for use by women who are trying to conceive as it has been used as a contraceptive in some cultures.

Additional uses and side effects may exist but further research is necessary to determine the exact properties and effects of use.

**General:** Indian Kamilla is native to Asia, Australia, and India where the oils are used as a wax product, cosmetic ingredient, or varnish. The glands & hairs are powdered as a dye product or for use as a traditional supplement. The fruit is harvested and skinned then the skins are dried and powdered for use in traditional supplements.

**Indian Madder, Madder, Manjistha, Tamaralli**
**Botanical Name:** Rubia cordifolia

**Properties:** Anodyne, Antibacterial, Antitussive, Astringent, Colorant, Diuretic, Emmenagogue, Expectorant, Febrifuge, Hypotensive, Styptic, Tonic, Vulnerary

**Traditional Use:** Indian Madder has been used as a traditional topical or supplement preparation to treat bacterial infections like pneumococci and staphylococcus.

**Part Used:** Root

**Side Effects:** Indian Madder is not recommended for use by women who are pregnant or nursing.

Indian Madder affects blood pressure.

Additional uses and side effects may exist but further research is necessary to determine the exact properties and effects of use.

**General:** Indian Madder is a perennial native to Africa, Asia, and Europe. Hardy to zone 6, it is not particular regarding soil composition but does prefer partial shade and consistent moisture. Indian Madder can be propagated by seeds sown when they are ripe or by division.

Indian Madder stems & roots yield a red colorant used as a cosmetic and textile dye. The leaves are eaten as a cooked vegetable and the fruits are eaten raw. The roots of mature plants are harvested in the fall, peeled, dried, and powdered for use as a traditional supplement.

**Indian Pipe, Ghost Plant**
**Botanical Name:** Monotropa uniflora

**Properties:** Anodyne, Antibacterial, Antispasmodic, Febrifuge, Hypnotic, Nervine, Sedative

**Traditional Use:** Indian Pipe has traditionally been applied as a poultice to help reduce infection, alleviate pain, and speed healing in skin sores, ulcers, & wounds.

**Part Used:** Leaf, Root, Stem

**Side Effects:** Indian Pipe is not recommended for use by women who are pregnant or nursing.

Indian Pipe acts as a sedative and is not recommended for use without the advice of a qualified herbalist or physician.

Additional uses and side effects may exist but further research is necessary to determine the exact properties and effects of use.

**General:** Indian Pipe is a perennial parasitic plant native to Asia, South America, and North America. It is not particular regarding soil composition but does prefer full or partial shade and consistent moisture. Indian Pipe is propagated by seed but is a difficult plant to cultivate. Some success has been had with rooting cuttings on host plants & trees growing in a warm, humid environment.

The plant is harvested for use as an asparagus like food or dried & powdered for use as a traditional supplement.

**Indigo – Wild, American Indigo, Baptista, False Indigo, Horsefly Weed, Indigo Broom, Rattlebush, Wild Indigo, Yellow Indigo**
**Botanical Name:** Baptisia tinctoria

**Properties:** Adaptogen, Antibacterial, Antiseptic, Antiviral, Astringent, Cholagogue, Colorant, Emetic, Estrogenic, Febrifuge, Immunostimulant

**Traditional Use:** A decoction of Wild Indigo root has traditionally been used as part of a topical ointment, wash, or poultice to treat infections like staphylococcus, reduce acne outbreaks, and speed healing in skin ulcers and wounds.

Wild Indigo has been used as a traditional supplement to stimulate the immune system against infection.

Wild Indigo has traditionally been used as an ointment or gargle to alleviate canker sores, throat infection, and mouth or throat inflammation.

Wild Indigo has been used as a traditional supplement to stimulate the immune system, help support antibody production, and ward off common infections.

**Part Used:** Root

**Side Effects:** Wild Indigo is not recommended for use by women who are pregnant or nursing.

Wild Indigo is not recommended for use in children's treatments.

Wild Indigo may cause skin irritation in some people.

Wild Indigo is not recommended for people with gastrointestinal disorders.

Overuse of Wild Indigo may cause diarrhea, difficulty breathing, increased heart rate, nausea, vomiting or even death.

Additional uses and side effects may exist but further research is necessary to determine the exact properties and effects of use.

**General:** Wild Indigo is a perennial native to eastern North America. Hardy to zone 5, it prefers sandy or loamy soil and has the ability top add nitrogen back into nutritionally poor areas. It does require full sun and prefers consistent moisture. It can be propagated by seed sown out as soon as it is ripe and it self-seeds readily. Wild Indigo can also be propagated by division of larger clumps early in the growing season.

Wild Indigo is related to Dyer's Indigo and has smaller concentrations of blue toned colorant valued in dyeing and can be used in larger quantity to achieve the same tones. The young shoots are sometimes eaten as a vegetable.

Wild Indigo root is harvested, dried and powdered for use in traditional supplement infusions up to 3 times daily or in ointment preparations at a rate of 1:1 in 60% alcohol.

**Iporoni, Iporuru, Ipurosa, Macochihua, Niando**
**Botanical Name:** Alchornea castaneifolia

**Properties:** Analgesic, Antibacterial, Antifungal, Anti-inflammatory, Antiparasitic, Aphrodisiac, Astringent, Diuretic, Hallucinogenic, Hypoglycemic, Psychedelic, Stimulant

**Traditional Uses:** Iporuru is used in traditional topical and supplement preparations to alleviate bacterial infections like e coli and staphylococcus, fungal infections like athlete's foot and parasitic skin infestations like scabies.

**Parts Used:** Bark, Leaf, Root

**Side Effects:** Iporuru is not recommended for use by women who are pregnant or nursing.

Additional uses and side effects may exist but further research is necessary to determine the exact properties and effects of use.

**General:** Iporoni is native to the Amazon rainforest where it has been harvested as a food product and traditional supplement for thousands of years.

## Jacote, Cajote, Mombin, Sineguela
**Botanical Name:** Spondias purpurea

**Properties:** Analgesic, Antibacterial, Antispasmodic, Astringent, Contraceptive, Diuretic, Laxative, Styptic

**Traditional Use:** Jacote has been used as a topical preparation to reduce bleeding, alleviate infection, and speed healing in skin sores, ulcers, and wounds.

Jacote fruit has traditionally been used as a gargle or spray to help speed healing in mouth ulcers and reduce infection & inflammation of the throat & mouth.

**Part Used:** Bark, Flower, Fruit

**Side Effects:** Jacote is not recommended for use by women who are pregnant or nursing.

Jacote is not recommended for use by women who are trying to conceive as it has been used as a contraceptive in some cultures.

Additional uses and side effects may exist but further research is necessary to determine the exact properties and effects of use.

**General:** Jacote is native to Central America and South America and cultivated in tropical regions throughout the world where the fruit is harvested as a food.

## Juniper, Guinevere, Ginepro, Juniper Berries, Zimbro
**Botanical Name:** Juniperus communis

**Properties:** Abortifacient, Analgesic, Antibacterial, Antifungal, Anti-inflammatory, Antiseptic, Antispasmodic, Antiviral, Aphrodisiac, Arthritis, Astringent, Cancer, Carminative, Circulation, Depurative, Diaphoretic, Disinfectant, Diuretic, Emmenagogue, Hypotensive, Insect Repellant, Nervine, Rubefacient, Sedative, Tonic, Vermifuge

**Traditional Use:**  Juniper berries are traditionally used to irrigate a urinary tract infection while acting to treat the underlying infection.

Juniper is used as an ingredient in disinfecting household cleaning products.

Juniper is traditionally used as a topical wash or ointment to speed healing of wounds and prevent infections.

**Part Used:**  Berry, Needles, Oil

**Side Effects:**  Juniper is not recommended for use by women who are pregnant or nursing.

Juniper berries are not recommended for use by women who suffer from heavy menstrual bleeding.  They have been used as a dietary abortifacient in some cultures and are known to increase menstrual bleeding.

Juniper is not recommended for use by people who have diabetes, intestinal disorders, high blood pressure, or kidney disease.

Juniper may increase bleeding and is not recommended for use by those who have a bleeding disorder.

Overuse of Juniper may cause urine to smell like violets.

Overdose of Juniper can cause kidney irritation, blood in the urine, and potential liver damage.

Juniper oil is for external use only.

Additional uses and side effects may exist but further research is necessary to determine the exact properties and effects of use.

**General:**  Juniper is an evergreen shrub native to Africa, Asia, and Europe and has been naturalized to parts of North America.  Hardy to zone 2, it is not particular regarding soil composition but does prefer full to partial sun.  It prefers consistent moisture but will tolerate drought once established.  Juniper can be propagated by seed but the hard seed coat may make germination difficult.  Propagation from cuttings taken late in the year or by layering is more successful.

Juniper branches and extractions are used as part of traditional insect repelling preparations.  The fruits are harvested in the fall and eaten raw or cooked as a flavoring in a variety of dishes.  The seeds are roasted and used as a coffee substitute.

Juniper berries are harvested for use as a diet or tea supplement while the oils are extracted from the needles.  Do not bruise or crush the berries until you are ready to use them.

**Jurema**
**Botanical Name:**  Mimosa hostilis

**Properties:** Antibacterial, Antimicrobial, Astringent, Emollient, Narcotic, Vulnerary

**Traditional Use:** Jurema has been used as a topical and traditional supplement to treat or prevent bacterial infections.

Jurema is traditionally used in topical preparations to reduce pain, treat infection, and speed healing in skin burns, sores, ulcers, and wounds.

**Part Used:** Leaf

**Side Effects:** Jurema is not recommended for use by women who are pregnant or nursing.

Jurema root bark may have narcotic properties and is banned for sale in the United States.

Additional uses and side effects may exist but further research is necessary to determine the exact properties and effects of use.

**General:** Jurema is an evergreen shrub native to Central and South America. Hardy to zone 9, it is not particular regarding soil composition and is known to fix nitrogen back into poor quality soils. It does prefer full to partial sun but is tolerant of dry conditions. Jurema can be propagated by seeds collected when the seedpods burst, air dried and then direct sown or by cuttings taken during the late spring and planted during any season except those that are extremely wet.

The wood is used to make fence posts and other construction products that will be exposed to the weather and the bark has been used in tanning and dyeing. The leaf has been harvested as a traditional supplement for thousands of years.

**Kava-Kava, Ava Pepper, Ava Root, Awa, Gea, Kao, Kavain, Kawa, Mulak, Maori Kava, Muruk, Sakau, Tonga, Waka, Yagona, Yaquon**
**Botanical Name:** Piper methysticum

**Properties:** Analgesic, Anesthetic, Anodyne, Antibacterial, Antifungal, Antioxidant, Antispasmodic, Aphrodisiac, Cancer, Cox-2 Inhibitor, Diuretic, Expectorant, Muscle Relaxant, Psychotropic, Sedative, Stimulant

**Traditional Use:** Kava-Kava has antibacterial and antifungal properties that have traditionally been used treat a variety of infections including internal and external bacterial infections like staphylococcus and fungal infections like athlete's foot.

Kava-Kava has traditionally been used as a chew to alleviate throat & mouth pain while treating infection.

**Part Used:** Rhizome, Root, Underground Stem

**Side Effects:** Kava-Kava is not recommended for use by women who are pregnant or nursing.

Kava-Kava is not recommended for use in children's treatments.

Kava Kava is not recommended for use with alcoholic beverages while using Kava-Kava.

Kava-Kava has been reported to cause liver damage or liver failure. The U.S. Food and Drug Administration (FDA) issued a warning that using kava supplements has been linked to a risk of severe liver damage.

Kava Kava acts as a sedative and users should not drive or operate heavy machinery while using Kava-Kava.

Long-term use of Kava-Kava can cause skin issues like scales, itchiness, ulcers, or yellowing of the skin or eyes.

Kava-Kava has been associated with involuntary muscle spasms and can interact with several drugs used for the treatment of Parkinson's Disease.

Additional uses and side effects may exist but further research is necessary to determine the exact properties and effects of use.

**General:** Kava Kava is native to Fiji, Hawaii, and Samoa. It is cultivated as a cash crop by some. It is not particular regarding soil composition but does prefer full to partial sun and consistent moisture. It is most commonly propagated by division of the rhizome or cuttings of the root taken during the growing season.

Kava-Kava rhizome, root, and underground stems are used in teas, extracts, and powder form. Kava-Kava is native to the South Pacific and is a member of the pepper family. Kava-Kava has been used in non-traditional and traditional medicine and ceremonies for centuries. Traditionally Kava has been administered for supplement purposes at a rate of 1 tbsp dried or powdered kava-kava root steeped in 1-cup boiling water for 30 minutes.

**Kino**
**Botanical Name:** Pterocarpus marsupium

**Properties:** Anodyne, Antibacterial, Anti-inflammatory, Astringent, Cholesterol, Hypoglycemic

**Traditional Use:** Kino bark infusions have traditionally been used to treat bacterial infections.

Kino leaves are used in traditional topical preparations to prevent infection and speed healing in skin sores, ulcers, and wounds.

Kino bark & heartwood have traditionally been used as a gargle to alleviate throat & mouth inflammation while treating related infections.

**Part Used:** Bark, Heartwood, Leaf

**Side Effects:** Kino is not recommended for use by women who are pregnant or nursing.

Kino affects blood sugar.

Additional uses and side effects may exist but further research is necessary to determine the exact properties and effects of use.

**General:**  Kino is a deciduous tree native to India where the bark and heartwood have been harvested, dried, and powdered for use in traditional supplements for thousands of years.

**Knotweed, Allseed, Anjubar, Armstrong, Beggarweed, Bird's Tongue, Birdweed, Centinode, Cow Grass, Crawlgrass, Doorweed, Hogweed, Knotgrass, Pigrush, Pigweed, Red Robin, Sanguinaria, Sparrow Tongue**
**Botanical Name:**  Polygonum aviculare

**Properties:**  Antibacterial, Anti-inflammatory, Astringent, Cardiotonic, Cholagogue, Diuretic, Emetic, Emollient, Expectorant, Febrifuge, Haemostatic, Styptic, Vasoconstrictor, Vulnerary

**Traditional Uses:**  Knotweed is traditionally used in gargle or spray preparations to help reduce gingivitis related to plaque and bacterial buildup on the teeth, to reduce bleeding from the gums, and to treat throat or mouth infection & inflammation.

Knotweed has been used as a traditional supplement to treat urinary tract infection and to ease irritation in conditions like irritable bladder.

Knotweed has traditionally been used in topical preparations to reduce infection and speed healing in skin sores, ulcers, and wounds.

**Parts Used:**  Leaf

**Side Effects:**  Knotweed is not recommended for use by women who are pregnant or nursing.

Knotweed is not recommended for use in children's treatments.

Additional uses and side effects may exist but further research is necessary to determine the exact properties and effects of use.

**General:**  Common Knotweed is native to Asia and Europe where it can be found growing wild in wastelands and untended areas.  Hardy to zone 5, it is not particular regarding soil composition but does prefer full to partial sun and consistent moisture.  Knotweed can be propagated by division or seeds sown in the spring and will self sow readily if given its own place in the garden.

Knotweed aerial parts yield a yellow to green toned colorant used as a textile dye.  Young Knotweed leaves and seeds are eaten raw or cooked. The grassy leaf is harvested at the end of the flowering season, dried, and powdered for use in traditional supplements.

**Kola Nut, Blissey Nut, Bissy Nut, Cola Nut, Guru Nut, Gworo, Soudan Coffee**
**Botanical Name:**  Cola acuminata

**Properties:**  Antibacterial, Antifungal, Antimicrobial, Aphrodisiac, Cancer, Cardiac, Stimulant

**Traditional Use:** Kola Nut extract is antibacterial and antifungal and have been used in traditional topical and supplement preparations to treat bacterial and fungal infections.

**Part Used:** Nut

**Side Effects:** Kola Nut is not recommended for use by women who are pregnant or nursing.

Kola Nut is not recommended for use by people who have anxiety disorders, bleeding disorders, heart conditions, diabetes, glaucoma, or high blood pressure.

Kola Nut may cause anxiety, headache, increased heart rate, insomnia, irritability, nausea, nervousness, restlessness, ringing in the ears, and vomiting.

Kola Nut is a stimulant and it affects the heart and metabolism. You should consult with a physician or qualified herbalist prior to incorporating Kola Nut into any treatment plan beyond kitchen consumption.

You should not stop using Kola Nut abruptly as withdrawal can cause anxiety, dizziness, headaches, irritation, and nervousness.

**General:** Kola Nuts are native to Africa where the nuts are used as part of traditional ceremonies, commercial supplements, and traditional supplements.

**Larch, Larix**
**Botanical Name:** Larix decidua

**Properties:** Antibacterial, Antiseptic, Antiviral, Astringent, Binding Agent, Cholesterol, Diuretic, Emollient, Expectorant, Haemostatic, Immunostimulant, Laxative, Stabilizer, Starch, Vulnerary

**Traditional Use:** Larch is a fiber and is used as a traditional supplement to increase good intestinal bacteria that helps to even out the digestive processes and may be beneficial in treating digestive ailments like IBS.

Larch is traditionally used to help boost the immune system and is frequently used as a prophylactic against common infections.

**Part Used:** Outer Bark

**Side Effects:** Larch is not recommended for use by women who are pregnant or nursing.

Larch is an immunostimulant and is not recommended for use by people with an immunoreactive disease like Multiple Sclerosis or Lupus.

Additional uses and side effects may exist but further research is necessary to determine the exact properties and effects of use.

**General:** Larch is native to Europe and has been naturalized in North America. Hardy to zone 4, it prefers sandy to loamy soil, full sun, and moist to wet conditions. Larch can be propagated by seeds cold stored and then sown in the spring.

Larch wood resin is used to preserve wood and the wood itself is used in construction. The inner bark is eaten or dried and ground into flour. The bark is also harvested, dried, and powdered for use in traditional supplements.

## Lavender
**Botanical Name:** Lavandula angustifolia, Lavandula officinalis

**Properties:** Analgesic, Antibacterial, Anti-inflammatory, Antifungal, Antioxidant, Antiseptic, Antispasmodic, Antiviral, Cancer, Colorant, Cardio-Tonic, Carminative, Deodorant, Diuretic, Emmenagogue, Hypotensive, Insect Repellant, Muscle Relaxant, Nervine, Sedative, Vermifuge

**Traditional Use:** Lavender oil has been used as a cleaning agent to kill bacterial, fungal, and viral infections.

Lavender is traditionally added to topical preparations to help reduce inflammation, prevent infection and speed healing of skin sores, skin ulcers, and wounds.

Lavender is added to traditional gargle preparations to reduce mouth & throat inflammation, prevent or treat infection and speed healing of mouth ulcers.

**Part Used:** Flower, Leaf, Stem

**Side Effects:** Lavender is not recommended for use by women who are pregnant or nursing.

There have been reports that topical use of lavender oil can cause breast growth in boys, men, and young women.

Lavender may cause changes in appetite, constipation, headaches, and drowsiness in some people.

Lavender can cause skin irritation in some people.

Lavender is not recommended for use with anti-anxiety, antidepressants, antihistamines, or sedatives.

Overuse of lavender oil for internal supplements can be toxic if taken by mouth. Oils are for external use only. The leaves have been ingested.

Additional uses and side effects may exist but further research is necessary to determine the exact properties and effects of use.

**General:** Lavender is native to the Mediterranean and was used in supplements and ceremonial treatments in ancient Egypt, Greece, and Rome. Hardy to zone 5, it is cultivated worldwide for use as a traditional aromatherapy, supplement tea, or extract. Lavender is not particular regarding soil composition but does prefer full sun, well-drained soil, and consistent moisture. It can be propagated by seed sown out in the spring or by cuttings taken in the mid-summer with a heel of the previous year's growth.

Lavender essential oil is used in a variety of cosmetic, perfumery, and aromatherapy recipes. The oil is used as an insect repellant ingredient. The flowers are harvested as soon as the blooms begin to fade and the oils steam extracted. The flower, leaf, and stem are harvested for use fresh or dried and powdered for use in traditional topical, aromatherapy and supplemental treatments.

## Lemon, Lemon Oil
**Botanical Name:** Citrus limonum

**Properties:** Adaptogen, Antibacterial, Anti-inflammatory, Antimicrobial, Antioxidant, Antiviral, Astringent, Carminative, Diuretic, Homeostatic, Immunostimulant, Rubefacient, Stimulant

**Traditional Use:** Lemon oil has natural antibacterial properties and a refreshing scent that makes it a good choice in natural house cleaning products.

Lemon oil has been used as an antibacterial & antiviral supplement and topical preparation to treat infections like streptococcus, staphylococcus, and MRSA.

Lemon is high in vitamin C and is traditionally used in immunity building programs helping the body to fight off infections.

Lemon juice is used as a traditional gargle or spray to treat throat & mouth infection while reducing the related inflammation.

Lemon is traditionally included in vapor treatments to disinfect the air and provide an uplifting and refreshing scent.

**Part Used:** Juice, Rind - Oil

**Side Effects:** Lemon is not recommended for use beyond dietary by women who are pregnant or nursing.

Lemon oil is phototoxic increasing the effect of sunlight on the skin.

Lemon oil should be diluted when using in any remedy as it may irritate the skin.

Additional uses and side effects may exist but further research is necessary to determine the exact properties and effects of use.

**General:** Lemon is native to India but has been cultivated in other parts of the world. Hardy to zone 9, it prefers loamy or heavy, well-drained soils with full sun and consistent moisture. Lemon can be propagated by seed, rinsed and sown as soon as it is ripe or by cuttings taken in the mid-summer.

Lemon rind oils are used as a flavoring, perfume component, and household cleaner. Lemon seed oil has been used in soap making and the oils from the leaves are commonly called petitgrain oil in aromatherapy though the Bitter Orange is the source of true petitgrain. Lemon juice is used as a cleaning and bleaching product.

Lemon fruits are eaten raw, cooked, or as a beverage. Lemon oil is extracted from the rind or seed for use in traditional and topical preparations. It is harvested for use in culinary, supplement, cosmetic, and cleaning recipes.

## Lemongrass, Citronella, Fever Grass, Lemon Grass, Oil Grass
**Botanical Name:** Cymbopogon citratus

**Properties:** Analgesic, Antibacterial, Antidepressant, Antifungal, Anti-inflammatory, Antimicrobial, Antioxidant, Antiseptic, Astringent, Deodorant, Digestive, Diuretic, Emmenagogue, Febrifuge, Hypotensive, Insect Repellant, Nervine, Nutritive, Tonic, Sedative, Vasodilator, Vermifuge

**Traditional Use:** Lemongrass has illustrated antibacterial and antifungal effects and is often included in household cleaning preparations to inhibit the growth of bacteria and fungus.

**Part Used:** Leaf, Stalk, Oil

**Side Effects:** Lemon grass is not recommended for use by women who are pregnant or nursing.

Lemon grass may cause an allergic reaction or skin irritation.

Lemongrass may lower blood pressure.

Additional uses and side effects may exist but further research is necessary to determine the exact properties and effects of use.

**General:** Lemongrass is native to Asia but is now cultivated in many tropical and sub-tropical regions of the world or as an indoor plant in colder climates. Hardy to zone 9, it is easily propagated by seed and will self-seed readily. Lemongrass can also be divided anytime during the growing season. Some success has been had by water rooting lemongrass stalks. Lemongrass prefers nitrogen rich soil and consistent moisture.

Lemongrass stalks are harvested for use as a highly nutritious raw or cooked food. Lemongrass discourages flea infestations and mosquitoes making it a common additive in natural insect treatments for the home and pets.

Lemongrass stalks are harvested for use fresh or dried as a traditional infusion or the essential oils are steam extracted for use in topical or aromatherapy preparations.

## Licorice, Black Sugar, Gan-Cao, Licorice, Licorice Root, Liquorice, Sweet Root
**Botanical Name:** Glycyrrhiza glabra

**Properties:** Antibacterial, Antifungal, Antiinflammatory, Antiperspirant, Antitussive, Antiviral, Cancer, Deodorant, Depurative, Demulcent, Detoxification, Diuretic, Emollient, Expectorant, Laxative, Liver Function, Phytoestrogen, Tonic

**Traditional Use:** Licorice root has traditionally been used to soothe the mucus membranes and expel excess mucus in congestive conditions like asthma, bronchitis, colds, and influenza while acting to treat any underlying infection.

Licorice root is used as a traditional supplement to speed the healing of many disorders of the gastrointestinal tract including heartburn, IBS, intestinal ulcers, gastric reflux, and duodenal, gastric, and peptic ulcers and to treat any underlying viral or bacterial infection.

**Part Used:** Root

**Side Effects:**  Licorice root is not recommended for use by women who are pregnant or nursing.

Licorice root is not recommended for use in children's treatments.

Licorice root containing glycyrrhizin can cause high blood pressure, elevated sodium levels, low potassium levels, and water retention in some people.

Licorice root is not recommended for long-term use.

Licorice is not recommended for use with diuretics, corticosteroids, or other medicines that reduce the body's potassium levels.

Licorice is not recommended for use by those with heart disease or high blood pressure.

Licorice root can affect the body's levels of cortisole.

Licorice root might affect estrogen and is not recommended for use by women who have an estrogen related condition.

Licorice root can cause fatigue, headache, menstrual irregularity, water retention and a decrease of sexual function and interest.

Additional uses and side effects may exist but further research is necessary to determine the exact properties and effects of use.

**General:**  Licorice root is native to Asia, Greece, and Turkey and has a long history of supplement use in both eastern and western medicine.  Hardy to zone 8, it prefers sandy or loamy soil, full or partial sunlight and consistent moisture.  Licorice can grow in poor quality soils and is known to fix nitrogen back into the soil.  It can be propagated by seeds that are soaked in warm water and then sown in a controlled environment or by division or the root buds in the spring.

The root is harvested when it is mature, peeled, dried, and powdered or made in to an extract for use in topical preparations, traditional supplements, or culinary products.  Licorice root sometimes has glycyrrhizin removed.  Licorice with glycyrrhizin removed will not have the same supplemental benefits.

**Lime**
**Botanical Name:**  Citrus x aurantifolia

**Properties:** Antibacterial, Antispasmodic, Antiviral, Appetite Stimulant, Arthritis, Astringent, Depurative, Disinfectant, Febrifuge, Immunostimulant, Styptic, Tonic

**Traditional Use:** Lime is a good source of Vitamin C and is traditionally used to help enhance immunity.

Lime is included in traditional spray treatments for relief from the infection, inflammation, and pain of a sore throat.

**Part Used:** Oil, Peel

**Side Effects:** Lime is not recommended for use beyond dietary by women who are pregnant or nursing.

Lime oil may cause photosensitivity in some people.

Additional uses and side effects may exist but further research is necessary to determine the exact properties and effects of use.

**General:** Lime is native to Asia but is cultivated in other semi-tropic regions including South America and southern North America. They have also been cultivated as container trees in colder climates. Seeds are harvested, washed, and then sown out immediately. Lime can also be propagated by cuttings taken in the early summer.

Lime it is harvested and eaten raw or used in beverages, culinary, topical, and dietary supplements.

**Liverwort – Common**
**Botanical Name:** Marchantia polymorpha

**Properties:** Antibacterial, Antifungal, Anti-inflammatory, Antimicrobial, Anti-inflammatory, Hepatic, Vulnerary

**Traditional Use:** Common Liverwort has traditionally been used to treat bacterial infections like e coli, proteus mirabilis, and staphylococcus aureus as well as fungal infections like aspergillus flavus, a. niger, candida albicans, and trychophyton mentagrophytes.

Common Liverwort has been used as a traditional topical ointment ingredient to reduce infection and inflammation while speeding healing in skin sores, ulcers, and wounds.

**Part Used:** Leaf

**Side Effects:** Common Liverwort is not recommended for use by women who are pregnant or nursing.

Additional uses and side effects may exist but further research is necessary to determine the exact properties and effects of use.

**General:** Common Liverwort is found in moist, tropical zones where the leaves have been harvested, dried, & powdered for use as a traditional supplement. Do not confuse Liverwort Common - Marchantia polymorpha with Liverwort American - Hepatica americana.

**Lomatium, Indian Carrot**
**Botanical Name:** Lomatium dissecta

**Properties:** Antibacterial, Antifungal, Antimicrobial, Antiviral, Expectorant, Stimulant

**Traditional Use:** Lomatium is a stimulating expectorant, antibacterial and antiviral that is traditionally used to relieve congestion associated with conditions like asthma, bronchitis, colds, influenza, and pneumonia while helping to shorten the duration and lessen the severity of conditions caused by an infection.

Lomatium has traditionally been used to combat infection including viral infections like influenza, bacterial infections like streptococcus, and fungal infections like athlete's foot.

Lamotium has been added to cleaning preparations to kill surface bacteria, fungus, and viruses.

Lamotium has been used as a traditional gargle to alleviate throat & mouth infections.

**Part Used:** Resin, Root

**Side Effects:** Lomatium is not recommended for use by women who are pregnant or nursing.

Lomatium may cause a severe allergic skin reaction in some people.

Additional uses and side effects may exist but further research is necessary to determine the exact properties and effects of use.

**General:** Lomatium is native to North America where the roots are harvested, dried, and powdered for use as a traditional supplement.

**Loosestrife, Blooming Sally, Long Purples, Purple Loosestrife, Purple Willow Herb, Rainbow Weed, Spiked Loosestrife, Willow Sage**
**Botanical Name:** Lythrum salicaria

**Properties:** Antibacterial, Antibiotic, Anti-inflammatory, Antimicrobial, Astringent, Colorant, Hypoglycemic, Styptic, Vulnerary

**Traditional Use:** Loosestrife has traditionally been used as a gargle to treat bleeding gums, speed healing of mouth ulcers, and ease throat inflammation or infection.

Loosestrife has traditionally been used as a topical ointment or wash to prevent infection and speed healing of skin sores, ulcers, and wounds.

**Part Used:** Flower, Leaf, Stem

**Side Effects:** Loosestrife is not recommended for use by women who are pregnant or nursing.

Additional uses and side effects may exist but further research is necessary to determine the exact properties and effects of use.

**General:** Loosestrife is a native to Asia, Australia, and North America where the leaves are harvested for use as a calcium rich food, the flowers are used to make culinary colorants, or the flower, leaf, and stem are is harvested while flowering for use fresh or dried. They have been made into traditional infusions for internal use at a rate of up to 3 cups daily and for external washes.

## Lotus – White, Egyptian Lotus, Tiger Lotus, White Lotus, White Water Lily
**Botanical Name:** Nymphaea lotus

**Properties:** Antibacterial, Astringent, Diuretic, Nervine, Tranquilizing

**Traditional Use:** White Lotus has been used as a traditional supplement to treat bacterial infections like staphylococcus and antibiotic resistant strains like MRSA.

**Part Used:** Flower, Leaf, Seed

**Side Effects:** White Lotus is not recommended for use by women who are pregnant or nursing.

White Lotus may have narcotic properties, effect circulation, or cause other side effects and is not recommended for use without the advice of a qualified herbalist or physician.

Additional uses and side effects may exist but further research is necessary to determine the exact properties and effects of use.

**General:** The White Lotus is a perennial water plant native to Asia and has naturalized to Africa. It is cultivated as an ornamental water plant in other warmer regions or indoor aquariums. It is propagated as a water plant by seed or nurtured cuttings.

The essential oils of the flowers are used in porfumcry and the leaves have been eaten as a raw or cooked vegetable. The seeds are harvested for use as a food seasoning or ground & powdered for use as a flour product. The leaves, flower, and seeds are used as a traditional supplement tea.

## Ma Dou Ling
**Botanical Name:** Aristolochia contorta

**Properties:** Antibacterial, Anti-inflammatory, Antimicrobial, Antioxidant, Antiseptic, Antitussive, Astringent, Cancer, Expectorant, Hypotensive, Purgative, Sedative

**Traditional Use:** Ma Dou Ling has traditionally been used to treat bacterial infections like bacillus dysentericae, pneumococci, and staphylococcus aureus.

**Part Used:** Fruit, Root

**Side Effects:** Ma Dou Ling is not recommended for use by women who are pregnant or nursing.

Ma Dou Ling root may cause kidney damage and is not recommended for use without the advice of a qualified herbalist or physician.

Additional uses and side effects may exist but further research is necessary to determine the exact properties and effects of use.

**General:** Ma Dou Ling is native to Asia where it can be found growing wild on mountainous slopes. It is not particular regarding soil composition but does prefer full to partial sun and consistent moisture. Ma Dou Ling can be propagated by seeds sown out as soon as they are ripe, fall division, or winter root cuttings.

Ma Dou Ling leaves are eaten as a cooked vegetable and the fruit & root are harvested, dried, and powdered for use in traditional and commercial preparations.

**Ma Dou Ling**
**Botanical Name:** Aristolochia debilis

**Properties:** Anodyne, Antibacterial, Antifungal, Anti-inflammatory, Antimicrobial, Antioxidant, Antitussive, Cancer, Carminative, Diuretic, Expectorant, Hypotensive, Purgative, Sedative

**Traditional Use:** Ma Dou Ling has traditionally been used to treat bacterial infections like bacillus dysentericae, pneumococci, and staphylococcus aureus.

**Part Used:** Fruit, Root

**Side Effects:** Ma Dou Ling is not recommended for use by women who are pregnant or nursing.

Ma Dou Ling root may cause kidney damage and is not recommended for use without the advice of a qualified herbalist or physician.

Additional uses and side effects may exist but further research is necessary to determine the exact properties and effects of use.

**General:** Ma Dou Ling is native to Asia where it can be found growing wild in thickets and meadows. Hardy to zone 8, it is not particular regarding soil composition but does prefer full to partial sun and consistent moisture. Ma Dou Ling can be propagated by seeds sown out as soon as they are ripe, fall division, or winter root cuttings.

Ma Dou Ling leaves are eaten as a cooked vegetable and the fruit & root are harvested, dried, and powdered for use in traditional and commercial preparations.

**Magnolia, Beaver Tree, Ho No Ki, Holly Bay, Hou Po, Indian Bark, Japanese Whitebark, Red Bay, Red Magnolia, Swamp Laurel, Swamp Sassafras, Sweet Bay, White bay, White Laurel, Xin Ye, Hua**
**Botanical Name:** Magnolia officinalis

**Properties: Bark** – Antiseptic, Antispasmodic, Aphrodisiac, Diuretic, Diaphoretic, Expectorant, Hypotensive, Stimulant, Vulnerary **Flower** - Analgesic, Anti-inflammatory, Colorant, Digestive, Emmenagogue, Nervine, Sedative **Oil** – Antibacterial, Antiseptic, Stimulant

**Traditional Uses:** Magnolia bark and petal oils are traditionally used in topical washes or ointments to reduce itchiness in contact dermatitis and to reduce infection while speeding healing in skin sores, ulcers, & wounds.

Magnolia flower has been used as a traditional supplement snuff to treat sinus congestion, infection, inflammation, and headaches.

**Parts Used:** Bark, Flower Bud

**Side Effects:** Magnolia is not recommended for use by women who are pregnant or nursing.

Magnolia may cause heartburn, headaches, sleepiness, or tremors.

Additional uses and side effects may exist but further research is necessary to determine the exact properties and effects of use.

**General:** Magnolia is a scented ornamental native to Asia and cultivated in many warmer areas of the world. It is not particular regarding soil composition but does prefer good drainage, full to partial sunlight, and consistent moisture. Magnolia can be propagated by seeds sown out as soon as they are ripe or by spring layering.

The petals & buds are harvested for use as a cooked or raw vegetable. The petals are also harvested at the beginning of the flowering season, dried, in the sun, and powdered for use in traditional supplements. The oil is commonly extracted from the petals by steam distillation for use in aromatherapy and traditional supplements. The bark is harvested in the fall for use in an alcohol extraction.

### Mangosteen, Queen of Fruits
**Botanical Name:** Garcinia mangostana

**Properties:** Antibacterial, Antifungal, Antihistamine, Anti-inflammatory, Antioxidant, Antiviral, Astringent, Cancer, Diuretic, Immunostimulant

**Traditional Uses:** Mangosteen has traditionally been used to treat bacterial and fungal infections.

Mangosteen has been used as a traditional supplement to treat urinary tract infections.

Mangosteen is available in a variety of commercial preparations.

**Parts Used:** Fruit, Heartwood, Leaf, Juice, Rind

**Side Effects:** Mangosteen is not recommended for use by women who are pregnant or nursing.

Additional uses and side effects may exist but further research is necessary to determine the exact properties and effects of use.

**General:** Mangosteen is an evergreen tree native to the tropical areas of the world. It is cultivated for its fruits in the southern United States. Hardy to zone 9, it is propagated by seeds, cuttings taken in mid-summer or by division of the suckers early in the growing season.

The wood is used in some small woodcraft projects. The rind of the fruit is high in tannins and has been used in tanning. The fruit is eaten cold or cooked but is also used in commercial health drinks & supplements and traditional supplement preparations.

**Mastic**
**Botanical Name:** Pistacia lentiscus

**Properties:** Analgesic, Antibacterial, Antibiotic, Antifungal, Antioxidant, Antitussive, Cancer, Carminative, Cholesterol, Diuretic, Expectorant, Hypotensive, Insecticide, Stimulant

**Traditional Use:** Mastic has traditionally been used as an ointment or supplement to treat bacterial infection like staphylococcus and fungal infections like athlete's foot.

Mastic resin has been used in traditional gargles or as a gum to reduce plaque and has been shown to reduce bacterial plaque by as much as 40%.

**Side Effects:** Mastic is not recommended for use by women who are pregnant or nursing.

Additional uses and side effects may exist but further research is necessary to determine the exact properties and effects of use.

**General:** Mastic is an evergreen shrub native to Greece but cultivated as a scented ornamental in other regions. Hardy to zone 9, it is not particular regarding soil composition but does require full sun and consistent moisture. Mastic can be propagated by seeds soaked and then sown in the spring, cuttings taken in mid-summer or layering.

Mastic root resin is used as a spice, gum product, fixative in perfumes, or as a glue or varnish component. The seed oils are used in soap making and lighting. The trunk resin has an anise like flavor used as a culinary additive. The resin or leaves are harvested, dried, and powdered for use as a traditional supplement.

**Meadowsweet, Bridewort, Dolloff, Dropwort, Lady of the Meadow, Meadow Wort, Mead Wort, Quaker Lady, Queen of the Meadow, Ulmaria**
**Botanical Name:** Filipendula ulmaria

**Properties:** Analgesic, Anti-inflammatory, Antimicrobial, Antiseptic, Astringent, Colorant, Depurative, Diaphoretic, Diuretic, Expectorant, Febrifuge, Tonic

**Traditional Use:** Meadowsweet has been used as a traditional treatment against bacterial infections like diphtheria and pneumonia.

Meadowsweet has traditionally been used as a topical preparation to reduce inflammation and pain while speeding healing and deterring infection in skin sores, ulcers, and wounds.

Meadowsweet has been used as a traditional supplement to treat urinary tract infections.

**Part Used:** Flower, Leaf, Stem

**Side Effects:** Meadowsweet is not recommended for use by women who are pregnant or nursing.

Meadowsweet is not recommended for use in children's treatments.

Meadowsweet contains substances similar to aspirin and is not recommended for use by individuals with an aspirin sensitivity.

Meadowsweet may cause bronchial constriction, nausea, or rashes in some people.

Overuse of meadowsweet may cause blood in the stool, kidney problems, ringing in the ears, or vomiting.

Meadowsweet contains salicylic acid and is not recommended for use by people with an allergy to aspirin, who are on blood thinning medication or in children's treatments.

Additional uses and side effects may exist but further research is necessary to determine the exact properties and effects of use.

**General:** Meadowsweet is native to Asia and North America and can be found growing in boggy areas. Hardy to zone 2, it is not particular regarding soil composition but does prefer full to partial sun and moist to wet soil. Meadowsweet can be propagated by seeds sown as soon as they are ripe or division.

Meadowsweet roots yield a dark brown toned colorant and the aerial parts yield a yellow toned colorant. The flower yield an essential oil used in perfumery and the roots or young leaves are eaten as a cooked vegetable. The dried leaves are used as a flavoring or sugar alternative. The aerial parts are harvested during the flowering season and air-dried for use in traditional supplement infusions.

**Moneywort, Creeping Jenny, Creeping Joan, Herb Two Pence, Meadow Runagates, Running Jenny, Serpentaria, String of Sovereigns, Twopenny Grass, Wandering Jenny, Wandering Tailor**
**Botanical Name:** Lysimachia nummularia

**Properties:** Antibacterial, Astringent, Diuretic, Expectorant, Styptic, Vulnerary

**Traditional Use:** The antibacterial and astringent properties of Moneywort have made it a traditional supplement for treating diarrhea especially when it results from a bacterial infection.

Moneywort's most common traditional use is as an external wash or ointment component to treat conditions like eczema and psoriasis and to deter infection while helping to speed wound healing.

**Part Used:** Whole

**Side Effects:** Moneywort is not recommended for use by women who are pregnant or nursing.

Additional uses and side effects may exist but further research is necessary to determine the exact properties and effects of use.

**General:** Moneywort is native to Europe and has been naturalized to other parts of the world including North America and Japan. Hardy to zone 4, it is not particular regarding soil composition but does prefer full or partial sunlight and moist to wet soil. It can grow in water. The plant does not produce a large number of seeds so propagation is usually done by division during the spring or by water rooted cuttings taken any time during the growing season.

The entire plant is harvested while in bloom, dried, and powdered for use in a traditional supplement tea, which is taken internally up to 3 times daily or for incorporation into a topical preparation.

**Mountain Lovage, Bear Root, Chuchpate, Colorado Cough Root, Indian Parsley, Mountain Carrot, Osha, Porters Licorice, Wild Celery Root**
**Botanical Name:** Ligusticum porteri

**Properties:** Antibacterial, Antispasmodic, Antiviral, Astringent, Emmenagogue, Expectorant

**Traditional Uses:** Mountain Lovage is used as a traditional supplement to reduce inflammation and congestion associated with conditions like bronchitis, colds, influenza, and pneumonia and to help shorten the severity and duration of respiratory infection.

**Parts Used:** Root

**Side Effects:** Mountain Lovage is not recommended for use by women who are pregnant or nursing.

Mountain Lovage is not recommended for use in children's treatments, by people who have kidney disease, liver disease, and should only be used after consultation with a qualified herbalist or physician.

Additional uses and side effects may exist but further research is necessary to determine the exact properties and effects of use.

**General:** Wild Lovage is native to North America where it has been used as a traditional supplement for hundreds of years. The root and seed are harvested and the oils extracted or dried & powdered for use as a traditional supplement.

**Mugwort, Altamisa, Carline Thistle, Felon Herb, Sailor's Tobacco, St. John's Plant, Wild Wormwood**
**Botanical Name:** Artemisia vulgaris

**Properties:** Abortifacient, Antibacterial, Antifungal, Antimicrobial, Antiseptic, Carminative, Cholagogue, Diaphoretic, Digestive, Diuretic, Emmenagogue, Expectorant, Hypoglycemic, Insect Repellant, Insecticide, Narcotic, Nervine, Sedative

**Traditional Use:** Mugwort leaf has been used in traditional topical and internal preparations to treat bacterial infections like bacillus typhi, e coli, staphylococcus aureus, and streptococci.

Mugwort has been used in traditional ointments to alleviate the itching associated with healing skin especially burns while preventing bacterial infections in the wounds.

**Part Used:** Leaf, Root, Stem

**Side Effects:** Mugwort is not recommended for use by women who are pregnant or nursing.

Mugwort has been used as an abortifacient in some cultures.

Mugwort may cause an allergic reaction in some people.

Overuse of Mugwort may cause convulsions, dizziness, increased heart rate, increased perspiration, nausea, tremors, or permanent nerve damage.

Additional uses and side effects may exist but further research is necessary to determine the exact properties and effects of use.

**General:** Mugwort is native to Africa, Asia, Europe, and North America. Hardy to zone 3, it is not particular regarding soil composition but does prefer full or partial sun and consistent moisture though it can tolerate drought once established. Mugwort is easily propagated by seed and will self-sow readily if given its own place in the garden. It can also be propagated by division in the spring or by cuttings taken at the beginning of the summer.

Mugwort root is used in fresh or dried powder preparations to repel insects or made into a strong decoction for use as an insecticide.

The leaf & flowers are harvested while in bloom and the roots are harvested before first frost, dried, and powdered for use in a traditional supplement infusion or topical ointment.

**Mullein, Adam's Flannel, Beggar's Blanket, Blanket Herb, Candleflower, Candlewick, Duffle, Feltwort, Flannel Leaf, Flannelflower, Great Mullein, Woolen**
**Botanical Name:** Verbascum thapsus

**Properties:** Anodyne, Antibacterial, Anticoagulant, Anti-inflammatory, Antimicrobial, Antiseptic, Astringent, Antiviral, Astringent, Colorant, Demulcent, Diuretic, Emollient, Expectorant, Immunostimulant, Narcotic, Sedative, Vulnerary

**Traditional Use:** Mullein is traditionally infused in oils using a sunbath and 3 drops of the resulting oils are placed inside the ear canal 2-3 times a day to help sooth an earache and reduce infection.

Mullein oil has traditionally been used to reduce infection and inflammation in the mouth and throat while speeding healing of mouth ulcers.

Mullein has been used as a traditional topical preparation to reduce infection & inflammation while speeding the healing of skin sores, ulcers, and wounds.

**Part Used:** Leaf, Flower, Root

**Side Effects:**  Mullein is not recommended for use by women who are pregnant or nursing.

Mullein may interfere with the body's clotting ability and is not recommended for use without the advice of a qualified herbalist or physician.

Additional uses and side effects may exist but further research is necessary to determine the exact properties and effects of use.

**General:**  Mullein is native to Africa, Asia, and Europe but has been naturalized to North America where it is considered an invasive weed by some.  Hardy to zone 3, it is not particular regarding soil composition or moisture but does require full sun.  Mullein can be found growing wild in untended areas or propagated by seeds sown out in the spring.

The whole Mullein plant yields a yellow to green colorant used as a culinary or textile dye.  Mullein flowers yield a yellow toned colorant used as a textile dye or hair colorant.  The leaves are used to make a bland aromatic tea while the leaves and flowers make a sweeter tea.  The leaf, flower, and root are harvested at the beginning of the flowering season, dried, and powdered for use in traditional supplement tea preparations.

## Myrrh
**Botanical Name:**  Commiphora myrrha

**Properties:**  Anodyne, Antibacterial, Antifungal, Antimicrobial, Anti-inflammatory, Antiseptic, Astringent, Carminative, Emmenagogue, Expectorant, Hypoglycemic, Insect Repellant, Pulmonary Stimulant, Sedative, Tonic, Vulnerary

**Traditional Use:**  Myrrh resin is traditionally used as a topical preparation to treat infection and speed healing in skin ulcers, cold sores, & canker sores.

Myrrh has been used as a traditional supplement and is approved for commercial use in Europe to treat infection and speed healing of skin ulcers, mouth ulcers, and the throat.

Myrrh has antibacterial, antifungal, antiseptic, and astringent action that make it a traditional ingredient in mouthwashes, skin washes, and soaks for cleansing and treatments of bacterial infections, viral infections, and fungal diseases like athlete's foot and thrush.

**Part Used:**  Resin

**Side Effects:**  Myrrh is not recommended for use by women who are pregnant or nursing.

Overuse of Myrrh can cause nausea or vomiting.

Myrrh may affect the menstrual cycles in some women.

Individuals with diabetes should consult with a  qualified herbalist or physician before using myrrh as it may affect blood sugar.

Additional uses and side effects may exist but further research is necessary to determine the exact properties and effects of use.

**General:** Myrrh is native to the Mediterranean but is cultivated in other regions where the resin is harvested during the summer months for use in perfumery and traditional supplements. The bark is wounded to cause the formation of oily resin that is harvested and the oils extracted by steam distillation.

## Myrtle, Common Myrtle, Saharan Myrtle
**Botanical Name:** Myrtus communis

**Properties:** Antibacterial, Antibiotic, Antimicrobial, Antiseptic, Antiviral, Astringent, Cardiac, Carminative, Haemostatic, Rubefacient, Stimulant, Sedative, Tonic, Vermifuge

**Traditional Use:** An infusion of Myrtle has traditionally been used as a stimulating expectorant to help alleviate the congestion and constriction associated with respiratory ailments like asthma, bronchitis, colds, influenza, pneumonia and whooping cough and since myrtle has strong antibiotic properties it aids in reducing the length of the associated infection.

Mrytle has been used as a traditional preparation to treat bacterial infections.

Myrtle is used as a traditional preparation to treat urinary tract infections.

**Part Used:** Branch, Leaf, Twig

**Side Effects:** Myrtle is not recommended for use by women who are pregnant or nursing.

Additional uses and side effects may exist but further research is necessary to determine the exact properties and effects of use.

**General:** Myrtle is native to Asia but cultivated in other regions. Hardy to zone 8, it is not particular regarding soil composition but does prefer full sun and consistent moisture. Myrtle can be propagated by seeds soaked and sown in the spring, cuttings taken in mid summer or layering.

The aerial parts of the plant yield an essential oil used in perfumery, soap making, and natural care products. Myrtle fruits are eaten raw or cooked , the leaves are used as a flavoring, and the whole plant is harvested during the summer, dried, and powdered for use in traditional supplement infusions taken up to 3 times daily.

## Nasturtium, Grande Capucine, Indian Cress, Monks Cress
**Botanical Name:** Tropaeolum majus

**Properties:** Antibacterial, Antibiotic, Antifungal, Antioxidant, Antiseptic, Antiviral, Depurative, Diuretic, Emmenagogue, Expectorant, Laxative, Rubefacient, Vermifuge

**Traditional Use:** Nasturtium has traditionally been used to treat bacterial infections.

Nasturtium has been used in traditional topical ointments & washes to reduce infection and speed healing in skin sores, ulcers, and wounds.

Nasturtium has traditionally been used as a supplement to treat urinary tract infections.

**Part Used:** Flower, Leaf, Seed, Stem

**Side Effects:** Nasturtium is not recommended for use by women who are pregnant or nursing

Nasturtium is not recommended for use in children's treatments.

Nasturtium is not recommended for use by those with ulcers or with kidney disease.

Additional uses and side effects may exist but further research is necessary to determine the exact properties and effects of use.

**General:** Nasturtium is native to South America but has become naturalized to other regions as an ornamental plant. Hardy to zone 9, it prefers sandy to loamy soil, full sun, and consistent moisture. Nasturtium can be propagated by seeds sown in the spring.

Nasturtium seed oil is used in making paints and varnishes and the leaves are used in soap making. The flower, leaf, and stems are harvested, dried, and powdered for use in traditional supplement infusions and the seed is harvested and crushed for use in treating skin parasites.

**Neem, Arishtha, Beard Tree, Holy Tree, Indian Lilac, Margosa**
**Botanical Name:** Azadirachta indica

**Properties:** Antibacterial, Antifungal, Anti-inflammatory, Contraceptive, Detoxifier, Emollient, Hypoglycemic, Immunostimulant, Insect Repellant, Purgative, Tonic, Vermifuge, Viral Infection

**Traditional Use:** Neem oil has been used as a ccommercial and traditioanl topical preparation and cleaning agent against a variety of gram negative and gram-positive bacteria including salmonella typhora, streptococcus, streptomycin-resistant strains, and tuberculosis.

Neem leaf tea has traditionally been used as a preparation to treat bacterial infections like e. coli, salmonella, staphylococcus aureus, and streptococcus pyogenes.

Neem bark has been used as a traditional supplement to stimulate the immune system and help ward off infections or slow the progress of conditions like AIDS.

Neem has traditionally been used as a topical preparation to reduce infection while speeding healing of skin sores, ulcers, and wounds.

**Part Used:** Bark, Leaf, Seed Nut Oil

**Side Effects:** Neem is not recommended for use by women who are pregnant or nursing.

Neem is not recommended for use in children's treatments.

Neem is for external use only.

Neem is not recommended for use by people with an autoimmune disease like Multiple Sclerosis and Lupus.

Neem may lower blood sugar.

Large doses of Neem Oil can be toxic if taken internally.

Overuse of Neem may cause diarrhea, drowsiness, loss of consciousness, coma, and even death.

Additional uses and side effects may exist but further research is necessary to determine the exact properties and effects of use.

**General:** Neem is native to the tropical regions of Africa and Asia where all parts of the tree are harvested. Neem is hardy to zone 9 and has been grown as a container tree in other climates. It prefers a very high quality soil but is accepting of a wide ranger of soil composition. It can be propagated by seed. It requires well-drained soil and consistent watering.

The shoots & flowers of the Neem tree are harvested as a vegetable, the gum is used as a thickening agent, and the stems are used as a tooth cleaning brush. The seeds are harvested and the oil steam extracted or the barks & leaves are harvested, dried, & powdered for use in traditional supplements & cleaning products.

**Negrito, Bitterwood, Maruba, Paradise Tree**
**Botanical Name:** Simarouba glauca

**Properties:** Analgesic, Antibacterial, Antifungal, Antimicrobial, Antiviral, Astringent, Cancer, Vermifuge

**Traditional Use:** Negrito has been used as a household cleaner to neutralize bacteria, fungus, and viruses in the air and on hard or soft surfaces.

Negrito has been used as a household cleaner or traditional preparation to treat bacterial infections like e. coli, salmonella, staphylococcus aureus, and streptococcus pyogenes.

A decoction of Negrito bark is traditionally used to alleviate diarrhea, especially when caused by infections of the digestive tract.

Negrito has been used as a traditional topical preparation to reduce infection while speeding healing of skin sores, ulcers, and wounds.

**Part Used:** Bark, Wood

**Side Effects:** Negrito is not recommended for use by women who are pregnant or nursing.

Overuse of Negrito may cause nausea, perspiration, or vomiting.

Additional uses and side effects may exist but further research is necessary to determine the exact properties and effects of use.

**General:** Negrito is a flowering tree native to Central America and southern North America, especially along the coastal hammocks of Florida. Negrito is not particular regarding soil composition but does prefer full to partial sun and moist to wet soil. It can be propagated by seed collected early in the spring, dried, and then sown indoors. If the seed coat is removed, the seeds can be germinated inside a plastic bag in the sun and then the young plants removed for final placement.

The seed are harvested and the oils extracted as food oil and the bark is harvested, dried, & powdered for use as a topical or traditional decoctions given at a rate of 6 ounces 2 times daily.

### Nepitella, Lesser Calamint
**Botanical Name:** Calamintha nepeta

**Properties:** Antibacterial, Antifungal, Antimicrobial, Diaphoretic, Expectorant, Hepatic

**Traditional Use:** Nepitella infusions have traditionally been used to treat bacterial & fungal infections.

**Part Used:** Leaf

**Side Effects:** Nepitella is not recommended for use by women who are pregnant or nursing.

Additional uses and side effects may exist but further research is necessary to determine the exact properties and effects of use.

**General:** Nepitella is a member of the mint family native to Europe but naturalized in other regions including the United States where the leaves are harvested, dried, and powdered for use in traditional supplement infusions.

### Niauli Oil, Caje Oil, Huile, Paperbark
**Botanical Name:** Melaleuca viridiflora

**Properties:** Analgesic, Antibacterial, Anti-inflammatory, Antiseptic, Circulation, Expectorant, Insecticide, Nervine, Stimulant, Vermifuge, Vulnerary

**Traditional Uses:** Niauli Oil has been used in traditional topical preparations to clean oily skin and combat bacteria in certain types of acne and to prevent infection and speed healing in skin ulcers and wounds.

Niauli oils are traditionally used in a vapor, spray, or household cleaner to disinfect the air and surfaces.

Niauli oils are used in treatments to purify water.

Niauli oil is diluted and then applied directly to the throat, mouth, or skin to reduce inflammation and is traditionally believed to be most effective at treating bacterial infections and associated inflammation.

**Parts Used:** Leaf, Twigs - Oil

**Side Effects:** Niauli Oil is not recommended for use by women who are pregnant or nursing.

Niauli Oil is not recommended for use in children's treatments.

Niauli Oil may cause diarrhea, nausea, or vomiting.

Overuse of Niauli Oil may cause breathing problems, circulation problems, and low blood pressure.

Additional uses and side effects may exist but further research is necessary to determine the exact properties and effects of use.

**General:** Niauli Oil is extracted from the leaves of the Melaleuca viridiflora tree native to Australia. Do not confuse Niauli oil with Tea Tree oil or Cajuput oil that is taken from a different species of the Melaleuca plant.

The Melaleuca viridiflora tree is native to Australia where the bark is used as bedding, containers, and building shelter. The essential oil is extracted from young leaves and twigs for use in traditional supplement and disinfectant preparations.

## Ningpo, Chinese Figwort, Ningpo Figwort
**Botanical Name:** Scrophularia ningpoensis

**Properties:** Antibacterial, Antifungal, Cardiotonic, Diuretic, Febrifuge, Hypoglycemic, Hypotensive, Vasodilator

**Traditional Use:** Ningpo has been used as a traditional topical preparation to treat bacterial infections and fungal infections.

**Part Used:** Root

**Side Effects:** Ningpo is not recommended for internal use.

Ningpo is not recommended for use by women who are pregnant or nursing.

Ningpo can depress heart function and is not recommended for use without the advice of a qualified herbalist or physician.

Overuse of Ningpo depresses the heart function.

Additional uses and side effects may exist but further research is necessary to determine the exact properties and effects of use.

**General:** Ningpo Figwort is a perennial native to Asia. Hardy to zone 6, it is not particular regarding soil composition but does prefer full to partial sun and moist to wet conditions. Ningpo Figwort can be propagated by seeds sown as soon as they are ripe or by division.

Ningpo Figwort has been used as a traditional cardiac supplement for thousands of years. The root is harvested in the fall, dried, and powdered for use by herbalists.

**Oregano, Dostenkraut, Mountain Mint, Origan, Wild Marjoram, Winter Marjoram, Wintersweet**
**Botanical Name:** Origanum vulgare

**Properties:** Anodyne, Antibacterial, Antifungal, Antimicrobial, Antioxidant, Antiparasitic, Antispasmodic, Antiviral, Cancer, Carminative, Cox-2 Inhibitor, Diaphoretic, Emmenagogue, Expectorant, Immunostimulant, Nervine, Rubefacient, Sedative, Stimulant, Vermifuge

**Traditional Use:** Oregano is traditionally used to treat bacterial infections like pneumonia, staphylococcus, and streptococcus.

Oregano is used as a traditional supplement to help stimulate the immune system and ward off common infections.

Oregano oil has illustrated an ability to inhibit bacteria and other infectious microorganisms and is traditionally used in antibacterial, antifungal, and antiviral products.

**Part Used:** Leaf, Oil, Stem

**Side Effects:** Oregano is not recommended for use beyond dietary by women who are pregnant or nursing.

Oregano may cause an allergic reaction in some people.

Oregano may irritate the skin.

Additional uses and side effects may exist but further research is necessary to determine the exact properties and effects of use.

**General:** Oregano is cultivated worldwide for culinary use and harvested during the flowering season when the oils are extracted by steam distillation for use in traditional supplement preparations. Dried Oregano is used as a culinary seasoning but is typically not strong enough for use as a supplement.

**Palmarosa, Indian Geranium**
**Botanical Name:** Cymbopogon martinii

**Properties:** Antibacterial, Antifungal, Antiviral, Astringent, Insect Repellant, Vulnerary

**Traditional Use:** Palmarosa oil is used as a traditional topical wash, ointment, or soak to treat bacterial skin infections like staphylococcus and fungal conditions like athlete's foot.

Palmarosa oil is used in traditional topical preparations to reduce infection and speed healing of skin sores, ulcers, and wounds.

**Part Used:** Grass Oils

**Side Effects:** Palmarosa oil is not recommended for use by women who are pregnant or nursing.

Palmarosa oil is for external use only.

Additional uses and side effects may exist but further research is necessary to determine the exact properties and effects of use.

**General:** Palmarosa is a species of grass related to citronella grass. Native to Asia and India it is cultivated in other regions for its essential oil. Hardy to zone 9, it is not particular regarding soil composition but does prefer full to partial sun, good drainage, and consistent moisture. It can be propagated by seed with some effort but is more commonly divided in the spring.

The plant is used to deter insects from a particular area or placed with stored goods to deter infestations. The oil is extracted through steam distillation for use in cosmetics, perfumes, and supplements.

**Patchouli, Huo Xiang, Patchouly, Puthca Pat**
**Botanical Name:** Pogostemon cablin

**Properties:** Anodyne, Antibacterial, Antifungal, Appetite Suppressant, Aphrodisiac, Astringent, Diuretic, Insect Repellant, Sedative, Vulnerary

**Traditional Use:** Patchouli is used as a traditional topical preparation to stimulate cell regeneration, speed healing, treat infection, and reduce scarring of skin sores, ulcers, and wounds.

**Part Used:** Leaf Oil

**Side Effects:** Patchouli is not recommended for use by women who are pregnant or nursing.

Additional uses and side effects may exist but further research is necessary to determine the exact properties and effects of use.

**General:** Patchouli is native to India but can be cultivated in many regions as long as it is protected from frost. It is not particular regarding soil composition but does require full sun and consistent moisture. Patchouli can be propagated by seed or by cuttings taken in the spring or summer and water rooted.

Patchouli oil is valued for perfumery and incense. It has also been used as an insect repellant for people, animals, houses, and stored goods. Patchouli oil is extracted from the leaves for use in topical preparations.

**Pau D'Arco, Taheebo**
**Botanical Name:** Tabebuia avellanedae

**Properties:** Analgesic, Antibacterial, Anti-inflammatory, Antifungal, Antimicrobial, Antioxidant, Antiviral, Astringent, Cancer, Hypotensive, Immunostimulant, Laxative, Sedative, Tonic

**Traditional Use:** Pau D'Arco has been used as a traditional supplement to stimulate the immune system and prevent bacterial, fungal, and viral infections.

Pau D'Arco has traditionally been used as a topical preparation to treat infection and speed healing in skin sores, ulcers, and wounds.

**Part Used:** Inner Bark

**Side Effects:** Pau D'Arco is not recommended for use by women who are pregnant or nursing.

Pau D'Arco may lower blood pressure.

Additional uses and side effects may exist but further research is necessary to determine the exact properties and effects of use.

**General:** Pau D'Arco is a canopy tree native to the forests of Central and South America but has been naturalized to the southern parts of the United States. The bark has been harvested for thousands of years for use as a traditional supplement. Pau D'Arco is traditionally harvested, dried, shredded, and boiled for no less than 15 minutes prior to use as a traditional supplement.

**Peppermint, Black Peppermint, Bo He, Brandy Mint, Lamb Mint, Mentha, Mint, Mint Balm, Sentebon, White Peppermint**
**Botanical Name:** Mentha x piperita officinalis, Mentha x piperita vulgaris

**Properties:** Abortifacient, Adaptogen, Analgesic, Anodyne, Antibacterial, Antifungal, Antioxidant, Antispasmodic, Antiseptic, Antiviral, Astringent, Cancer, Cardiac, Carminative, Colorant, Cephalic, Cholagogue, Diaphoretic, Emmenagogue, Expectorant, Febrifuge, Hepatic, Insect Repellant, Muscle Relaxant, Nervine, Tonic, Vasoconstrictor, Vasodilator, Vermifuge

**Traditional Use:** Peppermint tea is traditionally used to stimulate the immune system & combat infectious agents. It has been used to help reduce the length of common infections when used as soon as symptoms appear.

**Part Used:** Leaf, Oil

**Side Effects:** Peppermint is not recommended for use beyond dietary by women who are pregnant or nursing.

High amounts of Peppermint have been as an abortifacient in some cultures.

Peppermint can cause headache, heartburn, nausea, and mouth sores in some people.

Peppermint may cause an allergic reaction in some people.

Peppermint oil may irritate the eyes, nose, or gastro-intestinal tract.

Do not ingest peppermint oil. Peppermint oil is for topical use only unless special coated tablets are used for delivery.

Additional uses and side effects may exist but further research is necessary to determine the exact properties and effects of use.

**General:** Peppermint is a cross between water mint and spearmint native to the Mediterranean but naturalized throughout much of the world. Hardy to zone 3, peppermint is a hardy perennial that spreads rapidly by runner in nearly any soil, sun, and water conditions and may become an invasive weed.

The leaves are eaten raw or cooked and have been used as a flavoring in a variety of beverage, culinary, and confectionary recipes. The whole plant is harvested before flowering and the essential oil extracted by steam distillation. The essential oil of peppermint is added to topical preparations. Peppermint leaves are traditionally used in a tea or powder form.

**Periwinkle, Church Flower, Lesser Periwinkle, Myrtle, Old Maid, Ram Goat Rose, Ratanjot**
**Botanical Name:** Vinca minor, Vinca rosea

**Properties:** Antibacterial, Antispasmodic, Astringent, Cancer, Carminative, Cephalic, Depurative, Detergent, Diuretic, Homeostatic, Hypotensive, Immunostimulant, Sedative, Styptic, Vasodilator

**Traditional Use:** Periwinkle has traditionally been used in a spray or gargle to alleviate throat & mouth inflammation and bacterial infection.

Periwinkle has been used as a traditional topical preparation to reduce infection, inflammation, and pain while speeding healing in skin sores, ulcers, and wounds.

**Part Used:** Flower, Leaf, Seed

**Side Effects:** Periwinkle is not recommended for use by women who are pregnant or nursing.

Periwinkle may lower blood sugar.

Periwinkle may lower blood pressure.

Overuse of Periwinkle may cause bleeding, dizziness, liver damage, low blood sugar, nausea, nerve problems, seizures, vomiting, or even death if ingested.

Additional uses and side effects may exist but further research is necessary to determine the exact properties and effects of use.

**General:** Periwinkle is an easily cultivated ground cover that spreads easily and rapidly in a variety of sun, soil, and water conditions. It is native to Spain, France, and Europe but is naturalized in North America.

Periwinkle stems have been used in weaving and basket making. The flower, leaf, and seeds are harvested during the flowering season for use in traditional supplement infusions used up to 3 times daily.

## Peyote, Devil's Root, Dumpling Cactus, Magic Mushrooms, Mescal Buttons, Mescaline, Pellote, Sacred Mushroom
**Botanical Name:** Lophophora williamsii

**Properties:** Analgesic, Antibacterial, Anti-inflammatory, Antimicrobial, Hallucinogenic, Nervine

**Traditional Uses:** Peyote has been used as a traditional supplement to treat bacterial and fungal infections.

**Parts Used:** Discs

**Side Effects:** Peyote is not recommended for use by women who are pregnant or nursing.

Peyote is a hallucinogenic drug.

Peyote may cause anxiety, dizziness, drowsiness, emotional instability, headache, nausea, paranoia, psychotic behavior, suicidal behavior, vision changes, and vomiting.

Additional uses and side effects may exist but further research is necessary to determine the exact properties and effects of use.

**General:** Peyote is a cactus with disc shaped buttons that are cut from the plant, sliced and chewed, dried and powdered, or made into an extract for use in traditional supplements and religious ceremonies.

## Picao Preto, Beggar's Tick, Broomstick, Spanish Needle
**Botanical Name:** Bidens pilosa

**Properties:** Antibacterial, Antifungal, Anti-inflammatory, Cancer, Diuretic, Styptic, Vulnerary

**Traditional Use:** Picoa has traditionally been used as a topical preparation to treat bacterial infections like staphylococcus.

Picoa has been used as a traditional topical wash or ointment to reduce infection, stop bleeding, and speed healing in skin sores, ulcers, and wounds.

**Part Used:** Whole

**Side Effects:** Picoa is not recommended for use by women who are pregnant or nursing.

Picoa may cause extreme photosensitivity.

Additional uses and side effects may exist but further research is necessary to determine the exact properties and effects of use.

**General:** Picao is an annual cultivated in many tropical regions. It is considered an invasive plant in some areas where it can be found growing wild in damp areas. It is not particular regarding soil composition but does require full sun and moist to wet soil. It will self-sow readily if given its own location or can be propagated by seeds direct sown as soon as they are ripe.

The shoots & leaves are eaten as a raw or cooked vegetable, or the whole plant is harvested for use as a traditional supplement infusion.

## Pimpernell, Bibernellkraut, Hollowstem Burnet, Pimpinella, Saxifage
**Botanical Name:** Pimpinella major

**Properties:** Antibacterial, Anti-inflammatory, Astringent, Diaphoretic, Diuretic, Expectorant

**Traditional Uses:** Pimpernell has been used as a traditional treatment to break up bladder & kidney stones and treat urinary tract infections.

Pimpernell has traditionally been used as a gargle to treat infection and alleviate throat & mouth inflammation.

**Parts Used:** Leaf, Root

**Side Effects:** Pimpernell is not recommended for use by women who are pregnant or nursing.

Additional uses and side effects may exist but further research is necessary to determine the exact properties and effects of use.

**General:** Pimpernell is a perennial native to Europe and naturalized to North America where it can be found growing in untended areas. Hardy to zone 5, it is not particular regarding soil composition but prefers full to partial sun and consistent moisture. Pimpernel can be propagated by seeds sown when they are fresh and will self-sow readily if given its own place in the garden.

The root & leaf are harvested at the beginning of the flowering season, dried, & powdered for use in traditional supplements.

## Plantain, Broadleaf Plantain, Erva De Orelha, Grand Plantain, Greater Plantain, Plantago, Ribwort, Snakeweed, Tanchagem
**Botanical Name:** Plantago major

**Properties:** Analgesic, Anodyne, Antibacterial, Antifungal, Anti-inflammatory, Astringent, Cancer, Demulcent, Diuretic, Expectorant, Haemostatic, Hypotensive, Laxative, Styptic, Vulnerary

**Traditional Use:** The fresh leaves and juice of Plantain are soothing and antibacterial making them a traditional ingredient in balms to sooth skin irritation, insect bites, and stings while combating infection.

Plantain is an antibacterial anti-inflammatory that contains phytochemicals that are believed to speed the healing process making it a traditional component of a poultice or balm to help sooth and heal skin sores, ulcers, and wounds while acting to combat infection.

Plantain's antibacterial, anti-inflammatory, and demulcent actions make it a traditional remedy for throat & mouth inflammation and treatment of related infections.

**Part Used:** Flower, Fruit, Leaf, Seed

**Side Effects:** Plantain is not recommended for use beyond dietary by women who are pregnant or nursing.

Plantain may cause an allergic reaction in some people.

Additional uses and side effects may exist but further research is necessary to determine the exact properties and effects of use.

**General:** Plantain is native to Asia and Europe. Hardy to zone 5, it is not particular regarding soil composition but does require full sun and consistent moisture. Plantain can be propagated by seeds sown in the spring.

The young leaves and seeds are eaten raw or cooked and the seeds have been ground for use as flour. The flower, fruit, leaf, and seed are all used in traditional supplements.

### Poke Root, Indian Poke
**Botanical Name:** Phytolacca acinosa

**Properties:** Antiasthmatic, Antibacterial, Antifungal, Anti-inflammatory, Antitussive, Antiviral, Diuretic, Emetic, Expectorant, Laxative, Vermifuge

**Traditional Uses:** Poke is being investigated for its potential benefit as a broad-spectrum antiviral and antibacterial and is considered potentially useful in treatments and preventatives for mutating viral infections. All parts of the plant are considered toxic and poke should only be used under the supervision of a qualified herbalist or physician.

**Parts Used:** Root

**Side Effects:** Poke is not recommended for use by women who are pregnant or nursing.

The entire poke plant may contain toxic compounds and should only be used under the supervision of a qualified herbalist or physician.

Additional uses and side effects may exist but further research is necessary to determine the exact properties and effects of use.

**General:** Poke is native to eastern Asia and has naturalized in other parts of the world including North America. Hardy to zone 7, it is not particular regarding soil composition but prefers full to partial sun and consistent moisture. Poke can be propagated by seed sown in the spring or division of the clump early in the growing season.

Poke leaves, shoots, and root have traditionally been eaten as a cooked vegetable but some reports indicate they may contain toxic compounds. The fruits yield a red toned colorant traditionally used as an ink. The root is harvested in the fall, dried, and powdered for use in traditional preparations.

## Pomegranate, Dadima
**Botanical Name:** Punica granatum

**Properties:** Antibacterial, Antioxidant, Antiviral, Astringent, Cardio-tonic, Colorant, Demulcent, Emmenagogue, Immunostimulant, Vermifuge

**Traditional Use:** Pomegranate bark extracts are traditionally used to treat bacterial and viral infections.

Pomegranate bark extract is used as a traditional as part of household vapor and spray disinfecting preparations.

Traditionally Pomegranate has been as part of a gargle for relief from the pain and inflammation of a sore throat and to treat related infection.

**Part Used:** Bark, Fruit, Oil, Rind, Seed

**Side Effects:** Pomegranate is not recommended for use by women who are pregnant or nursing.

Pomegranate bark extracts are very toxic. Do not use bark extracts.

Pomegranate may cause an allergic reaction in some people.

Overuse of Pomegranate may cause dizziness, gastric upset, vomiting, vision disorders, or even death.

Additional uses and side effects may exist but further research is necessary to determine the exact properties and effects of use.

**General:** Pomegranate is native to Africa, China, and India and has been naturalized to parts of California and Arizona. Hardy to zone 9, it is not particular regarding soil composition or moisture but does prefer full sun. Pomegranate is easily propagated by seed, mature cuttings, layering, or by division of the suckers.

The dried rind of the pomegranate fruit produces colors ranging from deep yellow to greenish-yellow tones. The age of the fruit affects the final color of the dye with the less ripe fruits containing more green tones used in textile dyeing. Iron mordant gives a deep mossy green color. The flowers and unripe fruit rind yield a red to reddish black toned colorant used in cosmetics, textile dying, and ink. The root bark yields a deep black colorant with high tannins giving it the ability to act as a self-mordant.

Pomegranate yields a durable, yellow toned wood used in small woodcraft projects. Pomegranate fruits are eaten as a raw food and the juice is used raw or in the creation of soups, jellies, and sauces.  Fresh seeds are eaten raw and the leaves are dried for use as a seasoning or eaten as a cooked vegetable.

Pomegranate has been harvested for use in traditional supplements for thousands of years.  The bark, fruit, oils, rind, and seeds are all used in traditional preparations.

## Pond Lily, Beaver Root, Cow Cabbage, Fragrant Water Lily, Water Cabbage, Water Lily, White Pond Lily
**Botanical Name:**  Nymphaea odorata

**Properties:**  Anodyne, Antibacterial, Anti-inflammatory, Antiseptic, Astringent, Cancer, Demulcent, Expectorant, Hypotensive, Vulnerary

**Traditional Use:**  Pond Lily is incorporated into a traditional gargle to treat diseases of the mouth and throat including bacterial infections, strep throat, canker sores, and severe inflammation.

Pond Lily is traditionally used in topical preparations to treat infection and speed healing in skin sores, ulcers, and wounds.

**Part Used:**  Rhizome, Flower - Seed

**Side Effects:**  Pond Lily is not recommended for use by women who are pregnant or nursing.

Pond Lily may lower blood pressure.

Additional uses and side effects may exist but further research is necessary to determine the exact properties and effects of use.

**General:**  Pond Lily is native to North America and is naturalized throughout the world where it can be found growing underwater.  Hardy to zone 5, it requires full sun and can be grown in boggy areas, ponds, or other water gardens.  Pond Lily can be propagated by seeds sown in water as soon as they are ripe or by spring division.

The leaves and flower buds are eaten as a raw or cooked vegetable and the roots & seeds are roasted and eaten or ground into flour.  The rhizome is harvested in the autumn, dried, and powdered for use in external wash, poultice, or ointment preparations of 1 part powder to 1 part ethanol or ¼-teaspoon powder to 1-teaspoon liquid base daily.  For acute conditions of the throat 5 drops of the external tincture is traditionally given up to 3 times daily.

## Pongam Tree, Honge Tree, Indian Beech
**Botanical Name:**  Pongamia pinnata

**Properties:**  Antibacterial, Anti-inflammatory, Antiseptic, Antiviral, Astringent, Digestive

**Traditional Use:**  The leaf oil is used in traditional topical preparations to reduce infection and speed healing in skin sores, ulcers, and wounds.

**Part Used:**  Leaf, Oil, Seed

**Side Effects:** Pongam is not recommended for use by women who are pregnant or nursing.

Additional uses and side effects may exist but further research is necessary to determine the exact properties and effects of use.

**General:** Pongam is a tree native to India and naturalized to Asia. Pongam is easily cultivated in warmer regions worldwide for its ability to amend the soil and for its attractive scented flowers. The bark is harvested to make rope and the seeds are used to make cosmetic products & the seeds & leaf are used in traditional supplements.

## Purslane, Ma Chi Xian, Pigweed, Pursley
**Botanical Name:** Portulaca oleracea

**Properties:** Antibacterial, Antibiotic, Anticoagulant, Anti-inflammatory, Astringent, Cholesterol, Depurative, Diuretic, Febrifuge, Hypotensive, Vermifuge, Vulnerary

**Traditional Use:** Fresh Purslane leaves are used as a traditional topical poultice to alleviate pain, infection, & inflammation while speeding healing in skin sores, ulcers, and wounds including burns.

Purslane is rich in omega 3 fatty acids and has been used as part of a traditional dietary treatment plan to stimulate immunity and help the body ward off common infections.

Purslane is used as a traditional supplement to alleviate irritable bladder, urinary tract infections, and difficulty passing urine.

**Part Used:** Leaf

**Side Effects:** Purslane is not recommended for use by women who are pregnant or nursing.

Purslane may lower the body's ability to clot and is not recommended for use by people who are taking a blood thinning medication or who have a bleeding disorder.

Purslane may lower blood pressure.

Additional uses and side effects may exist but further research is necessary to determine the exact properties and effects of use.

**General:** Purslane is a succulent native to Asia and southern Europe but it has been naturalized to southern North America. It is considered an invasive weed in some regions but cultivated in others as a groundcover or nutritive leafy green vegetable. It Is not particular regarding soil composition but does prefer good drainage, full sun, and consistent moisture. It can be propagated by seed and will self-sow readily if given its own area in the garden.

The leaves and stems are eaten as a raw or cooked vegetable and the seeds are eaten raw or cooked or ground into flour. The plant has also been burnt and the ashes used as a salt substitute.

The leaves are harvested and used fresh or dried as a traditional supplement.

**Rabbitbrush**
**Botanical Name:** Ericameria nauseosa

**Properties:** Antibacterial, Anti-inflammatory, Astringent, Colorant, Expectorant, Febrifuge, Hypotensive, Vulnerary

**Traditional Use:** Rabbitbrush has been used in traditional topical preparations to treat infection, reduce skin inflammations and speed healing of skin sores, ulcers, and wounds.

**Part Used:** Stems, Twigs

**Side Effects:** Rabbitbrush is not recommended for use by women who are pregnant or nursing.

Rabbitbrush is not recommended for internal use without the advice of a qualified herbalist or physician.

Overuse of Rabbitbrush may cause an extreme drop in blood pressure.

Additional uses and side effects may exist but further research is necessary to determine the exact properties and effects of use.

**General:** Rabbitbrush is a shrub native to western North America and cultivated elsewhere as an ornamental or as a forage plant. It is not particular regarding soil composition and can thrive in poor quality soil and water conditions. It can be propagated by seed and will self-sow readily if given the right conditions. Rabbitbrush can also be propagated by division of suckers and by layering in the spring.

The leaves have been used as a sanitary padding, the flower head as a stuffing material, and the root sap as a source of hypoallergenic rubber or gum product. The stems and twigs are harvested, dried, and powdered for use in traditional topical preparations.

**Radish**
**Botanical Name:** Raphanus sativus

**Properties:** Antibacterial, Antifungal, Antimicrobial, Antispasmodic, Antiviral, Astringent, Cancer, Carminative, Digestive, Diuretic, Expectorant, Hypo-thyroidic, Laxative, Stimulant

**Traditional Use:** The whole radish plant has been used to help treat bacterial infections like e. coli or streptococci.

**Part Used:** Leaf, Root, Seed

**Side Effects:** Radish is not recommended for use beyond dietary by women who are pregnant or nursing.

Radish skins may affect the thyroid gland.

Additional uses and side effects may exist but further research is necessary to determine the exact properties and effects of use.

**General:** Radish is cultivated as a food source worldwide and is harvested before flowering for traditional supplement use with 1 radish grated to a juice pulp and mixed in a base, steeped for 12-24 hours and used at a rate of 1 spoonful every hour until symptoms abate.

**Ravensara, Clove Nutmeg**
**Botanical Name:** Ravensara aromatica

**Properties:** Antibacterial, Antifungal, Antiseptic, Antiviral, Expectorant

**Traditional Use:** Ravensara is used in air inhalants and traditional supplements to alleviate the congestion associated with conditions like asthma, bronchitis, colds, influenza, and pneumonia and to help fight infection and shorten the length and severity of common respiratory infections.

Ravensara oils are traditionally used in vapor therapy and household cleaners to reduce bacterial, fungal, and viral infectious agents.

Ravensara is used in traditional preparations to reduce the likelihood of infections in skin wounds.

**Part Used:** Bark – Leaf – Oil

**Side Effects:** Ravensara is not recommended for use by women who are pregnant or nursing.

Additional uses and side effects may exist but further research is necessary to determine the exact properties and effects of use.

**General:** Ravensara is native to Madagascar and cultivated elsewhere for the essential oils extracted from the bark & leaves. The oils are extracted through steam distillation and used in topical and aromatherapy preparations.

**Red Rooted Sage, Chinese Red Sage, Chinese Salvia, Dan Shen, Danshen, Red Roots Salvia, Tan Seng**
**Botanical Name:** Salvia miltiorrhiza

**Properties:** Adoptogenic, Antibacterial, Anti-inflammatory, Antiseptic, Antispasmodic, Antithormbic, Antihypertonic, Antimicrobial, Astringent, Cardiotonic, Emmenagogue, Hepatic, Sedative, Styptic, Vasodilator, Vulnerary

**Traditional Use:** Red Rooted Sage has been used as a traditional treatment for bacterial infections like bacillus typhi, e coli, pseudomonas, shingella, and staphylococcus.

**Part Used:** Leaf, Root

**Side Effects:** Red Rooted Sage is not recommended for use by women who are pregnant or nursing.

Red Rooted Sage may cause dizziness, drowsiness, and increased bleeding.

Additional uses and side effects may exist but further research is necessary to determine the exact properties and effects of use.

**General:** Red Rooted Sage is native to Asia but has been cultivated in other areas. Hardy to zone 6, it prefers sandy to loamy soil, full sun, and consistent moisture. It can be propagated by seeds sown in the spring or by cuttings.

The root is harvested in the early fall, dried, and powdered for use in traditional tea and soak remedies.

**Redstem Wormwood, Yin Chen**
**Botanical Name:** Artemisia scoparia

**Properties:** Antibacterial, Antiseptic, Cholagogue, Diuretic, Hepatic, Vasodilator

**Traditional Use:** Redstem Wormwood is traditionally used to prevent or treat bacterial infection and laboratory research has illustrated an ability against bacillus dysenteriae, bacillus subtilis, bacillus typhi, pneumococci, staphylococcus aureus, and streptococci.

**Part Used:** Seed Oil, Whole

**Side Effects:** Redstem Wormwood is not recommended for use by women who are pregnant or nursing.

Redstem Wormwood may cause allergic reactions in some individuals.

Additional uses and side effects may exist but further research is necessary to determine the exact properties and effects of use.

**General:** Redstem Wormwood is native to Asia where it can be found growing wild in wasteland areas. Hardy to zone 3, it is not particular regarding soil composition but does require full sun and dry to moist conditions. It can be propagated by seeds sown out in the spring and will self sow readily if given its own place in the garden.

Redstem Wormwood seeds and flowering stem yield an essential oil used in perfumery and cleaning products and the whole plant is harvested for use in traditional topical preparations.

**Rosebay, Rhododendron, Snow Rose**
**Botanical Name:** Rhododendron aureum

**Properties:** Analgesic, Antibacterial, Anti-inflammatory, Antimicrobial, Astringent, Diaphoretic, Narcotic, Stimulant

**Traditional Use:** Rosebay oil has been used to reduce skin inflammation while treating or preventing bacterial infections like bacillus, staphylococcus, and other gram-positive strains.

**Part Used:** Flower, Leaf, Stem

**Side Effects:** Rosebay is not recommended for use by women who are pregnant or nursing.

Internal use of Rosebay may cause inebriation and is considered toxic.

Additional uses and side effects may exist but further research is necessary to determine the exact properties and effects of use.

**General:** Rosebay is a shrub native to Asia and cultivated in mountainous regions worldwide. Hardy to zone 2, it prefers sandy to loamy soil with good drainage, full to partial sun and consistent moisture.

The flowers are harvested during flowering & dried for use as a traditional supplement while the flowers, leaves, and stems are harvested and the oils extracted through steam distillation for use in topical preparations.

**Rosemary, Old Man, Romarin, Romero, Rusmari, Rusmary**
**Botanical Name:** Rosmarinus officinalis

**Properties:** Analgesic, Antibacterial, Antifungal, Antiinflammatory, Antimicrobial, Antioxidant, Antiseptic, Antispasmodic, Antiviral, Arthritis, Astringent, Cancer, Cardio-Tonic, Cephalic, Circulation, Colorant, Cox-2 Inhibitor, Diaphoretic, Digestive, Diuretic, Emmenagogue, Hepatic, Hypertensive, Insect Repellant, Muscle Relaxant, Nervine, Rubefacient, Stimulant, Vermifuge

**Traditional Use:**
Rosemary leaves are used as a traditional treatment for viral, fungal and bacterial infections of the skin.

The leaves are used as an air purification element especially in sick rooms where its antibacterial, antifungal and antiviral properties are considered effective.

**Side Effects:** Rosemary is not recommended for use beyond dietary by women who are pregnant or nursing.

Rosemary has been used as an abortifacient in some cultures.

Rosemary is not recommended for use in children's treatments.

Rosemary is not recommended for use by people who have epilepsy or a similar condition.

Rosemary is not recommended for use by people who have Crohn's disease, ulcerative colitis, or ulcers.

Rosemary oil is for external use only and can be toxic if taken internally.

Rosemary may affect diabetes, high blood pressure, or the effectiveness of medications to control blood pressure or diabetes,

Rosemary may cause an allergic reaction in some people.

Additional uses and side effects may exist but further research is necessary to determine the exact properties and effects of use.

**General:**  Rosemary is an evergreen shrub or herb native to Asia but has been naturalized in much of the world as a garden shrub and a kitchen herb.  Hardy to zone 6, it prefers sandy to loamy soil, full sun, and consistent moisture.

The young flowers, leaves, and shoots are eaten as a raw or cooked vegetable or dried for use as a seasoning.   The leaves and flowers yield a yellow toned colorant used in culinary, cosmetic and textile dying.  The oils from the leaves and stems are used in perfumery and soap making.  The leaves are used as an air purification element especially in sick rooms where its antibacterial, antifungal and antiviral properties are considered effective.

The leaves are harvested after flowering, dried in the sun and incorporated into supplement teas used up to 4 times a day or as a 1:5 tincture with 70% ethanol.  The oils are extracted through steam distillation for use in soap making, cosmetics, aromatherapy and topical preparations.

# Roselle
**Botanical Name:**  Hibiscus sabdariffa

**Properties:**  Antibacterial, Antimicrobial, Astringent, Cancer, Diuretic, Emmenagogue, Emollient, Laxative, Hypotensive, Stimulant, Vulnerary

**Traditional Use:**  Roselle has antimicrobial properties that have made it a traditional supplement to treat infections like e. coli.

Roselle has traditionally been used as a gargle preparation to speed healing of mouth sores and to reduce throat & mouth infection and inflammation.

Roselle has traditionally been used as a topical preparation to reduce infection and speed healing of skin sores, ulcers, and wounds.

Roselle has been used as a traditional supplement to alleviate urinary tract infections and to help reduce the size of kidney or bladder stones.

**Part Used:**  Flower, Leaf

**Side Effects:**  Roselle is not recommended for use by women who are pregnant or nursing.

Additional uses and side effects may exist but further research is necessary to determine the exact properties and effects of use.

**General:**  Roselle is a perennial shrub native to tropical and semi-tropical regions where the leaves and flowers have been harvested for use as in teas or eaten as a cooked or raw vegetable.  The plant is harvested to create a fiber similar to jute.

Roselle leaves & flowers have been harvested for use in traditional supplements and are being investigated for use as a hypertension drug alternative.

Roselle buds have been harvested, dried, and powdered for use in traditional supplement teas. Fresh buds tend to rot more quickly and are not often used in supplements.

**Rupturewort, Bruchkraut, Flax Weed, Herniary**
**Botanical Name:** Herniaria glabra

**Properties:** Antibacterial, Antispasmodic, Astringent, Diuretic, Expectorant, Vulnerary

**Traditional Uses:** Rupturewort has traditionally been used as a topical wash or poultice to prevent infection and speed healing of skin sores, ulcers, and wounds.

Rupturewort has been used in traditional supplements to treat urinary tract infections and to alleviate spasms associated with conditions like irritable bladder.

**Parts Used:** Whole

**Side Effects:** Rupturewort is not recommended for use by women who are pregnant or nursing.

Additional uses and side effects may exist but further research is necessary to determine the exact properties and effects of use.

**General:** Rupturewort is groundcover native to Europe that has been naturalized to other areas including North America. The whole plant is gathered while in bloom for use fresh or dried in traditional supplements.

**Sage, Dalmatian Sage, Garden Sage, Meadow Sage, Sauge, Scarlet Sage, Spanish Sage, True Sage**
**Botanical Name:** Salvia officinalis

**Properties:** Analgesic, Antibacterial, Antifungal, Anti-inflammatory, Antimicrobial, Antioxidant, Antiperspirant, Antiseptic, Antispasmodic, Astringent, Cancer, Carminative, Cholagogue, Colorant, Depurative, Emmenagogue, Estrogenic, Insect Repellant, Nervine, Preservative, Stimulant, Vasodilator

**Traditional Use:** Sage is traditionally burnt in a room to purify the air against common bacterial and viral infections.

Sage has been used as a tooth-cleaning rub in natural care products and is traditionally used as toothpaste to prevent infection in the mouth, heal inflamed gums, and treat tooth infections.

Sage oil has antimicrobial & antiseptic properties that are used in traditional skin washes or salves to treat bacterial infections of the skin and has shown high effectiveness in testing at treating ringworm.

Sage oil has natural antibacterial, antiseptic, and antimicrobial properties that make it a common ingredient in natural cleaning products.

The astringent, analgesic, and antibacterial properties of sage tea make it a traditional choice for soothing an inflamed throat and in reducing dental infection, inflammation, and pain while helping to speed healing of inflamed gums and mouth sores.

**Part Used:** Flower, Leaf, Stem

**Side Effects:** Sage is not recommended for use beyond dietary by women who are pregnant or nursing.

Sage is not recommended for use beyond dietary by people who have diabetes, high blood pressure, or seizure disorders.

Sage is approved by the U.S. Food and Drug Administration as a spice or seasoning.

Sage can cause an allergic reaction in some people and the oil can irritate the skin.

Sage powder dust may cause breathing difficulties in some people.

Sage oil is for external use only while sage tea can be taken as a tea.

Sage is not recommended for long-term use. Long-term use may cause liver damage, nervous system damage, or seizures.

Additional uses and side effects may exist but further research is necessary to determine the exact properties and effects of use.

**General:** Sage is native to the Mediterranean but has naturalized to Europe and is cultivated in North America. Hardy to zone 5, it prefers sandy or loamy soil, full sun, and consistent moisture. Sage can be propagated by seed sown out in the spring, cuttings taken at any time during the growing season or by spring layering.

Sage is cultivated as a culinary additive and has been used as an alternative toothpaste. The leaves or oils are used in natural hair care products to darken graying hair. Sage is grown in the garden to repel insects and the dried leaves are used in stored goods to deter insect and vermin infestations. Sage leaves & flowers are eaten raw or cooked and the dried leaves are a commonly used household seasoning.

Sage leaves are harvested just before the plant comes into flower and dried for use in traditional supplement teas, extracts, and powders and the oils are extracted through steam distillation for use in aromatherapy, cleaning sprays, and topical preparations. Sage has been used for centuries as a spice, seasoning and supplement throughout the world. Purple leaved sage is the most highly valued in traditional treatments.

The flowers of another species of sage the Perovskia atriplicifolia known as Russian Sage yield a blue toned colorant used as a cosmetic, culinary or textile dye.

**Sage Brush**
**Botanical Name:** Artemisia tridentate

**Properties:** Antibacterial, Antimicrobial, Antiseptic, Antiviral, Astringent, Colorant, Febrifuge, Sedative

**Traditional Use:** Sage Brush has been used as a disinfectant household cleaner.

Sage Brush leaves have traditionally been used in topical preparations to speed healing and disinfect sores, ulcers, and wounds.

**Part Used:** Leaf

**Side Effects:** Sage Brush is not recommended for use by women who are pregnant or nursing.

Additional uses and side effects may exist but further research is necessary to determine the exact properties and effects of use.

**General:** Sage Brush is an evergreen shrub native to Central & North America and cultivated in other regions. The bark is harvested for making baskets & other woven products or as an insulation. The seeds have been harvested for the popping effect they give when tossed into an open fire and the wood is used in construction and as a burning product. The leaves are harvested for use as a cooked vegetable or in traditional supplements.

**Sassafras, Ague Tree, Cinnamon Wood, Root Bear Tree**
**Botanical Name:** Sassafras albidum

**Properties:** Analgesic, Anodyne, Antibacterial, Antiseptic, Antiviral, Arthritis, Cancer, Colorant, Depurative, Diaphoretic, Diuretic, Emmenagogue, Febrifuge, Hypotensive, Insect Repellant, Vasodilator, Vermifuge

**Traditional Use:** Sassafras bark infusions have traditionally been used in topical wash preparations to reduce the risk of infection, ease pain, and speed healing in skin conditions like acne, contact dermatitis, skin sores, skin ulcers, and wounds.

Sassafras root and bark oil has been used as a traditional topical pain reliever and antiseptic agent especially in dental and wound care.

**Part Used:** Bark, Root

**Side Effects:** Sassafras is not recommended for use by women who are pregnant or nursing.

Sassafras is not recommended for use in children's treatments.

Sassafras is considered safe in food quantities but may not be safe in supplement quantity.

Studies indicate that compounds in sassafras may cause liver damage and it has been banned from use in food products by the FDA.

Safrole growth, transport, and use are monitored closely as it is a precursor to the creation of ecstasy.

Sassafras oils may be carcinogenic.

Sassafras oils may be harmful to the liver.

Additional uses and side effects may exist but further research is necessary to determine the exact properties and effects of use.

**General:** Sassafras is native to the eastern coast of North America and is generally found growing on hilltops and ridges in mountainous areas. Hardy to zone 5, it is not particular regarding soil composition but does prefer full to partial sunlight and consistent moisture. It is propagated by seeds sown as soon as they are ripe, by root cuttings taken in the late winter or by division of the suckers in the early spring.

Sassafras bark and wood yield a brown toned colorant that tends toward yellow or orange depending on the mordant. The oils are used to repel insects especially mosquitoes.

Sassafras root & bark are harvested, dried, and powdered for use in traditional topical and dietary supplement treatments. Sassafras tincture is used in most internal traditional preparations and has been given as 10 drops of tincture up to 3 times daily. The bark and root yield an essential oil extracted through steam distillation and used in aromatherapy, topical and medicinal preparations.

## Savory, Bean Herb, Savory, Summer Savory, Winter Savory
**Botanical Name:** Satureja montana

**Properties:** Antibacterial, Antioxidant, Antiseptic, Antiviral, Astringent, Carminative, Digestive

**Traditional Use:** Savory has carminative and antiseptic properties that make it a traditional treatment for bacterially related digestive problems  and astringent properties that help to alleviate mild to moderate diarrhea.

The antiseptic and astringent properties of savory make it a traditional spray or gargle for the treatment of mouth & throat inflammation or infection.

**Part Used:** Flower, Leaf, Stem

**Side Effects:** Savory is not recommended for use beyond dietary by women who are pregnant or nursing.

Savory may cause an allergic reaction or skin irritation.

Additional uses and side effects may exist but further research is necessary to determine the exact properties and effects of use.

**General:** Savory is native to Africa and parts of Europe but is cultivated in many regions of the world where it is harvested during flowering and dried for use as a seasoning, tea product, or traditional supplement infusion up to 3 times daily.

## Scurvy Grass, Scrubby Grass, Spoonwort

**Botanical Name:** Cochlearia officinalis

**Properties:** Antibacterial, Antioxidant, Antiseptic, Antiviral, Astringent, Diuretic, Laxative

**Traditional Use:** Scurvy Grass juice has traditionally been used as a gargle to help heal mouth sores and to treat throat & mouth inflammation and infection.

Scurvy Grass has been used as a traditional topical preparation to help speed healing and prevent infection in skin sores, ulcers and wounds.

**Part Used:** Flower, Leaf

**Side Effects:** Scurvy Grass is not recommended for use by women who are pregnant or nursing.

Additional uses and side effects may exist but further research is necessary to determine the exact properties and effects of use.

**General:** Scurvy Grass is common to salt marshes & cliff areas where it is harvested in the spring and dried for use in traditional topical preparations or as a Vitamin C rich food source.

## Sea Grape, Bay Grape
**Botanical Name:** Coccoloba uvifera

**Properties:** Antibacterial, Antifungal, Anti-inflammatory, Antioxidant, Antiseptic, Astringent, Hypo-Glycemic, Vulnerary

**Traditional Use:** Sea Grape has been used in traditional topical and supplement preparations to treat bacterial infections like e coli.

Sea Grape has traditionally been used as a topical preparation to speed healing and reduce the likelihood of infection in skin sores, ulcers, and wounds.

**Part Used:** Bark – Gum, Fruit, Leaf,

**Side Effects:** Sea Grape is not recommended for use by women who are pregnant or nursing.

Sea Grape lowers blood sugar and should not be used without the advice of a qualified herbalist or physician.

Additional uses and side effects may exist but further research is necessary to determine the exact properties and effects of use.

**General:** Sea Grape is a small shrub or tree native to the shoreline in Central America, South America, and North America. Hardy to zone 9, it can be propagated by seeds sown out as soon as they are ripe or by cuttings taken in the spring.

Sea Grape is cultivated as an ornamental plant in the south and to help stabilize loose, sandy soils. The wood is used in woodcraft and the fruit is eaten raw or cooked. Sea Grape fruits are used to make wine and vinegar and the sap is used in tanning. The bark, leaf, and fruit are harvested for use in supplement or topical decoctions.

**Shan Zhu Yu, Japanese Cornel**
**Botanical Name:** Cornus officinalis

**Properties:** Antibacterial, Antiseptic, Astringent, Diuretic, Hypotensive

**Traditional Use:** Shan Zhu Yu has traditionally been used to treat bacterial infections like staphylococci.

Shan Zhu Yu is used as a traditional gargle or spray to treat throat & mouth inflammation & infection.

Shan Zhu Yu is traditionally used to treat urinary tract infections.

**Part Used:** Fruit

**Side Effects:** Shan Zhu Yu is not recommended for use by women who are pregnant or nursing.

Additional uses and side effects may exist but further research is necessary to determine the exact properties and effects of use.

**General:** Shan Zhu Yu is native to Asia where it has been harvested for thousands of years as a traditional treatment. The fruit is harvested when ripe and the stem bark is harvested at the end of the season, dried, and powdered for use in traditional topical and supplement preparations.

**Shepherd's Purse, Blind Weed, Caseweed, Casewort, Lady's Purse, Mother's Heart, Pick Pocket, Rattle Pouches, Shovelweed, St. James Weed, Toywort, Witches Pouch**
**Botanical Name:** Capsella bursa

**Properties:** Antibacterial, Anti-inflammatory, Astringent, Cancer, Diuretic, Emmenagogue, Febrifuge, Hypotensive, Styptic, Vasodilator

**Traditional Use:** Shepherd's Purse is traditionally placed in the nose or applied directly to wounds to stop bleeding and prevent infection.

Shepherd's Purse is an antibacterial and anti-inflammatory with diuretic properties that does not deplete the potassium levels in the body making in a traditional choice for the treatment of urinary tract infection.

**Part Used:** Whole

**Side Effects:** Shepherd's Purse is not recommended for use by women who are pregnant or nursing.

Shepherd's Purse is not recommended for use by people with a kidney or liver disease.

Shepherd's Purse is not recommended for use by people on blood thinning medications.

Shepherd's Purse coagulates the blood and you should consult with a qualified herbalist or physician before using it as a supplement.

Overuse of Shepherd's Purse may cause changes in blood pressures, breathing difficulties, drowsiness, hart palpitations, thyroid changes, or even death.

Additional uses and side effects may exist but further research is necessary to determine the exact properties and effects of use.

**General:**  Shepherd's Purse can be found in many regions around the world and is adaptable to a variety of soil, sun, and water conditions.  It is harvested, dried, and included in traditional supplement infusions.

## Snake Needle Grass
**Botanical Name:**  Hedyotis diffusa

**Properties:**  Analgesic, Antibacterial, Anti-inflammatory, Diuretic, Febrifuge, Hepatic, Immunostimulant

**Traditional Use:**  Snake Needle Grass has been used as a traditional supplement treatment for bacterial infections like staphylococcus.

Snake Needle Grass has traditionally been used in topical preparations to reduce infection, inflammation, and pain in skin sores, ulcers, and wounds.

Snake Needle Grass has been used as a traditional gargle to reduce throat or mouth pain, inflammation and infections.

Snake Needle Grass has traditionally been used to treat urinary tract infection.

**Part Used:**  Whole

**Side Effects:**  Snake Needle Grass is not recommended for use by women who are pregnant or nursing.

Additional uses and side effects may exist but further research is necessary to determine the exact properties and effects of use.

**General:**  Snake Needle Grass is native to Asia where it has been used in traditional Chinese medicine for thousands of years.  The whole plant is harvested for use in tinctures or dried and powdered for use as a traditional supplement or topical preparation.

## Sorrel, Acedera, Azeda Brava, Common Sorrel, Field Sorrel, Garden Sorrel, Sorrel Dock, Sour Dock
**Botanical Name:**  Rumex acetosa

**Properties:**
Antibacterial, Antioxidant, Antiseptic, Astringent, Colorant, Diuretic, Laxative, Nutritive, Tonic

**Traditional Use:** Sorrel has traditionally been used to treat topical and internal bacterial infections.

**Part Used:** Flower, Leaf, Stem

**Side Effects:** Sorrel is not recommended for use by women who are pregnant or nursing.

Sorrel is not recommended for use in children's treatments.

Sorrel can cause gastrointestinal upset.

Sorrel can cause an allergic reaction or skin irritation.

Sorrel may cause or aggravate kidney stones in some people.

Additional uses and side effects may exist but further research is necessary to determine the exact properties and effects of use.

**General:** Sorrel is native to Europe and has been cultivated in other areas. The roots, leaves, and stems have been used as a traditional dye product while infusions of the stem are used as a furniture or silver polish. The juice of the sorrel plant is used as a stain remover. The leaves and flowers are eaten as a raw or cooked vegetable. The leaves are dried as a culinary seasoning and the roots have been dried and powdered for use as pasta flour and the seeds are ground for baking flour.

**Spearmint, Curled Mint, Fresh Mint, Garden Mint, Green Mint, Lamb Mint, Mackerel Mint, Our Lady's Mint, Pahari Pudina, Sage of Bethlehem, Spire Mint, Yerba Buena**
**Botanical Name:** Mentha spicata

**Properties:** Analgesic, Anti-inflammatory, Antifungal, Antimicrobial, Antioxidant, Antiseptic, Antispasmodic, Aphrodisiac, Astringent, Carminative, Digestive, Diuretic, Expectorant, Febrifuge, Insecticide, Insect Repellant, Nervine, Stimulant, Vermin Repellant

**Traditional Use:** Spearmint is traditionally used to help treat bacterial and fungal infections and as part of a cleaning agent to reduce bacteria & fungus in the home.

**Part Used:** Leaf, Oil

**Side Effects:** Spearmint is not recommended for use by women who are pregnant or nursing.

Spearmint essential oils should be diluted prior to use.

Additional uses and side effects may exist but further research is necessary to determine the exact properties and effects of use.

**General:** Spearmint is native to Europe and naturalized to many countries of the world. Hardy to zone 3, it is not particular regarding soil composition but does prefer full to partial sun and consistent moisture. Spearmint can be propagated by seeds sown in the spring or division though it will spread rapidly on its own if given its own place in the garden. It is considered an invasive weed by some.

Spearmint oil is extracted from the flower, leaf, and stem harvested during the flowering season and is used as an insect or vermin repellant, an aromatic, or flavoring. The leaves are used as a raw or cooked flavoring, tea alternative, aromatherapy agent, or traditional preparation.

## Spicebush, Benjamin Bush, Northern Spicebush, Wild Allspice
**Botanical Name:** Lindera benzoin

**Properties:** Antibacterial, Antiseptic, Antiviral, Astringent, Diaphoretic, Disinfectant, Febrifuge, Insect Repellant, Stimulant, Tonic, Vermifuge

**Traditional Use:** Spice Bush bark and bark oils have traditionally been used as an air inhalant, spray cleaner, or infusion to disinfect sick rooms.

Spice Bush bark decoctions are used as a traditional treatment for bacterial and viral infections.

**Part Used:** Bark, Leaf, Leaf Oil

**Side Effects:** Spice Bush is not recommended for use by women who are pregnant or nursing.

Additional uses and side effects may exist but further research is necessary to determine the exact properties and effects of use.

**General:** Spice Bush is native to North America where it can be found growing wild along streams and in swampy areas. Hardy to zone 5, it is not particular regarding soil composition but does require partial shade and constantly wet soils. Spice Bush can be propagated by seeds sown out as soon as they are ripe, air layering, or cuttings taken in the mid summer.

Spice Bush leaves and leaf oils have been used to repel insects and the twigs and bark yield a mint-scented oil.

## Spruce, Fir Tree, Spruce, Spruce Fir, Norway Spruce
**Botanical Name:** Picea abies

**Properties:** Antibacterial, Antiseptic, Antiviral, Astringent, Febrifuge, Hyperemic, Rubefacient

**Traditional Use:** Spruce oil has been approved in Europe for use as a treatment for bronchitis, colds, congestion, coughs, and fevers. Fir helps to reduce mucus production in the airways while acting as a mild antibacterial & antiviral.

**Part Used:** Needles - Oil

**Side Effects:** Spruce is not recommended for use by women who are pregnant or nursing.

Spruce is not recommended for individuals suffering from bronchial asthma as it may make symptoms worse.

Spruce should not be applied to broken skin or over large areas of skin.

Additional uses and side effects may exist but further research is necessary to determine the exact properties and effects of use.

**General:** Spruce is an evergreen tree native to Europe but is cultivated in other regions of the world as an ornamental. Spruce oil is extracted from the branches and needles where it is traditionally taken as an infusion at a rate of 4 drops up to 3 times daily, an inhalant, or as an external ointment at a rate of 25% overall mixture.

### St. John's Wort, Amber, Goatweed, Tipton Weed
**Botanical Name:** Hypericum perforatum

**Properties:** Abortifacient, Analgesic, Anodyne, Antibacterial, Ant-Inflammatory, Antidepressant, Antifungal, Antimicrobial, Antioxidant, Antiseptic, Antispasmodic, Antiviral, Astringent, Cholagogue, Colorant, Digestive, Diuretic, Expectorant, Nervine, Sedative, Stimulant, Vermifuge, Vulnerary

**Traditional Use:** St. John's Wort tea is used as a traditional skin wash for to reduce scarring, speed healing, and disinfect skin sores, ulcers and wounds.

**Part Used:** Flower, Leaf

**Side Effects:** St. John's Wort is not recommended for use by women who are pregnant or nursing.

St. John's Wort is not recommended for use by women who are trying to conceive.

St. John's Wort has been used as an abortifacient in some cultures.

St. John's Wort may cause skin irritation.

St. John's Wort is not recommended for use by people with Bipolar Disorder, Schizophrenia, or Severe Depression.

St. John's Wort may interfere with the function of a variety of supplement and prescription products.

St. John's Wort is not recommended for use by people who are on prescription antidepressants.

St. John's Wort may cause increased sensitivity to sunlight.

St. John's Wort may cause dizziness, dry mouth, fatigue, gastrointestinal upset, headache, and sexual dysfunction in some people.

Additional uses and side effects may exist but further research is necessary to determine the exact properties and effects of use.

**General:**  St. John's Wort is native to Africa, Asia, and Europe and is cultivated in other regions for supplemental purposes.  Hardy to zone 3, it is not particular regarding soil composition but does prefer good drainage, full to partial sun and consistent moisture.  It can be propagated by seeds sown out as soon as they are ripe or by division in the spring.

The flowering tops of the St. John's Wort are harvested during the flowering season, dried, and used in traditional supplement teas, extracts and in powdered form for both internal and topical applications.

**Star Anise**
**Botanical Name:**  Illicium verum

**Properties:**  Antibacterial, Antifungal, Antispasmodic, Antiviral, Carminative, Expectorant, Phytoestrogen, Relaxant, Stimulant

**Traditional Use:**  Star Anise fruits have traditionally been used to treat bacterial infections.

**Part Used:**  Fruit, Seed - Oil

**Side Effects:**  Star Anise is not recommended for use by women who are pregnant or nursing.

Star Anise is not recommended for use in children's treatments.

Star Anise is not recommended for use by people who have a hormone sensitive disorder like endometriosis, fibroids, or cancer.

Star Anise may cause an allergic reaction or skin irritation in some people.

Additional uses and side effects may exist but further research is necessary to determine the exact properties and effects of use.

**General:**  Star Anise is native to Asia and cultivated in other areas.  Hardy to zone 8, it prefers sandy to loamy soil, full to partial sun and consistent moisture.  Star Anise can be propagated by seed sown out in the spring, layering during the growing season, or cuttings taken in the late summer.

Star Anise bark is pounded and burnt for the scent and the fruit is used as a flavoring or harvested when nearly ripe used fresh, dried, or as an essential oil in traditional supplements.

**Stonecrop, Bird Bread, Biting Stonecrop, Creeping Tom, Gold Chain, Golden Moss, Jack of the Buttery, Mousetail, Prick Madam, Stonecrop, Wall Ginger, Wallpepper**
**Botanical Name:**  Sedum acre

**Properties:**  Analgesic, Antibacterial, Astringent, Cathartic, Diuretic, Hypotensive, Laxative, Rubefacient, Vermifuge, Vulnerary

**Traditional Uses:**  Stonecrop is traditionally used in ointments or applied as a fresh poultice to help ease pain, reduce infection, and speed healing of burns, eczema, hemorrhoids, wounds, and ulcers and to aid in the removal of warts.

**Parts Used:** Leaf, Stem

**Side Effects:** Stonecrop is not recommended for use by women who are pregnant or nursing.

Stonecrop may cause skin irritation or blistering in some people.

Internal use of Stonecrop may cause severe gastrointestinal upset.

Additional uses and side effects may exist but further research is necessary to determine the exact properties and effects of use.

**General:** Stonecrop can be found throughout the northern hemisphere where it grows wild or is cultivated as an ornamental. It is not particular regarding soil composition but does prefer full sun and dry to moist soil. It can be propagated by seed or division and can become very aggressive in sunny positions.

The leaves are eaten as a raw or cooked vegetable and the leaf has been dried and powdered for use as a pepper like flavoring.

The leaf and stem are harvested for use fresh, as a tincture, or dried and powdered for use in traditional preparations.

### Storax, Copalm, Gum Tree, Liquid Amber, Oriental Sweetgum, Sweet Gum, Turkish Sweetgum, White Gum
**Botanical Name:** Liquidambar orientalis

**Properties:** Antibacterial, Anti-inflammatory, Diaphoretic, Expectorant, Stimulant, Vulnerary

**Traditional Use:** Storax has traditionally been included in topical preparations to prevent infection and speed healing of skin sores, ulcers, and wounds.

**Part Used:** Inner Bark, Resin

**Side Effects:** Storax is not recommended for use by women who are pregnant or nursing.

Storax may cause diarrhea.

Storax may cause an allergic reaction or skin irritation.

Additional uses and side effects may exist but further research is necessary to determine the exact properties and effects of use.

**General:** Storax is native to Asia and has been naturalized to other parts of the world including North America. Hardy to zone 8, it is not particular regarding soil composition but does prefer full to partial sun and consistent moisture. Storax can be propagated by seeds sown as soon as they are ripe, cuttings taken in mid-summer or layering.

Storax resins are used in incense, as a gum alternative or to flavor foods. The resin is extracted and then inner bark harvested and boiled to create a supplement decoction for use as part of an inhalation or topical preparation.

**Smooth Sumac**
**Botanical Name:** Rhus glabra

**Properties:** Antimicrobial, Astringent, Colorant, Diuretic, Vulnerary

**Traditional Use:** Smooth Sumac has been used as a traditional topical or supplement preparation to treat both gram positive and gram-negative bacterial infections.

Smooth Sumac bark has traditionally been used to reduce inflammation, prevent infection, and speed healing of skin sores, ulcers, and wounds.

Smooth Sumac bark has been used as a traditional gargle to treat infection and reduce inflammation of the throat or mouth.

**Part Used:** Bark

**Side Effects:** Smooth Sumac is not recommended for use by women who are pregnant or nursing.

Additional uses and side effects may exist but further research is necessary to determine the exact properties and effects of use.

**General:** Smooth Sumac is native to North America where the bark is harvested for use in traditional topical preparations.

**Sundew, Dew Plant, Lustwort, Red Rot, Youthwort**
**Botanical Name:** Drosera rotundifolia

**Properties:** Antibacterial, Antimicrobial, Antispasmodic, Antitussive, Expectorant, Immunostimulant

**Traditional Use:** Sundew has traditionally been used as a topical or supplement preparation to treat bacterial infections like pneumococcus, staphylococcus, and streptococcus.

**Part Used:** Whole

**Side Effects:** Sundew is not recommended for use by women who are pregnant or nursing.

Additional uses and side effects may exist but further research is necessary to determine the exact properties and effects of use.

**General:** Sundew is native to China, Europe, India, and North & South America where it is harvested for use in strong traditional supplement infusions up to 4 times daily.

**Swallowroot, Madina, Makli Beru, Nannari**

**Botanical Name:** Decalepis hamiltonii

**Properties:** Antibacterial, Anti-inflammatory, Antioxidant, Appetite Stimulant

**Traditional Uses:** Swallowroot has been used as a traditional topical or supplement to treat bacterial infections like e. coli, pseudomonas, and salmonella.

**Parts Used:** Root

**Side Effects:** Swallowroot is not recommended for use by women who are pregnant or nursing.

Additional uses and side effects may exist but further research is necessary to determine the exact properties and effects of use.

**General:** Swallowroot is a native to India where the root is harvested, dried and powdered or made into a tincture as a traditional supplementary treatment.

### Sweet Rush, Dwarf Sedge, Japanese Rush, Sweet Flag
**Botanical Name:** Acorus gramineus

**Properties:** Anodyne, Antibacterial, Antifungal, Antispasmodic, Cardiotonic, Carminative, Diaphoretic, Diuretic, Emmenagogue, Expectorant, Febrifuge, Insect Repellant, Sedative, Tonic, Vermifuge

**Traditional Use:** Sweet Rush has been used as a traditional treatment to treat bacterial infections like staphylococcus and streptococci.

**Part Used:** Root

**Side Effects:** Sweet Rush is not recommended for use by women who are pregnant or nursing.

Additional uses and side effects may exist but further research is necessary to determine the exact properties and effects of use.

**General:** Sweet Rush is native to Asia and cultivated as an ornamental in other regions. Hardy to zone 5, it is not particular regarding soil composition but does require full sun and moist to wet soil. Sweet Rush can be propagated by seeds sown as soon as they are ripe or division in the spring.

Sweet Rush root is dried and used in stored goods to repel insects or eaten as a raw or cooked vegetable. The root has also been dried for use as a spice or used fresh or dried and powdered in traditional preparations.

### Tain Nan Xing
**Botanical Name:** Arisaema consanguineum

**Properties:** Anodyne, Antibacterial, Antifungal, Anti-inflammatory, Antispasmodic, Expectorant, Sedative

**Traditional Use:** Fresh Tain Nan Xing root is used as a traditional topical preparation to treat bacterial and fungal infections.

Fresh Tain Nan Xing root has traditionally been used as a wash to reduce inflammation, ease pain, and prevent bacterial infections in skin sores, ulcers, and wounds.

**Part Used:** Leaf

**Side Effects:** Tain Nan Xing is not recommended for use by women who are pregnant or nursing.

Fresh Tain Nan Xing is not recommended for internal use and may cause numbness or a tingling sensation in the lips, mouth, tongue, or throat.

Additional uses and side effects may exist but further research is necessary to determine the exact properties and effects of use.

**General:** Tain Nan Xing is native to Asia where it can be found growing wild in damp forests. It is cultivated in other regions as an ornamental and traditional supplement. The root is harvested in the fall and used fresh in topical preparations or dried and powdered for use in traditional supplements.

**Tamanu, Alexandrian Laurel, Indian Laurel, Kamani Punna, Palo Maria**
**Botanical Name:** Calophyllum inophyllum

**Properties:** Antibacterial, Antifungal, Anti-inflammatory, Antimicrobial, Cancer, Deodorant, Emollient, Vermifuge, Vulnerary

**Traditional Use:** Tamanu oil has significant antibacterial, antifungal, and antimicrobial qualities that make it a traditional treatment for a variety of infections.

**Part Used:** Seed Oil

**Side Effects:** Tamanu Oil is not recommended for use by women who are pregnant or nursing.

Tamanu Oil may cause dizziness, headache, and nausea.

Additional uses and side effects may exist but further research is necessary to determine the exact properties and effects of use.

**General:** Tamanu is an evergreen shrub or tree native to Africa, Asia, and Australia but has been naturalized to other parts of the world as a fragrant ornamental. It is not particular regarding soil composition but does prefer full to partial sun and consistent moisture. It can be propagated by seed or by division of the suckers in the spring.

The wood has been used in woodcraft, especially water related construction and the seed oil is used as a fuel alternative, in natural hair & skin care recipes or in traditional topical preparations.

Tamanu seeds are harvested and the oils extracted by steam distillation for use in traditional topical and supplement preparations.

**Tamarind, Imlee, Tintiri**
**Botanical Name:** Tamarindus indica

**Properties:** Antibacterial, Antifungal, Anti-inflammatory, Antimicrobial, Antiseptic, Digestive, Immunostimulant, Laxative, Vermifuge, Vulnerary

**Traditional Use:** Tamarind has traditionally been used to stimulate the immune system and to prevent common infections.

Tamarind has been used as a traditional poultice, ointment, or wash to reduce inflammation & infection while speeding healing in skin sores, ulcers, and wounds.

**Part Used:** Fruit, Seed

**Side Effects:** Tamarind is not recommended for use by women who are pregnant or nursing.

Additional uses and side effects may exist but further research is necessary to determine the exact properties and effects of use.

**General:** Tamarind is a large evergreen native to Africa and has been naturalized to North & South America where the fruit is harvested when ripe for use as a food. The oil is extracted from the seed through steam distillation for use in topical preparations, cosmetics, and supplements.

**Tarragon, Little Dragon, Mugwort**
**Botanical Name:** Artemisia dracunculus

**Properties:** Antibacterial, Antifungal, Antispasmodic, Appetite, Astringent, Carminative, Diuretic, Emmenagogue, Insect Repellant, Sedative, Vermifuge

**Traditional Use:** Tarragon has been used in traditional skin washes or ointments to reduce seepage, prevent infection and speed healing in skin sores, ulcers, and contact dermatitis pustules.

**Part Used:** Leaf

**Side Effects:** Tarragon is not recommended for use by women who are pregnant or nursing.

Tarragon is not recommended for long-term use.

Tarragon may cause an allergic reaction in some people.

**General:** Tarragon is native to Germany, Russia, and Southern Europe but is cultivated in many regions of the world. Hardy to zone 3, it prefers sandy to loamy soil, full to partial sun and consistent moisture. Tarragon can be propagated by seed sown in the late winter or early spring.

Tarragon is grown to repel insects from planting beds. The leaves are harvested when in bloom, air dried, and used for culinary and supplement purposes or the oils are extracted through steam distillation for use in topical and aromatherapy preparations.

**Tartarian Aster**
**Botanical Name:** Aster tataricus

**Properties:** Antibacterial, Antifungal, Antitussive, Expectorant, Stimulant

**Traditional Use:** Tartarian Aster has been used as a traditional treatment for bacterial infections like bacillus, e. coli, and staphylococcus.

**Part Used:** Roots

**Side Effects:** Tartarian Aster is not recommended for use by women who are pregnant or nursing.

Additional uses and side effects may exist but further research is necessary to determine the exact properties and effects of use.

**General:** Tartarian Aster is native to Asia where it has been used as a traditional treatment for thousands of years. The root is harvested in the fall, dried, and powdered for use as a traditional supplement preparation

**Tea, Black Tea, Chinese Tea, English Tea, Green Tea**
**Botanical Name:**
Camellia sinensis

**Properties:** Analgesic, Anti-inflammatory, Antioxidants, Antispasmodic, Antiviral, Appetite Depressant, Astringent, Cancer, Cardio-tonic, Colorant, Cox-2, Diuretic, Inhibitor, Hypoglycemic, Hypotensive, Nervine, Stimulant

**Traditional Use:** Black tea is traditionally used as a gentle eyewash treatment for conjunctivitis and as a traditional wash to reduce inflammation, fight viral infection like herpes infection.

**Part Used:** Leaves

**Side Effects:** Tea is not recommended for use in women who are pregnant or nursing.

Tea is not recommended for use by people who have anemia, anxiety, bleeding disorders, diabetes, glaucoma, heart problems, high blood pressure, osteoporosis, or an overactive thyroid.

Tea is not recommended for use in women who have a hormone sensitive condition like endometriosis, fibroids, and cancer.

Overdose of tea may cause confusion, convulsions, diarrhea, dizziness, headache, heartburn, irregular heartbeat, nervousness, sleep problems, tremor, and vomiting.

Green tea contains compounds that may make anticoagulant drugs less effective.

Tea does contain caffeine and overuse may lead to anxiety, frequent urination, irritability, insomnia, restlessness, and upset stomach.

There have been reports of liver problems in some people taking a concentrated tea extract over an extended period.

Tea may be addictive.

Additional uses and side effects may exist but further research is necessary to determine the exact properties and effects of use.

**General:** Tea is cultivated in many parts of the world as a commonly consumed beverage. Hardy to zone 8, it prefers sandy to loamy soils with good drainage, partial sun, and consistent moisture. Tea can be propagated by seeds sown out as soon as they are ripe or by cuttings taken at any time during the growing season.

Black, brown, and green teas come from the same plant and the difference in coloring is a result of a change in the way that the tea is handled during processing. The more extensive the handling, the darker the tea product and resulting colorant. Brown Tea is only partially fermented while Black Tea is fully fermented and Green Tea is not fermented.

Tea leaves yield an essential oil used in perfumery and as a culinary flavoring. The seeds yield oil used in manufacturing. Tea flower petals yield a greenish gray to black toned colorant used as a textile dye. The leaves yield a tan to deep brown toned colorant used as a culinary, cosmetic, or textile dye. The wood is used to make small woodcraft.

Tea is typically brewed and consumed as a beverage but is available in extract form. Therapeutic doses are traditionally believed to be reached by drinking 1 teaspoon of green tea leaf in 1-cup boiling water 5 times or more daily.

**Tea Tree**
**Botanical Name:** Melaleuca alternifolia

**Properties:** Analgesic, Antibacterial, Antifungal, Anti-inflammatory, Antimicrobial, Antiseptic, Antiviral, Expectorant, Immunostimulant, Insecticide, Vulnerary

**Traditional Use:** Tea tree oil is traditionally used in aromatherapy to reduce air borne infectious agents.

Tea Tree has been blended at a rate of 5% oil, 5% peroxide, to 90% base to create a traditional topical treatment for bacterial infections.

Crushed Tea Tree leaves have traditionally been used as a snuff like inhalant to reduce the duration of respiratory infections like the common cold, influenza, and pneumonia.

Tea tree oil is traditionally used as a broad-spectrum antimicrobial against a wide variety of bacterial, fungus, and viruses. It is traditionally included in salves and ointments, and natural cleaning products.

In addition to its own infection fighting properties, Tea Tree leaves are used as a traditional infusion to stimulate the body's own immune system.

An infusion of Tea Tree leaves has traditionally been used as a treatment for urinary tract infections.

Tea Tree oil has been incorporated into traditional topical creams and lotions to minimize the risk of infection in skin sores, ulcers, and wounds.

**Part Used:** Branch Tips, Leaf - Oil

**Side Effects:** Tea Tree Oil is for external use only.

Tea Tree Oil is not recommended for use by women who are pregnant or nursing.

Tea Tree Oil may not be recommended for use in topical preparations for young children.

Tea Tree Oil should is not recommended for use on deep wounds.

Tea Tree oil should not be used near the eyes, ears, or nose.

Tea Tree Oil can cause skin burning, dryness, irritation, itching, redness, or stinging in some people.

Ingestion of Tea Tree Oil may cause diarrhea, coma, and death.

Additional uses and side effects may exist but further research is necessary to determine the exact properties and effects of use.

**General:** Tea Tree oil comes from the leaves of an evergreen shrub commonly called Tea Tree. It is native Asia and Australia but cultivated in other regions. Hardy to zone 9, it is not particular regarding soil composition but does prefer good drainage, consistent moisture, and full sun. It can be propagated by seed sown indoors in the fall or by cuttings taken in the mid summer that contain a heel of the previous year's growth.

Tea Tree has been used for centuries by the aborigines as a topical treatment and traditional supplement. Tea Tree oil is extracted from the leaves by steam distillation and is used topically and in cleaning products.

**Thyme, French Thyme, Garden Thyme, Red Thyme, Rubbed Thyme, Spanish Thyme, Tomillo, Van Ajwayan, White Thyme**
**Botanical Name:** Thymus vulgaris

**Properties:** Analgesic, Antibacterial, Antifungal, Antioxidant, Antiperspirant, Antiseptic, Antispasmodic, Antitussive, Antiviral, Aphrodisiac, Cancer, Carminative, Depurative, Diaphoretic,

Digestive, Emmenagogue, Expectorant, Hypertensive, Insect Repellant, Nervine, Sedative, Vermifuge

**Traditional Use:** Thyme has been used in traditional air purification and disinfectant treatments.

Thyme is often used as part of a household cleaner disinfectant recipe.

Thyme is traditionally used in gargles to treat throat or mouth inflammation and infection and is included in many commercial mouth and throat preparations.

**Part Used:** Flower, Leaf, Stem

**Side Effects:** Thyme is not recommended for use by women who are pregnant or nursing.

Thyme can cause an allergic reaction in some people.

Thyme oil may elevate the blood pressure.

Overuse of thyme can effect the menstrual cycles in some women

The oils isolated from the Thyme plant can be toxic and should not be ingested but the herb itself is generally considered safe.

Additional uses and side effects may exist but further research is necessary to determine the exact properties and effects of use.

**General:** Thyme is native to the Mediterranean but is cultivated in many areas of the world. Hardy to zone 7, it is grown in containers in cooler regions. It prefers sandy or loamy soil, good drainage, and full sun. It can be propagated by seed, spring division, cuttings in the mid summer that contain a heel of the last years growth or by layering at any time during the growing season.

Thyme is harvested as a culinary seasoning and as a liquid extract for use in traditional supplements. The oils are used in perfumery or in traditional topical preparations. The leaves and flowers are eaten as a raw vegetable or added to recipes as a flavoring.

The oils are extracted through steam distillation for use in aromatherapy. Red Thyme and White Thyme oil come from the same plant. The alteration in coloring is due to oxidation during the extraction and methods used when processing of the oils. Red Thyme oil contains stronger antiseptic properties and is traditionally used for disinfection. White Thyme oil has more of the impurities removed and tends to have a milder action making it preferred in many traditional treatments.

**Tree of Heaven, Ailante, Ailanto, Chinese Sumach, Copal Tree, Heaven Tree, Indian Tree of Heaven, Paradise Tree**
**Botanical Name:** Ailanthus altissima

**Properties:** Antibacterial, Antispasmodic, Astringent, Cardiotonic, Colorant, Diuretic, Emetic, Emmenagogue, Expectorant, Febrifuge, Insect Repellant, Insecticide, Rubefacient, Tonic, Vermifuge

**Traditional Uses:** Tree of Heaven extracts are used in traditional preparations and cleaning products to reduce infectious bacteria.

**Parts Used:** Bark, Root

**Side Effects:** Tree of Heaven is not recommended for use by women who are pregnant or nursing.

Tree of Heaven flowers may cause an allergic reaction is some individuals.

Overuse of Tree of Heaven may cause diarrhea, headache, nausea, and tingling in the arms or legs.

Additional uses and side effects may exist but further research is necessary to determine the exact properties and effects of use.

**General:** Tree of Heaven is native to the northeast and central Asia and has been naturalized to Europe and the United States. Hardy to zone 7, it prefers sandy or loamy soil, full to partial sun and moist to wet conditions. Tree of Heaven can be propagated by seeds sown out as soon as they are ripe, division of the suckers in the spring or root cuttings taken in mid-winter.

Tree of Heaven leaves yield a yellow toned colorant used as a traditional dye product and the wood is used in papermaking. The leaves and flowers are used in dry insect repellant preparations and the oils are water extracted for use in spray repellant and insecticide preparations. Tree of Heaven is known to reduce soil moisture content and is traditionally grown in bog like or marshy areas to reduce moisture and related insect infestations.

Tree of Heaven leaves are harvested for use as a food source or the bark and roots are harvested for use In traditional supplements.

**Tribulus, Bindii, Bullhead, Caltrop, Cat's Head, Devil's Eyelashes, Devil's Thorn, Devil's Weed, Gouthead, Puncturevine, Puncture Weed**
**Botanical Name:** Tribulus terrestris

**Properties:** Abortifacient, Androgen Production, Antibacterial, Antiviral, Aphrodisiac, Astringent, Cardiac, Carminative, Demulcent, Diuretic, Estrogenic, Galactogogue, Hypotensive, Steroidal Saponins, Stimulant

**Traditional Use:** Tribulus has been shown to have antibacterial and antiviral properties that make it a traditional tea for use in treating internal and external bacterial and viral infections.

**Part Used:** Fruit, Leaf, Seed

**Side Effects:** Tribulus is not recommended for use by women who are pregnant or nursing.

Tribulus seed has been used as an abortifacient in some cultures.

Tribulus is not recommended for use by people who are taking nitroglycerine or have a heart condition.

Tribulus may act on the hormones and is not recommended for use by men who have prostate problems.

Tribulus may affect blood sugar levels.

The fruit of the Tribulus is not for internal use.

Additional uses and side effects may exist but further research is necessary to determine the exact properties and effects of use.

**General:** Tribulus is native to Europe and has been naturalized to other parts of the world where it is considered an invasive weed by some. It is not particular regarding soil composition but does prefer full sun and consistent moisture. Tribulus can be propagated by seeds and will self sow readily if given its own place in the garden.

Tribulus leaves and shoots are eaten as a cooked vegetable and the seeds are ground into flour. The whole plant is harvested, dried, and powdered for use as a traditional supplement.

**Umckaloabo**
**Botanical Name:** Pelargonium sidoides

**Properties:** Analgesic, Antibacterial, Antibiotic, Expectorant, Immunostimulant

**Traditional Use:** Umckaloabo has traditionally been used to treat bacterial infections like staphylococcus.

Umckaloabo has been used as a traditional supplement to treat chronic infections like ear and throat infections.

**Part Used:** Root

**Side Effects:** Umckaloabo is not recommended for use by women who are pregnant or nursing.

Additional uses and side effects may exist but further research is necessary to determine the exact properties and effects of use.

**General:** Umckaloabo is native to Africa and is cultivated elsewhere. The root is traditionally harvested for use in an alcohol extraction that is used as a traditional supplement and commercial preparation to combat infection.

**Usnea, Beard Moss, Old Man's Beard, Tree Moss, Tree's Dandruff, Usnia, Women's Long Hair**
**Botanical Name:** Usnea barbata

**Properties:** Analgesic, Antibacterial, Antibiotic, Antifungal, Anti-inflammatory, Antiviral, Expectorant, Febrifuge

**Traditional Uses:** Usnea has traditionally been used as a topical and supplement preparation to treat infections including fungal and bacterial infections like yeast, impetigo, staphylococcus and streptococcus.

Usnea has traditionally been used to provide general pain relief and helps to alleviate congestion in conditions like asthma, bronchitis, colds, and influenza. Usnea also has antibacterial and antiviral properties that make it a traditional supplement to shorten the length of common infections including bronchitis, colds, influenza, and pneumonia.

Usnea has traditionally been used in sprays & gargles to help alleviate throat pain, infection, & inflammation.

**Parts Used:** Whole

**Side Effects:** Usnea is not recommended for use by women who are pregnant or nursing.

Usnea may cause abdominal pain, nausea, fatigue, muscle weakness, and liver damage.

Additional uses and side effects may exist but further research is necessary to determine the exact properties and effects of use.

**General:** Usnea is a type of algae and fungus combination that grow together on trees and are often termed lichen. The whole plant is used in traditional supplements and is most frequently used as an alcohol extract.

**Uva Ursi, Arberry, Bearberry, Bearsgrape, Manzanita, Mountain Box, Mountain Cranberry, Ptarmigan Berry, Redberry, Rockberry, Sadberry**
**Botanical Name:** Arctostaphylos uva-ursi

**Properties:** Antibacterial, Ant-Inflammatory, Antiseptic, Astringent, Colorant, Diuretic, Hypnotic, Narcotic

**Traditional Use:** Uva Ursi has shown itself to be effective against e. coli and is traditionally used to treat bacterial infections.

Uva Ursi leaf infusions have been used in traditional gargles to reduce infection and speed healing in canker sores, mouth ulcers and tooth abscesses.

Uva Ursi leaves have traditionally been used in infusion washes and poultice preparations to reduce infection and inflammation while speeding healing in conditions like contact dermatitis, skin sores, ulcers, and wounds.

Uva Ursi leaf is used as a traditional tincture to alleviate urinary tract infection.

Uva Ursi has shown itself to be effective against E. Coli in laboratory studies.

**Part Used:** Leaf

**Side Effects:** Uva Ursi is not recommended for use by women who are pregnant or nursing.

Uva Ursi is not recommended for use by people who have kidney disease.

Uva Ursi is not recommended for use in children's treatments.

Uva Ursi may cause nausea and vomiting in sensitive individuals.

Overuse of Uva Ursi may cause breathing problems, eye problems, liver damage, convulsions, and even death.

Uva Ursi is not recommended for use with cranberry juice or vitamin C, as these are known to minimize the effectiveness of Uva Ursi.

Additional uses and side effects may exist but further research is necessary to determine the exact properties and effects of use.

**General:** Uva Ursi is native to Asia, Europe, and North America. Hardy to zone 4, it prefers sandy or loamy soil, full to partial sun and consistent moisture. Uva Ursi can be propagated by seeds sown out as soon as they are ripe, cuttings taken in the late spring or division in the early spring.

Uva Ursi leaves yield a self-mordanting yellow to brown toned colorant used as a textile dye product while the fruits yield a grayish brown tone. The berries are crushed and used as a waterproofing coating and the dried fruits are used as beads.

Uva Ursi fruits are eaten raw or cooked, brewed as a beverage or preserved for use as jelly. Uva Ursi leaves are harvested in the early fall while they are still green for use in traditional tinctures or powders. Uva Ursi is impervious to water but can be incorporated into a tincture or powdered for use in treatments.

**Vietnamese Balm**
**Botanical Name:** Elsholtzia ciliata

**Properties:** Antibacterial, Antihistamine, Antiviral, Astringent, Carminative, Depurative, Diaphoretic, Diuretic, Stimulant

**Traditional Use:** Vietnamese Balm has traditionally been used as a broad-spectrum antibacterial agent.

**Part Used:** Whole

**Side Effects:** Vietnamese Balm is not recommended for use by women who are pregnant or nursing.

Additional uses and side effects may exist but further research is necessary to determine the exact properties and effects of use.

**General:** Vietnamese Balm is native to Asia and commonly considered an invasive weed though it is sometimes cultivated as an ornamental in other areas. Hardy to zone 5, it is not particular regarding soil composition but does require full sun and moist conditions. It is easily propagated by seeds and will self-sow readily if given its own place in the garden.

Vietnamese Balm leaves are eaten raw or cooked and the seeds have been dried and powdered for use as a seasoning. The oils are extracted from the plant for use in traditional topical and aromatic preparations. The whole plant is harvested, dried, and powdered for use as a supplemental preparation.

**Wafer Ash, Hop Tree, Pickaway Anise, Prairie Grub, Scrubby Trefoil, Stinking Ash, Stinking Prairie Bush, Swamp Dogwood, Wingseed**
**Botanical Name:** Ptelea trifoliata

**Properties:** Antibacterial, Antifungal, Antimicrobial, Stomachic, Tonic

**Traditional Use:** Wafer Ash has been used as a traditional topical preparation to reduce the likelihood of infection in wounds.

**Part Used:** Root Bark

**Side Effects:** Wafer Ash is not recommended for use by women who are pregnant or nursing.

Wafer Ash may cause photosensitivity.

Additional uses and side effects may exist but further research is necessary to determine the exact properties and effects of use.

**General:** Wafer Ash is native to Central and North America but is cultivated as an ornamental in Europe. Hardy to zone 5, it is not particular regarding soil composition but prefers full to partial sun and consistent moisture. Wafer Ash can be propagated by seeds sown as soon as they are ripe, layering or cuttings taken in mid-summer.

Wafer Ash fruits are eaten raw or used as a hop substitute in beer making. The bark, leaf, and root have been harvested for use as a supplement extract.

**Water Plantain, Mad Dog Weed**
**Botanical Name:** Alisma plantago

**Properties:** Antibacterial, Astringent, Contraceptive, Diaphoretic, Diuretic, Hepatic, Hypoglycemic, Hypotensive, Rubefacient

**Traditional Use:** Water Plantain root oil has traditionally been used to treat bacterial infections like pneumococci and staphylococcus.

Water Plantain has traditionally been used as a gentle diuretic and antibacterial in the treatment of urinary tract infection.

**Part Used:** Leaf, Root, Root Oil, Seed

**Side Effects:**  Water Plantain is not recommended for use by women who are pregnant or nursing.

Water Plantain seed has been used as a contraceptive in some cultures and is not recommended for use by those trying to conceive.

Water Plantain may affect blood sugar.

Water Plantain may affect blood pressure.

Additional uses and side effects may exist but further research is necessary to determine the exact properties and effects of use.

**General:**  Water Plantain is a flowering plant native to Asia, Europe, and North America where it can be found growing along the shores or in the edges of fresh water.   It is not particular regarding soil composition but does require full sun and high moisture to thrive.  Water Plantain can be grown entirely in water.   It can be propagated by seed sown out as soon as it is ripe or by division in the spring or fall.

The root is eaten as a starchy cooked food and the leaves are eaten as a boiled vegetable. The leaf or root is harvested at the beginning of the growing season, dried, and powdered for use in traditional supplement infusions or the oil extracted for use in topical and internal preparations.

**Wild Garlic, Ramsons**
**Botanical Name:**  Allium ursinum

**Properties:**  Antibacterial, Antifungal, Antimicrobial, Antioxidant, Antiseptic, Antiviral, Antiseptic, Antispasmodic, Astringent, Cholagogue, Cholesterol, Depurative, Diaphoretic, Diuretic, Emmenagogue, Expectorant, Febrifuge, Hypotensive, Immunostimulant, Insect Repellant, Rubefacient, Stimulant, Vermifuge

**Traditional Uses:**  Wild Garlic contains antibacterial and antifungal compounds that make it a traditional ingredient in topical treatments for bacterial and fungal infections

Wild Garlic contains a broad spectrum antimicrobial and has been used in traditional supplements to shorten the length of infections.

The juices of the Wild Garlic have been used as disinfecting agent in household cleansing products.

Wild Garlic has traditionally been used in dietary plans to boost the body's immune response helping to ward off common infections.

Wild Garlic juice is used as a traditional topical poultices or washes to disinfect wounds.

**Parts Used:**  Bulb, Whole

**Side Effects:**  Wild Garlic is not recommended for use beyond dietary by women who are pregnant or nursing.  Wild Garlic is a known uterus stimulant.

Wild Garlic is not recommended for use beyond dietary in children's treatments.

Overuse of Wild Garlic may cause heartburn in some people.

Overuse of Wild Garlic may burn the skin in some people.

Garlic may cause bad breath, body odor, upset stomach, and rarely allergic reactions in some people.

Wild Garlic may reduce the blood clotting ability.  Do not use garlic supplements if you are planning to have surgery, dental work, or have a bleeding disorder.

Additional uses and side effects may exist but further research is necessary to determine the exact properties and effects of use.

**General:**  Wild Garlic is a bulb plant native to Western Asia and Europe but cultivated elsewhere for its ability to deliver higher potency than commonly cultivated garlic with less aroma.  Hardy to zone 5, Wild Garlic is not particular regarding sun conditions but does prefer sandy or loamy soil and consistent moisture.  It can be propagated by seed or by bulb division.

The juices of the Wild Garlic have been used as an insect repellant primarily against insects like moths.  The bulbs, leaves, and flowers are eaten as a raw or cooked vegetable though the aroma increases as the plant ripens.

Wild Garlic is similar in composition and uses to cultivated Garlic but has a milder aroma and weaker action making it more common for use in traditional treatments given over a longer period.

**Wintergreen – Round Leaved, Pyrola, Round Leaved Wintergreen**
**Botanical Name:**  Pyrola rotundifolia

**Properties:**  Antibacterial, Antiseptic, Antispasmodic, Astringent, Cardio-Tonic, Contraceptive, Diuretic, Nervine, Sedative, Tonic

**Traditional Use:**  Round Leaved Wintergreen has been used as a traditional topical wash or ointment to reduce infection and speed healing in skin sores, ulcers, and wounds.

Round Leaved Wintergreen has traditionally been used as a gargle to alleviate throat inflammation and infection.

Round Leaved Wintergreen has been used as a traditional supplement to treat urinary tract infection.

**Part Used:**  Leaf

**Side Effects:** Round Leaved Wintergreen is not recommended for use by women who are pregnant or nursing.

Additional uses and side effects may exist but further research is necessary to determine the exact properties and effects of use.

**General:** Round Leaved Wintergreen is native to the United States where it is cultivated as a groundcover. The leaves are harvested during flowering and used fresh or dried and powdered for use in traditional supplements or topical preparations.

**Wintergreen – Spotted, Spotted Wintergreen, Striped Wintergreen**
**Botanical Name:** Chimaphila maculata

**Properties:** Analgesic, Antibacterial, Antiseptic, Astringent, Diuretic, Febrifuge, Stimulant, Tonic

**Traditional Use:** Spotted Wintergreen has been used as a traditional topical wash or ointment to reduce infection and speed healing in skin sores, ulcers, and wounds.

Spotted Wintergreen has traditionally been used as a gargle to alleviate throat inflammation and infection.

Spotted Wintergreen has been used as a traditional supplement to treat urinary tract infection.

**Part Used:** Leaf

**Side Effects:** Spotted Evergreen is not recommended for use by women who are pregnant or nursing.

Additional uses and side effects may exist but further research is necessary to determine the exact properties and effects of use.

**General:** Spotted Wintergreen is an evergreen perennial groundcover native to Central America and North America where it is cultivated as an ornamental. The leaves are harvested for use in alcohol extraction or dried and powdered for use in topical and supplement treatments.

**Woad, Ben Lan Gen, Chinese Indigo, Dyer's Woad, Farberwaid, Glastum, Hierba Pastel, Indigo Woad, Isatis, Quing Dai**
**Botanical Name:** Isatis tinctoria

**Properties:** Analgesic, Antibacterial, Antibiotic, Anti-inflammatory, Antiviral, Cancer, Colorant, Febrifuge, Immunostimulant

**Traditional Use:** Woad is traditionally used as a short-term antibiotic to treat a wide range of infections including bacterial and viral infections.

**Part Used:** Leaf, Root

**Side Effects:** Woad is not recommended for use by women who are pregnant or nursing.

Woad is not recommended for use in children's treatments.

Woad contains aspirin like substances and is not recommended for use by people with an allergy to aspirin.

Woad is not recommended for people on blood thinning medication.

Additional uses and side effects may exist but further research is necessary to determine the exact properties and effects of use.

**General:** Woad is native to Asia but is naturalized to Europe and North America where it has been cultivated as a blue dye product for thousands of years.

The leaf and root are harvested for use fresh or dried in traditional supplements. Alcohol extracts are undergoing study as a potential treatment for slowing the growth of cancer cells.

**Wood Rose, Hawaiian Woodrose, Baby Woodrose, Elephant Climber, Elephant Creeper, Silver Morning Glory, Woolly Morning Glory**
**Botanical Name:** Argyreia speciosa

**Properties:** Analgesic, Antibacterial, Antioxidant, Hallucinogenic, Hepatic

**Traditional Uses:** Woodrose root and seed has traditionally been used to treat bacterial infections like e. coli and staphylococcus.

**Parts Used:** Flower, Leaf, Root, Seed

**Side Effects:** Woodrose is not recommended for use by women who are pregnant or nursing.

Woodrose is not recommended for use by people with a mental illness especially those with psychotic tendencies.

Woodrose may cause blurred vision, dilated pupils, dizziness, hallucinations, increased blood pressure, increased heart rate, nausea, rapid eye movement, and vomiting.

Additional uses and side effects may exist but further research is necessary to determine the exact properties and effects of use.

**General:** Woodrose is cultivated as a perennial ornamental vine in Asia, Europe, and North America. The seeds have been harvested for use in traditional supplements.

**Woodruff, Sweet Woodruff**
**Botanical Name:** Asperula odorata

**Properties:** Abortifacient, Antibacterial, Anticoagulant, Anti-inflammatory, Antispasmodic, Astringent, Cardiac, Colorant, Diaphoretic, Digestive, Diuretic, Nervine, Sedative

**Traditional Uses:** Woodruff is used in traditional topical ointments and washes to reduce infection and inflammation while speeding healing in skin sores, ulcers, and wounds.

**Parts Used:** Leaf, Stem

**Side Effects:** Woodruff is not recommended for use by women who are pregnant or nursing.

Woodruff has been used as an abortifacient in some cultures.

Woodruff may decrease the body's ability to clot and increase bleeding.

Additional uses and side effects may exist but further research is necessary to determine the exact properties and effects of use.

**General:** Woodruff is native to Africa and Europe but is cultivated in other areas. Hardy to zone 5, it is not particular regarding soil composition, but does prefer full or partial shade and consistent moisture. Woodruff can be propagated by seeds sown out as soon as they are ripe, spring division, or by cuttings taken after flowering.

Woodruff root yields a red toned dye product and the stems and leaves yield a greenish gray toned colorant used in textile dying. The dried plant is used as an aromatic decoration or to add scent to stored goods. The leaves are eaten as a raw or cooked vegetable or harvested just before the plant comes into flower, dried & powdered for use as a traditional supplement.

**Wormwood, Absinth, Armoise, Arttemisia, Chiu In Chen, Green Ginger, Inchinki, Injin, Kawara Yomogi, Kyunchinho, Rumput Roma, Shih Yin Chen**
**Botanical Name:** Artemisia absinthium

**Properties:** Abortifacient, Analgesic, Antibacterial, Anti-inflammatory, Antiseptic, Antispasmodic, Astringent, Cancer, Carminative, Cholagogue, Depurative, Digestive, Emmenagogue, Febrifuge, Hypnotic, Hypoglycemic, Insect Repellant, Nervine, Vermifuge

**Traditional Use:** Wormwood has been used as a traditional topical preparation to reduce the likelihood of infection while reducing inflammation and speeding healing of wounds.

**Part Used:** Flower, Leaf, Stem

**Side Effects:** Wormwood is not recommended for use by women who are pregnant or nursing.

Wormwood may lower blood sugar.

Wormwood may slow heart rate.

Wormwood is not recommended for long-term use. Long-term use of Wormwood can be toxic so use care when incorporating it into a pet plan.

Wormwood may cause an allergic reaction in some people.

Wormwood is considered safe as a dietary component but is considered toxic in large doses.

Wormwood may cause dizziness, headache, intestinal cramps, stomach pain, or vomiting.

Overuse of Wormwood may cause dizziness, numbness of the arms & legs, paralysis, restlessness, or death.

Wormwood should only be used under the guidance of a qualified herbalist or physician

Additional uses and side effects may exist but further research is necessary to determine the exact properties and effects of use.

**General:** Wormwood is native to Asia, Africa, and Europe but can now be found throughout the world. Hardy to zone 4, it prefers sandy to loamy soil, full to partial sun and dry to moist conditions. Wormwood is easily propagated by cuttings or root division but prefers shaded areas for optimal growth.

Wormwood is a strong pest repellant and will deter garden infestations and is sometimes incorporated into a repellant spray or lotion. Wormwood is grown as a perimeter guard and the fresh or dried flowers are used to deter insects, mice, and other vermin away from the house. The leaves are used as a seasoning and the flowers & leaves are harvested during flowering, dried, and powdered for use in traditional supplement extracts or infusions.

**Wormwood – Sweet, Absinthe, Ajenjo, Annual Mugwort, Annual Wormwood, Artemisia, Chinese Wormwood, Huang Hua Guo, Quing Hao, Sweet Annie, Sweet Wormwood**
**Botanical Name:** Artemisia annua

**Properties:** Antibacterial, Antibiotic, Antifungal, Antiparasitic, Antiviral, Sedative, Vermifuge

**Traditional Uses:** Sweet Wormwood is traditionally used in topical and supplement preparations to treat bacterial, fungal, parasitic, and viral infections.

**Parts Used:** Leaf, Flower, Stem

**Side Effects:** Sweet Wormwood is not recommended for use by women who are pregnant or nursing.

Sweet Wormwood may cause an allergic reaction in some people.

Additional uses and side effects may exist but further research is necessary to determine the exact properties and effects of use.

**General:** Sweet Wormwood is native to Asia but has naturalized throughout much of the world. The flower, leaf, and stem are used in traditional treatments.

**Yarrow – Siberian, Siberian Yarrow**
**Botanical Name:** Achillea sibirica

**Properties:** Antibacterial, Anti-inflammatory, Carminative, Diaphoretic, Emmenagogue, Tonic

**Traditional Use:**  Siberian Yarrow infusions have traditionally been used to reduce infection and speed healing in the teeth and mouth or for skin sores, ulcers, and wounds.

**Part Used:**  Flower, Leaf, Stem, Whole

**Side Effects:**  Siberian Yarrow is not recommended for use by women who are pregnant or nursing.

Additional uses and side effects may exist but further research is necessary to determine the exact properties and effects of use.

**General:**  Siberian Yarrow is native to Asia and has been naturalized other parts of the world including North America where it can be found growing in grassy meadows and dry, sunny slopes.  Hardy to zone 6, it is not particular regarding soil composition but does require full sun and dry to moist soil.  It can be propagated by seed but is more commonly propagated by spring division or cuttings.

Siberian Yarrow is harvested while in bloom and the leaves are eaten as a cooked vegetable or the whole plant is dried, and powdered for use in traditional infusions.

**Yellow Dock, Acedera, Amalvelas, Broad Leaved Dock, Curled Dock, Field Sorrel, Narrow Dock, Rumex, Sheep Sorrel, Sour Dock**
**Botanical Name:**  Rumex crispus

**Properties:**  Antibacterial, Anti-inflammatory, Antioxidant, Astringent, Cancer, Cholagogue, Depurative, Detoxification, Diuretic, Hepatic, Laxative, Tonic

**Traditional Use:**  Yellow Dock has been used as a traditional treatment for bacterial infections like e. coli, salmonella, and staphylococcus.

Yellow Dock has traditionally been used as a supplement to treat a urinary tract infection and to aid in reducing the size of bladder or kidney stones.

Yellow Dock has been used as a traditional snuff or infusion to reduce chronic or sudden inflammation of the nasal passages related to allergies and infection.

**Part Used:**  Root

**Side Effects:**  Yellow Dock is not recommended for use by women who are pregnant or nursing.

Overuse of Yellow Dock may cause potassium depletion.

Overuse of Yellow Dock may cause cramps, diarrhea, excessive urination, nausea, and skin irritation.

Overuse of Yellow Dock may irritate the mucus membranes and it should not be used by people with ulcers.

Yellow dock may cause or aggravate kidney stones in some individuals.

Yellow Dock may cause allergies in some people.

Yellow Dock may speed clotting.

Additional uses and side effects may exist but further research is necessary to determine the exact properties and effects of use.

**General:** Yellow Dock is native to Africa and Europe but has naturalized to other areas including the United States where some consider it an invasive weed. Hardy to zone 5, it is not particular regarding soil composition but does prefer full or partial sunlight and consistent moisture. It is easily propagated by seed and will self-sow readily if left alone.

The young leaves and shoots are used as a raw vegetable and the seeds have been eaten raw or cooked or ground for use as a coffee or flour alternative.

Yellow Dock root is harvested in the spring, dried, and powdered for use in traditional supplement teas and topical preparations. It is traditionally given at a rate of 15 drops of yellow dock tincture to 1-cup water taken up to 3 times daily.

**Yellow Elder, Rohi, Rohida, Rohitaka, Trumpet Bush, Yellow Bells, Yellow Trumpet**
**Botanical Name:** Tecoma stans

**Properties:** Antibacterial, Antifungal, Antimicrobial, Antioxidant, Hypoglycemic

**Traditional Uses:** Yellow Elder has traditionally been used to treat fungal & bacterial infections including e. coli, pseudomonas, and staphylococcus.

**Parts Used:** Flower, Leaf, Stem

**Side Effects:** Yellow Elder is not recommended for use by women who are pregnant or nursing.

Yellow Elder can affect blood sugar.

Additional uses and side effects may exist but further research is necessary to determine the exact properties and effects of use.

**General:** Yellow Elder is a flowering shrub related to the Trumpet Vine. It is native to Central, North, and South America but is cultivated in other parts of the world.

**Yellowhead, Yellow Starwort, Xuan Fu Hua**
**Botanical Name:** Inula britannica

**Properties:** Antibacterial, Anti-inflammatory, Cancer, Carminative, Cholagogue, Depurative, Diuretic, Expectorant, Laxative, Vulnerary

**Traditional Use:** Yellowhead has been used as a traditional topical preparation to reduce inflammation, speed healing, and prevent bacterial infections in skin sores, ulcers, and wounds.

**Part Used:**  Flower, Leaf

**Side Effects:**  Yellowhead is not recommended for use by women who are pregnant or nursing.

Additional uses and side effects may exist but further research is necessary to determine the exact properties and effects of use.

**General:**  Yellowhead is native to Asia and Europe but has been naturalized to North America. Hardy to zone 7, it is not particular regarding soil composition but does prefer full sun and moist to wet soil.  It is often cultivated in bog gardens and can be grown from seed sown out in the fall or by spring division.

The flowers and leaves are harvested during blooming, dried, and powdered for use as a traditional supplement.

## Using Natural Ingredients

The barks, flowers, leaves and roots that have been used for centuries as traditional supplements are still easily obtainable from health food stores, organic growers, and even in the wild. Many of plants used in traditional supplements are also easy to grow. Whether you have a windowsill garden or acreage waiting to be farmed, you can selectively grow, harvest, and process many of the traditional supplements successfully used for thousands of years to treat common ailments.

There are numerous ways of using plant products as supplements. You can use plant products as a drink, flavoring, culinary seasoning, aromatherapy treatment, and so forth. Nearly any supplement preparation you purchase at the store can be made from scratch using fresh plant products from sources you know you can trust to grow them without the addition of harmful chemical treatments. There are numerous natural product recipe guides available, including my Green & Natural book series that include simple recipes you can create to replace almost every supplement that you use.

The first step in making natural supplements is to know the type of supplements you need. The second step is to obtain the plant parts that you will use in the creation of the supplements. Most people quickly decide they want to create their own supplements starting at the beginning. That means growing their own plants to harvest, process, and use.

Each type of flower, herb, shrub, or tree will need a slightly different environment and handling for optimal growth. Propagation of plants is another entire subject that cannot be completely addressed here. If you are interested in propagating many types of plants using different methods, you should obtain a guide to help you along the way. Seed propagation is among the most common and cost effective ways to get a garden started so we will illustrate how easily you can cultivate your own supplement garden from seeds.

To create the perfect supplement garden for your needs, you must decide what plants you want to include. The compendium provides details about plants that have traditionally been used as supplements to address common conditions. You should compile a list of your preferred plants from the pages of the compendium.

As a starting organic grower, you will want to narrow the list to include those plants that fit within your climate and the space that you have available for growing.

You will want to consider the growth patterns of the plants you select for your supplement garden. Planning the types of plants included in the garden helps to ensure you have an adequate harvest during each season and do not need to replace exhausted plants. The two most common classifications of plants you will encounter are the annual and the perennial.

Some plants are annual plants. An annual plant is one that completes its entire life cycle in one year and then dies. Annuals usually grow quickly. When growing annuals for supplement use, you can harvest the entire plant each season. You will start the next season with a new plant. You can even harvest the seeds and process them yourself for next year.

If you live in a warmer climate, you should remember that a plant that is considered an annual in most regions might actually be a perennial in your area. You will want to confirm how the particular plants you select grow in your region before completely harvesting it in case the plant might yield more growth.

A perennial plant is a plant that continues to grow year after year. Many of the plants in the compendium are perennial plants. In some regions, perennial plants will simply continue to grow, going through slower and faster cycles of growth depending on the season. In other regions, perennial plants may enter a period of dormancy followed by a period of new growth. You will usually not want to harvest all of the parts of a perennial plant. You should take only as much as you need from the plant and leave the rest so the plant can continue to grow, regularly producing new crops for you to use.

Once you have a compiled a listing of the plants that you want to cultivate, you can obtain seedlings from a grower or purchase seeds from a reputable supplier. Most home supplement growers prefer to grow their plants from seeds.

The cost of growing a plant from seed is often much lower than the cost of purchasing seedlings or adult plants. In addition, when you grow a plant yourself, you know the exact history of the plant. You can feel confident that no chemicals were used during the growing process and that the plant you will be using as a supplement is healthy.

If you are growing from seed, you will need to gather a few items.

Seeds
Potting Medium
Coverage
Light Source

You will want to obtain containers that are safe for plant growth. There are many available growing containers. All natural, biodegradable plant starters are among the most environmentally friendly and chemical free options. These tend to be more costly than some other options and may not be worthwhile if you are keeping the mature plants indoors instead of transferring them to an outside space. There is a wide variety of seeding options available and you should select the one that will be most useful in your garden plan. The biggest consideration when selecting containers for supplement growing is to ensure that they are not made of a plastic product that can degrade and cause damage to your plants or cause the plant to ingest chemicals that will then contaminate any products you make from that plant.

The container you select should allow for water drainage. Commercially sold planting cups are usually created with a drainage feature. If you are making your own planting cups, you will want to put a few small holes in the bottom to allow excess water to drain away from the roots.

You will need to purchase pre-mixed seeding medium or harvest your own from a nutrient rich area of your yard. If you are a regular gardener, you know where the best potting soil can be found. If you are a beginner, purchasing pre-mixed organic seed starter is typically a better choice. Seeding mix should be light enough to allow for good air circulation but not so light that it creates an unsustainable rooting medium for the plants as they grow.

Fill each of your seed cups ¾ of the way full with seeding mix. Gently tap or press the soil to ensure there are no air pockets. Air pockets can cause the seed to drop too deeply into the soil and may make it difficult for young roots to find sufficient nutrients. A young root that encounters an air pocket is likely to wither and die weakening the plant.

Most seeds do best if you soak them in water for a few hours before planting. You may want to soak my seeds and filled soil cups at the same time. Make certain all of the products you will be using are well saturated with clean water.

The water that you use should be as free of chemicals as possible. If you have access to a clean stream or spring, this is an excellent place to obtain planting water. You could also collect rainwater to use in your garden. If necessary, most stores sell natural spring water.

After your seeds and soil are well moistened, you will sow the seeds. Most seeds do well with just a light covering of potting medium. A standard guide is to place the seed 3 times deeper than the size of the seed. Very tiny seeds are just barely placed into the soil while larger seeds are as much as ¼ inch into the medium.

Your seeds will need moisture protection during the early stages of development. You can purchase pre-made mini greenhouses or make a plastic tent to protect the seeds during germination and early development.

The seeds are now ready to do their job. You should place them in a warm area where they will not be disturbed. Seeds germinate at different rates so you will want to check on the seedlings often. A germinating seed requires warmth and moisture but does not need large amounts of light. Once the seedling emerges, it will require much more light.

If you are lucky enough to have a sunny area, natural light works well for most seedlings. Most indoor locations do not receive an adequate amount of light for new seedlings. You can use growing bulbs to provide light supplementation during the first weeks of seedling development. Each seedling will have varying light needs and you will want to check the exact growth requirements of the plants you have selected for your supplement garden.

A simple way to determine if your seedlings are getting enough light is to watch how they grow. Plants that are not receiving sufficient light will begin to become leggy as they search for a light source. That means they will grow tall, weak stems in an attempt to capture more light. If you notice your plants are growing tall but not thickening, chances are good that they are not receiving adequate light and you will need to add supplemental lighting.

Over the first few weeks, you will want to make sure that your seedlings stay moist but not saturated. The easiest way to keep the seedlings moist but not saturated is through bottom watering. If you have not already placed your growing cups on a tray, you will want to do so now.

The tray should have edges about as high as a cookie sheet. Pour water into the tray around the potting cups. This allows the soil to absorb the water the plant needs through the drainage holes in a cup or through the cup itself if you are using biodegradable planting cups. Watering from the top increases the likelihood of washing the seeds too deeply into the soil or damaging the newly emerged plants.

Each morning and afternoon, check the water level in the seedling tray. If too much water remains in the bottom of the pan, you will need to lessen the amount you give at each watering. If the pan becomes dry too quickly, you will either need to give more water at each watering or water more frequently. The goal is to provide enough moisture to keep the soil damp but not soggy.

If you live in a very moist climate, you may want to remove the germinating plastic once the seedlings emerge. If you live in a dry climate, are propagating during a cold month, or are growing delicate plants, you may want to leave the germinating plastic on the plants until they have developed their second set of leaves. By the time the second set of leaves has developed, the root system is typically strong enough to support the plant. If you do choose to leave the moisture retaining cover on the plants, you will need to create vents to ensure that your seedlings and potting medium are not too wet.

Once the second set of leaves have developed on your seedling it is time to begin "hardening" the plant. If you are planning to transplant the seedling outdoors, hardening is a critical step. If you are planning to maintain an indoor garden, hardening is still important but not critical to the success of your seedling.

Hardening means giving your seedlings the opportunity to become strong enough to survive natural environmental changes. A nice first step to begin hardening your plants is to open a nearby window or allow a fan to blow close to but not directly at the plants. This gives the plants to chance to adapt to changes in airflow and temperature.

If the seedlings are going to be indoor plants, you can gradually increase the number of hours that they are exposed to the airflow.

If you will be transplanting the seedlings to an outdoor garden, you will need to adapt them to the outside conditions. Once they seem to be bearing up well to indirect air and alterations in temperature, you should take seedlings outdoors for a few hours at a time. Spend a week or two gradually increasing the amount of time the plants stay outdoors. Once they are spending most of the day outside and any chance of extremely cold temperatures or severe storms have passed, you can transplant the seedlings to their permanent home.

Select the strongest seedlings to transplant. Some people pull out the hardier seedlings for transplanting and give the less hardy seedlings a bit more time to strengthen while others simply discard the weaker seedlings. Both methods have their positive points so you should do what works best for your ultimate growing plans.

Before you plant your seedling, you will want to pinch off the lowest set or sets of leaves. These nodes will grow roots once the plant is placed in the deeper soil of the permanent planting location.

You will pre-dig the holes for your seedlings whether you are planting them indoors or out. The hole should be deep enough to cover the bottom nodes you exposed when pinched the lower leaves. This deep planting will create a stronger plant and compensate for any legginess the plants developed reaching for light as seedlings.

176

You will want to ensure that the transplant soil is free of chemicals, weeds, and other contaminants. You will also want to use the best potting soil for your seedlings. A good mixture is 1 part vermiculate, 1 part perlite and 1 part potting mix.

If you have planted the seedlings in biodegradable grow cups, you will likely pull out all of the weaker plants and place the grow cup in your prepared location.

If you have planted the seedlings in a home made grow cup, you will need to turn the cup to release the seedling for transplant. You should use care to not to tug on the stems or leaves when removing the plant from the cup. Pulling on the plant during transplant will harm the delicate structures that the plant needs to survive. You might need to use a knife or spoon to help release the plant and lever it out of the cup.

You might notice the roots of the seedling are tightly bound in the shape of the planting cup. If the roots are tightly bound, you may want to loosen them before placing the plant into its permanent location. You can take your finger and gently tug the roots loose the same way you would untangle long hair. You can also take a clean pair of gardening scissors and make a straight cut on the four sides of the root ball by beginning at the bottom and working toward your seedling. This process helps to agitate the roots and encourages new growth. It also helps to spread the roots so that they grow outward from the plant, penetrating the soil in every direction. Penetration in all directions helps to give your plant the highest potential for gathering nutrients and water from the surrounding soil.

After you have worked the roots, place the selected seedling into the prepared hole and backfill with the potting mixture you have selected. You will want to pat the soil around the plant to remove any air pockets. You may want to mulch around outdoor plants to help them retain moisture and discourage weed growth.

Water the soil around the plants at least once a day for the first couple of weeks. The amount of water necessary will vary depending on the location, climate, type of plant, and soil conditions. The plants should stay moist but not soggy during the first weeks outdoors. Watering the soil instead of the plant helps prevent damage to the seedling. Think of it as a method similar to the bottom watering you completed on your newly emerged seedlings.

**Harvesting & Drying Herbs**

One of the biggest questions about homegrown plants is when to harvest. Many plants can be harvested at the beginning of the flowering season, though some are better in the middle or end of the season. Each entry gives a general idea on appropriate harvest times for a particular plant.

In general, if you are harvesting for the leaves or buds, you should harvest the plant before it blooms. If you are harvesting for the flowers & petals, you should harvest the plant in the middle of the growing season. If you are seeking seeds or roots, harvest them after the blooms have died off.

If you observe your plants, you should be able to begin to recognize the peak time for harvesting. Like a ripe tomato, all plant parts have a point where they are perfect for harvesting. This peak point is when the beneficial compounds are at the highest concentration.

The time of day you harvest can change the success of the supplement you are making. Some plants are at their richest early in the morning while others become richer as the warmth and moisture of the day give them the strength they need.

You will want to observe the specific type of plant you are harvesting to determine what time of day might be the peak time for that plant. The default time to harvest when you are not sure is mid-morning. This is the time after the dew has evaporated but before the plants begin to wilt from the heat of the day.

You will decide how to harvest based on the type of plant, method of drying you plan, and ultimate use of the plants.

If you are primarily interested in only the flowers & leaves of the plant, you can pluck these off the mother plant and allow the remainder to continue growing in the hopes of getting another harvest later in the season. If the plant is an annual or you need the roots, you will harvest the whole plant. If the plant is a perennial, you should use care not to over harvest since this increases the risk of killing the plant.

Once you have harvested the plant parts you will use, you should clean them. If you have purchased plants from another grower, you will want to make certain any chemicals used during the growing process are cleaned off your plant parts. Even if you grow the plants yourself, you will want to wash the plants to remove any bugs, eggs, soil, and other contaminants that might have gotten in with your plants.

You can pat the plants dry with a clean, soft cloth or simply shake the excess water off the plant and allow them to finish drip-drying while you prepare whatever next step you will take with your plants.

One of the most common methods of using plants as supplements is as a dried product that will be made into teas, infusions, decoctions, or other products. The purpose of drying your plant products is to remove the fluids, preserve the beneficial compounds and extend the useful life of the plant parts.

There is some confusion related to using fresh or dried plant parts when making products like extracts, oil infusions, and other supplements. All fresh plant products will contain some amount of water. The type of plant part you are using will dictate how much of the part is fluid and how much is plant. The presence of water will dilute the potency when you make supplements like an extract or tincture. You can use fresh plant parts but most people find they attain a higher efficiency and need less storage room when they dry the plant matter before processing it into various supplements.

There are many ways to dry plant parts. Each of them has benefits and drawbacks. The three basic methods that are most often used for drying plants are air-drying, speed drying, and hang drying.

## Air Drying Plants

Air-drying is exactly how it sounds. You will expose the parts of the plant to the air to allow the moisture to evaporate. A few plants do well when air and sun are combined during the process but most should be kept out of direct sunlight since it can evaporate or damage the beneficial compounds you are trying to obtain.

Air-drying is the slowest method of drying plant products but it often allows the plant parts to retain more beneficial compounds.

Before starting the air-drying process, you should decide where you are going to dry the plants. If the weather is just right, you may be able to dry the plants outside away from direct sunlight and the elements. More often, you will want to select an area inside the home where the plant will not be disturbed during drying.

The biggest consideration is that the area you select must be very dry. Plants will not dry properly in a space with high humidity.

The second consideration is that the area should not get extreme air movement from nature, fans, door closures, people, or another source. As the plant parts dry, they will become light. A good breeze will scatter the plants and ruin the project.

You should also consider the container you will use to dry your plants. There are many different types of air-drying racks available for purchase. Many of these allow you to stack the plants for drying. These are very convenient and some are even pretty. Depending on the amount of air-drying you will do, purchasing drying racks can become costly. If you want to keep costs low or will only be drying plants occasionally, you can make your own drying bins. A simple rack can be made by layering a clean cotton towel or waxed paper inside a shallow cookie sheet or even a cardboard box. Whatever bins you choose must not be able to absorb the compounds from your plant, must not contaminate the plant, must allow you to dry the plant parts in one layer not a pile, and must be durable enough to withstand the turning or agitation of the plant parts.

Once you have selected the container for your drying processes, you will need to finish preparing the plant parts.

The cleaned, dried herbs will need to be broken down into smaller pieces. It is often beneficial to break the plants into smaller pieces prior to drying. This not only saves you time later, it speeds the drying process since smaller parts give more air exposure and thus a faster drying process. You can pull the leaves, flowers, and stems apart with your hands or use a pair of clean shears to achieve the right size.

Place the plant pieces into the prepared container in one thin layer. This helps ensure more plant parts are exposed to the air. The more parts exposed to the air, the faster the plant materials will dry. The faster the plant materials dry, the less likely they are to develop mold growth.

Different plants will dry at different rates. You will want to agitate or turn your plant parts at least one time each day. The more moisture you have in the air or in the plant, the more frequently you will want to turn the mixture. The goal with agitating the plant parts is to ensure that everything dries evenly and quickly.

It is important that the plants dry as quickly as possible. If you enter a very humid period during the drying process, you may need to place the drying containers in the oven to help prevent excess moisture build up and mold growth.


## Oven Assisted Plant Drying

You can speed dry the plant parts in the oven. This is not one of my favorite methods because you run the risk of cooking the plant parts instead of simply drying them. There are times when oven drying may be the only logical solution like when a high humidity day hits in the middle of the drying process. It may be a better choice to risk cooking the herbs rather than risk losing the entire batch to mold.

If you choose to use the oven assist drying method, you need to make certain your oven is clean and free of chemicals. Any chemicals in the oven may pollute your plant products.

You should turn the oven on to its lowest setting and leave the door open to its first 'notch' or about 4 inches. This helps to allow air into the drying process and to keep the oven from becoming too warm.

You will need to array your plant parts as thinly as possible on the drying mat. A perforated oven-safe tray works best for oven assist drying. If you do not have an oven-safe tray, you can layer clean cotton or paper towels across the oven racks. Place the plant products onto the chosen holder.

The herbs will dry very quickly in the oven so you should check them every couple of minutes to ensure they do not over dry or 'cook'. The amount of time you will need to dry the plants will depend on the type of plant product you are using, the amount of moisture remaining in the plants, the humidity in the air, and other factors.

When you check the plants you will want to agitate them like you would during air-drying. This will help the plant parts to dry more evenly. If you are using a soft cloth and can safely pick up the drying tray, just bouncing the plant parts a few times may be a sufficient method of agitation. If you are using a solid rack, turn the herbs every few minutes.

## Speed Drying Herbs

Food dehydrators have completely changed the way some people dry their herbs. A dehydrator follows the same basic concept as air-drying it just does the job much more quickly. The dehydrator forces warm, dry air around the plant parts. This helps to remove the moisture from the plants more quickly and actually makes a more pleasing final product for some plant parts like oily fruit rinds, wood bark, and nuts.

The dehydrator must have a fan and allow you to set the heat setting extremely low or else you will cook your plants just as you would in an overheated oven. If the dehydrator you are using has a recommendation in the manual for drying herbs, you should start with those instructions and then adapt the settings to suit your particular needs. If there are no recommendations, start the process with the temperature on the lowest setting, usually around 90°, and gradually increase the temperature if you feel the plants are drying too slowly.

You will spread the plant parts onto the dehydrator trays in a single layer. You should make your layer loose so there is plenty of room for airflow to reach all sides of the plants.

The dehydrator will complete the drying process much more quickly than air-drying. You should check the plants every 15 – 20 minutes. At each check, you may want to rotate the trays. The plant parts closest to the heat source will dry more quickly and rotating the trays helps to distribute the airflow & heat. You should remove the plant parts as they become dry enough for use.

## Hang Drying Plants

Hang Drying is an easy way to dry plants that works well if you have plenty of space and a controlled room where you can hang the plants. Hang drying also helps to produce a stronger final product when you are going to be using only the flowers & leaves.

You will want to be certain there are no contaminants in the room for the plants to absorb during drying and that the air is very low in humidity. I use hang drying in the winter months since heating the house often serves a dual purpose of removing humidity from the air. Drying herbs in a closed house also helps to brighten and freshen the house naturally.

When you harvest for hang drying, you will leave longer stems on the plants. The stems will be used for the hanging. Cut each plant as close to the same length as you can.

Gather the ends of the stems together. You can use a pasta measure to judge how much you have gathered clumping about 1 serving worth per hanging group. If you make the hanging group too large, it will take longer to dry and you risk ruining the batch if the air cannot reach the middle plants.

Tie the gathered stems into a bouquet about 2 inches from the ends using natural string or jute. You will want to tie the stems tightly enough that they do not fall out of the clump but not so tightly that you break the stem. Leave an extra length of string to hook the clump to your hanger.

The stems will shrink as they dry so you may want to check the bundle occasionally to ensure that the tie has not loosened so much that you are losing stems.

Hang the herbs upside down with the cut stems facing toward the ceiling. This helps the compounds in the plant travel toward the leaves & flowers strengthening the final product.

Hang drying makes seed capture easy if you plan to propagate a new batch of plants. Place a bin, paper bag, or cardboard box underneath the hanging plant. The bin will capture any plant parts or seeds that fall off when the plant becomes dry enough to release them.

The amount of time necessary for hang drying will depend on the temperature of the area, humidity in the air, moisture in the plant, density of the plant, and other factors. You should check the plants regularly to see if they are ready for storage.

## Storing Dried Herbs

Each plant product will dry at a different rate and you should check often to see if any of the matter is ready for use or storage. You will become adept at judging the progress of the drying by sight. You should be able to see & feel a gradual reduction in the moisture of the plant parts.

Select a leaf or flower and hold it between your thumb and forefinger. Gently rub your fingers back and forth. The leaf or flower will break into tiny pieces without much effort. It should not powder. If the plant parts powder as soon as you touch them, they are too dry. Over-drying the plant parts diminishes the power of the active compounds.

At times, you will be drying flower buds or berries. These will appear different when dry from a leaf or flower petal. Select a berry or flower bud and look at it closely. It should look and feel like a hardened raisin. When it feels like a hardened raisin, it is ready for storage or use.

Stems and twigs dry differently than other plant parts. Select a stem or twig that appears to be dry and try to snap it into smaller pieces. Fully dried stems & twigs will snap easily much like a piece of uncooked spaghetti.

Seeds and nuts can be dried and broken to check their readiness for storage. Select a nut or seed and place it on a hard surface like a cutting board and then attempt to crush it with a kitchen mallet, the bottom of a ceramic cup, or the side of your shears. Nuts & seeds should break into a powder that does not clump easily. If the powder is still clumping, there are likely too many oils in the nut or seed and you should allow them to dry further before storage. If the powder is fine and easily sifted, the seeds or nuts are ready to be ground into flour for storage or use or stored whole until you are ready for them.

If you are still not certain your plant parts are ready for storage, you can select a small amount of the plant and place it in a clean, dry glass jar. Seal the lid tightly and place the jar in a warm, sunny location. If moisture condenses inside the jar over the first few hours, the plant is not ready for storage. If no moisture appears, the plant part is dry enough for storage.

You should store your newly dried plant product in a way that will not allow moisture or contaminants to permeate back into the dried goods. Some people use special stainless steel storage cans while others make "bags" from waxed paper. Porcelain, ceramic, and glass are other common choices.   You should choose whatever storage method works best in your household.  You do need to select a storage container that blocks moisture, light, and chemical contaminants.

Most correctly dried pant parts will retain many of their beneficial compounds for 1 year after the harvesting and storage date.

## Freezing Plants

Sometimes, plant parts need to be harvested at a time that is not conducive to drying or the parts just do not dry properly.  When this happens, another option is to freeze the plants.

Some people make freezing their primary method of storage for all of their harvests.  If you do not have a dry room, live in a moist climate, or are unable to air dry the plant parts for another reason, freezing may be an alternative for you.   You should remember that freezing is not technically a drying method and a great deal of the moisture will remain in the plant parts making any supplement made from freeze-dried plants weaker than their traditionally dried counterparts do.

Freezing is actually a simpler method of storing.  You will harvest and clean the plant parts the same way that you do in any storage process.  After the excess water has been removed, strip the leaves, petals, and any other plant parts you plan to save.  Place the usable pieces in the freezer storage container you have selected.  The faster you freeze the parts the better, so a deep freezer or the quick freeze shelf in some side-by-side freezers is a good choice.  The plant parts should be good for use for 3-4 months.

## Delivery Mediums

### Herbal Tea & Infusions

Once you have dried your plant parts, you will want to decide how to use them. Teas and infusions are two of the most common methods of using dried supplements. Making a natural tea or infusion allows you to obtain the benefits of the plant compounds while enjoying a variety of flavor sensations.

Infusions are not just for ingesting. You can use an infusion in the bath, in creams or lotions, as a wash, for cleaning, or for almost any other activity that can benefit from the compounds contained in the plants and can support a liquid medium.

An infusion is made using the soft plant parts. These are parts like the flower or leaf.

You will need to decide the source of the water you will use to make your tea or infusion. Filtered water, spring water, and rainwater are all good choices. The primary concern with water is to ensure it has as few contaminates as possible.

You will want to choose a teapot or kettle for heating water that is not going to degrade and release chemicals into the final product. Glass, stainless steel, and ceramic are all common choices.

Warm the water to boiling in the kettle and then remove it from the heat.

You will want to get a tea ball to contain your plant parts or tea strainer to help you remove the plant parts from the finished drink.

Tea balls tend to keep the plant parts together and leave far fewer 'clumps' in the finished drink but they also tend to compress the plant parts and make releasing the beneficial compounds more difficult.

Tea strainers allow the plant parts to move freely in the water, releasing more of their compounds but also tend to allow small plant parts to escape into the finished drink.

Either option works well and the one you choose will be based on your personal preference and needs.

You will choose the plant or combination of plants that provide the benefits you want from a supplement. These will vary greatly between people. You can even add a base tea just for the flavor! Regardless of the type of plants you are using, you will need between ¾ and 1 teaspoon of dried plant product per cup of liquid.

If you have not crumbled the plant parts before, you will want to break them into smaller pieces now. Smaller pieces gives the water more access to the plant parts and helps the compounds to release more easily.

You can add the dried pieces directly to your kettle as long as it has been removed from the heat source or place them in a cup and pour the water from the kettle on top.

Placing the herbs into the kettle, whether loose or in the tea ball, helps to prevent the oils from evaporating during steeping but also leaves residue inside the kettle that may interfere with the next supplement you make if you do not clean the kettle well after each use.

Pouring the water over the leaves in the cup allows more of the beneficial compounds to escape into the air but helps to prevent cross contamination between supplement usages since cups will usually be easier to wash than a kettle.

Either method of getting plant parts into contact with the water works and you should choose the option that suits you the best.

Allow the leaves to steep in the water for between 5 minutes and 6 hours depending on the supplement you are trying to create. A traditional tea is not as strong as an infusion and often an ingested supplement will be weaker than a topical preparation.

Once your drink is steeped to your desired strength, remove the plant parts from the liquid, flavor to taste, and enjoy.


### Cold Infusion

Many plants release their compounds best to warm water. Occasionally you may want to use a plant that does not release as well to heat. Some plants that are high in mucilage content or bitter compounds seem to do better when the compounds are infused in cold fluid. These are often referenced as digestive in descriptions.

A cold infusion is made by soaking the selected plant parts in room temperature or cooler liquid instead of hot water. You do not need to limit yourself to water. Some cold infusions are made with milk, juices, or another preferred liquid.

You will use the same proportions of plant parts and liquid as you do for a hot infusion. You will prepare the plant parts following the same processes. You will even consume the cold infusion the same way you do a hot infusion. The two major differences when making a cold Infusion are that you will use cold water, milk, or another liquid instead of hot and you will allow the plant parts to steep for a longer period than you do with a warm infusion.


### Decoction

A decoction is made with plant parts that are simmered in water. A decoction is usually used to extract the compounds from tougher plant parts like barks, roots, seeds, and wood. These plant parts are tougher than leaves or flowers and tend to require more heat to release the beneficial compounds.

The amount of plant product to water will vary depending on the plant you are using and the desired results. An average is 3 teaspoons of dried plant pieces for each 1 cup of water. You will want to adjust this ratio to suit the plant parts you are using and the results you need.

Tougher plant parts should be chopped finer when you begin. It is common to grate or powder decoction components before adding them to the water.

185

When making a decoction, you will simmer the plant parts instead of adding the plants to the water once it is already hot. This helps to force the tougher plants to release their compounds.

Add the plant parts and water to your simmering pot. A glass, stainless steel, or ceramic pot works well. You should place a lid on the pot to help prevent more loss of active compounds than necessary.

Simmer the decoction, keeping the heat just below a boil. The amount of time you will simmer the plant parts depends on a variety of factors including the plant's toughness and the strength you want from the finished product. Your goal is to reduce the fluids in the mixture. A traditional decoction is complete when the water has been reduced by ½. In other words, if you start with 1 cup of water, you will finish with ½ cup.

Strain the plant parts from the fluid as soon as you remove the mixture from the heat. Some decoctions may separate when cooled. Straining the plant parts while the mixture is hot allows you to retain the compounds. You may want to wear gloves and squeeze the excess fluids from the plant parts to reduce loss.

Since decoctions tend to be stronger than infusions because of the evaporation of some of the liquids, you will use less at a time. You can store extra liquids from your decoction in the refrigerator, often for 2-3 days depending on the plants that you have selected. You will want to store the decoction in a safe container like a stainless steel or glass bottle. Allow the mixture to cool before storage.

Shake or stir the decoction before each use. This ensures that any compounds that have separated are re-distributed.

### Syrup

A decoction or infusion can sometimes be bitter or more liquid in nature than the treatment requires so it is a common practice to make it into syrup. Syrups are especially useful when dosing will be by the teaspoon or tablespoon instead of by the cup. Making an infusion or decoction into syrup may also help to extend the shelf life.

The amount of sweetener product like Agave, sugar, or honey used to make syrup will vary depending on the personal preference of the user.

Traditional syrup is made using about 8 ounces of herbal fluid to 4 ounces of liquid honey, sweetener, or sugar. This amount will vary depending on personal preference and type of sweetener being used.

Heat the sweetener you have selected until it becomes liquefied. Remove the sweetener from the heat and add the plant infusion, powder, or decoction. Blend the ingredients well.

You may want to alter the mixture depending on the eventual use of the syrup. The thicker the syrup the better it "sticks". An example of a time when you want syrup to adhere well is if the syrup will be used as a treatment for a sore throat.

When you have attained the consistency you want, pour the finished syrup into a sterile, dark container. Refrigerating the syrup will help to extend the shelf life further. You can also add a natural preservative if you wish but research any preservatives carefully because some may interfere with or even destroy the beneficial compounds of the syrup. Typical syrup will keep usable for between 8 to 16 weeks.

## Electuary

The terms electuaries and syrups are used interchangeably by some people but are actually two different products. An electuary is a paste made of powdered plant products mixed with a base.

Powdered plant products are traditionally mixed with sweeteners like syrup, honey, berry jam or sugar and water. The powders and base are blended to make a paste. A paste is thicker than syrup.

The plant products used to make an electuary should be powdered as finely as possible. A coffee grinder, food processor, or mortar and pestle all work well for powdering dried plant parts.

The composition of an electuary can be as basic as one part powdered plant product mixed with two parts honey and as complex as dozens of types of plant product mixed with multiple sweetening agents and carriers. Honey is a good choice as a base for many people since it can actually help to extend the usable life of the finished product. The powdered plants that are used will depend entirely on the supplement you need. You can use as few or many plant powders and you want when making an electuary.

You will want to vary the balances of powder to carrier agent to suit your needs. Some powders are heavier and will require more carriers while others are lighter, and will need less. Common electuaries can range from 1 part powder to 3 parts carrier to 1 part powder to ½-part carrier.

When you have all of your components measured, heat the carrier or base slightly and blend in the powdered herbs. Store an unused electuary in a sterile, glass or metal container with a tight fitting lid.

## Extracts

An extract is a product made by separating the active compounds of a plant into a condensed state. Extraction is traditionally accomplished using a solvent, expressing the compounds, or reducing a decoction to a thickened state.

### Alcohol Extract or Tincture

An extract or tincture is made using plant parts and a solvent. Common solvents are grain alcohol, vodka, or wine. A simple explanation of the differences between extracts and tinctures is that an extract is traditionally made using 1 part plant matter to 1 part liquid while a tincture is made using 1 part plant matter to 3, 4, or even 5 parts liquid.

Alcohol extracts require three basic ingredients. You will need a glass or ceramic jar with a tightly fitting lid, a solvent like alcohol, and the desired plant products.

You will harvest and clean the plant parts according to the standard harvesting practices. Cut the plant parts into finely chopped pieces. You can use a blender or food processor to chop the plant parts. Make certain you do not grind them into such fine pieces you cannot strain the plant parts from the liquid when your extract is complete.

Place the plant parts into the jar. Fill the jar with the selected alcohol, making certain all of the plant parts are covered.

There are commercially and traditionally established ratios of alcohol, water, and plant materials for each type of plant you might process. You can refer to specific entries for the particular plant product or to commercial preparation standards to determine what is best for the particular plant you are extracting. In general, the higher the oil contents of the plant material, the higher the alcohol necessary to extract the beneficial compounds.

Once the jar is filled, seal the jar. Shake the jar to agitate the materials and to ensure that as much of the plant product is in contact with the alcohol as possible. Place the jar in a cool, dark place where it will not be disturbed. Every morning and night, shake the jar to agitate the mixture and distribute the plant parts in the alcohol.

The amount of time you will need to make an extract depends on the type of plant materials you are using. Soft leaves and petals yield more quickly than hard seeds & barks. Most extracts take between 2 and 8 weeks.

The final content of the alcohol extract should be approximately 25% alcohol. This helps to inhibit bacterial and fungal growth. Bacteria and fungus will still grow in an alcohol tincture but this ratio helps to slow the process.

When the extract has reached the strength you want, strain the plant products out of the liquid. You will want to squeeze all of the fluid out of the plant materials.

Alcohol extracts and tinctures should be stored away from light.

You can use a preservative to extend the shelf life of your tincture though it is not necessary. Some plant parts are natural preservatives.

Finished alcohol extracts or tinctures should be stored in dark glass containers to prevent the loss of active compounds. A finished alcohol extract will keep for as much as 3 years.


### Expressed Extract

You can make an expressed extract by pressing the juice out of certain types of plant parts. Not all plants can be juiced. If you are working with a plant part that can be juiced, you will express the liquid using a plant press, juicer, or simply by squeezing the applicable part.

Some juices can be used as a remedy in their own right. You will want to save every usable part of the plants you buy, grow, or harvest.

Typical extract treatments would use the plant part that is left after the excess juices are expressed. You will apply the plant parts to the affected area or prepare it according to the supplement instructions for ingestion.

## Simmer Extract

Some extracts are made through simmering. Much like a decoction, you will simmer the plant parts to condense the beneficial compounds down to their most potent form. Extracts can be made using oil, alcohol, vinegar, or water. You will follow the same steps as you do when making a decoction but you will reduce the fluid to ¼ or less of its original liquid volume. In other words, if you start with 1 cup of fluid, you will finish when you have ¼ cup or less of fluid.

## Infusion Flavoring

Sometimes the flavor of liquids like vinegar, oils, and alcohol can be enhanced by the addition of plant parts. Infusion flavorings provide not only the flavor and aroma but also the compounds of the plant parts selected for the process.

## Alcohol Infusion

Flavored alcohol has become very popular in recent years. You can make your own flavored, custom blends at home and add beneficial compounds customized to your specific wants & needs.

You can make flavored alcohol infusions using the same barks, flowers, fruits & leaves that you use to make your other products. Many available recipes include popular flavor combinations. You can use these if you just want to make flavored cocktails. Since this is all about obtaining the benefits of plant products, you may want to experiment with your own custom blends that not only taste great but also provide the healthy supplemental benefits that suit your personal situation.

You can make an alcohol infusion out of almost any liquor but most people prefer vodka. Vodka has a neutral flavor that can easily be changed through plant infusions. Rum, gin, whiskey, almost any alcohol you prefer will take flavor from a plant infusion. Select the alcohol that suits your preferences.

The biggest difference in this type of infusion is that fresh flowers, fruits, leaves, and other parts work better than the dried variety when making a flavored infusion. You will clean the plant parts you have selected. You should remove any damaged or spoiled pieces. You will also want to remove and discard any plant parts you do not want in your final product. For example, if you are using berries as part of your mixture, you may want to remove any leaves and stems attached to the berry. These will have different properties and give the final infusion a different taste.

You will need to chop or grind the plant parts. The finer you chop the plant parts, the better the flavor will infuse. Unless you are using the plant parts as a dressing, you will not want to chop them so fine that they are difficult to remove from the finished product.

The amount of plant parts to alcohol you are using, the exact plant parts you select, and the flavor you want from your finished product all influence the ratio of plant to alcohol you will use. A good guideline is ½ part plant parts to 1 part alcohol. You can adjust this as you become more familiar with the flavors of the plant parts you select.

Since this instructional is not dealing with very specific ingredients but rather generalities of processes, it is impossible to predict exactly what the balance will be for your particular recipe. Some plant products like juicy fruits yield flavor more quickly than some tougher plant products like nuts. You may need more or less alcohol to extract the flavor depending on exactly what you are using and how you want your drink to taste.

When you feel the mix you have created is likely to yield the strength and flavor you desire, seal the infusion jar with a tight fitting lid and place it in a warm area of your home. Some people find that the flavor infuses more quickly when the jar is placed in a sunny location. This may lower the beneficial effects of the plant compound but since flavored alcohol is as much about taste as it is about benefits, you may want to consider using sunlight as a tool. A more pure method of infusing is to keep light away from the mixture to help protect as many of the beneficial compounds as possible.

No matter what plant products you are using as a flavoring, you will want to keep a close taste watch on your infusion. The flavor is going to be custom suited to your tastes and needs so sample a few drops of the infusion every couple of days. When the flavor mix reaches your preference, the infusion is done. If the flavor mix becomes too strong, you can always dilute it with extra alcohol.

After your flavor has reached its peak, you will strain the plant parts from the alcohol base. A coffee filter, cheesecloth, or fine kitchen strainer all work well for removing plant parts.

Store the liquid in a clean, airtight container and enjoy. Just remember that you have transferred the active compounds of the plant parts into your alcohol and read the maximum daily limits and potential side effects before using your new product.


### Vinegar Infusion
Many people enjoy the flavor and aroma of a custom vinegar blend. Flavored vinegars are made following the same processes as flavored alcohol. You simply replace the alcohol with vinegar.

There are two important considerations regarding infused vinegar that you should remember. The vinegar will contain the compounds of the plants used during the process. Most people tend to use vinegar more freely in the family diet than they do alcohol. You should always review the potential effects, good and bad, of any plant materials before adding them to your diet. The infused vinegar will also be prone to the same type of spoilage as any other vinegar product.


### OILS
Oil extracts, oil flavorings, and essential oils are very different products. Each of them can be made at home but they do require slightly different processes. The processes for aromatic,

supplement, and flavored oils are similar to making other supplements & flavorings. The differences between one method of extraction and the next is the strength of the finished product.

## Cold Oil Infusion

An oil infusion is used to extract the oil soluble compounds in plant parts for use as a flavoring, aroma element, and supplement product.

You can infuse oil using the same processes you would use for alcohol and vinegar flavorings. You will harvest, clean, and prepare the plant parts you want in your oil according to the standard harvest instructions. Many people find that dried plant parts work better in oil infusions than fresh plant parts. Dried plant parts have had most of the water removed from the plant and may blend with oils better than fresh plants.

You should select the oils that work best for your personal situation and your taste preference. Olive oil is the most commonly selected flavored oil base but other oils work equally well. If you will be using your oil as a supplement instead of a flavoring, you will want to modify the oil selection accordingly. If you are planning to use the finished product in a topical treatment, jojoba oil is a nice choice. You should spend some time considering the uses you plan for your finished product and research the best oils for your purposes.

When making the oil infusion, follow the alcohol infusion instructions but replace the alcohol with oil. Just like with any infusion, it is important to remember that the oil will contain the active compounds of the plant parts you selected. Make certain you use oil according to the correct daily dosing limits and consider the potential effects of the plant parts before serving the oil product to others.

## Sun Oil Bath

One of the most common methods of extracting essential oils from a plant is to use an oil bath. You will select the plant materials to be used. Chop them into fine pieces. Place the chopped materials in a glass jar. Add a carrier oil with a long shelf life like jojoba until the plant matter is completely covered. Seal the jar and place it in the sun.

Direct sunlight may heat the oils too much so you should select an area that receives diffused sunlight. Windowsills are the most commonly chosen location. Allow the oil bath to heat throughout the day. Shake the jar each night to speed the process.

Continue to allow the oil bath to extract the essence until you feel that no further progress is being made. Strain the plant materials out of the oils. The resulting oil will not be as strong as the oils you obtain through distillation or solvent extraction.

You can re-infuse the oils to make them stronger. Simply repeat the process using the same oils as you did during the first sunbath but use fresh plant products. Each time you repeat the process with the same oil, the resulting product will be stronger.

The stronger the oil becomes, the higher the likelihood of a reaction. You should make sure you protect your skin from the oils and plant parts to minimize the likelihood of irritation and have a comprehensive understanding of the maximum dosage and effects of any plants you used in your bath.

## Using Infused Oils

Infused oils are frequently used in culinary and supplemental preparations. Infused oils are also used to make lotions, creams, and other topical preparations. You can find a variety of natural product recipes for the hair, lips, nails and skin. The infused oils you have made using the appropriate plant parts can be used in replacement for the liquid in your selected recipe.

There are two important considerations regarding infused oils you should remember. The oils will contain the compounds of the plants used during the process. You should always review the potential effects, good and bad, of any plant materials before adding them to your diet or personal care products. You should also remember that products made with infused oils will be prone to the same type of spoilage as any other oil product.

## Essential Oils

An essential oil is much stronger than infused oil. When you make an infusion, you are diluting the compounds with the alcohol, vinegar, or oil base. When making an essential oil, you are capturing the concentrated plant essences in their pure form and not diluting the results.

Essential oils are most frequently used for topical and aromatherapy treatments. Essential oils are often very powerful and should not be applied directly to the skin. Essential oils must be diluted before use.

The method of extraction you use to garner essential oils will depend on the specific plant, ultimate use, and desired strength of the oil.

## Distillation

The most common method of commercial essential oil extraction is by distillation. Distillation uses water to help extract the oils. There are different methods of distillation. You can purchase a distillation unit for personal use, make your own distillation unit using a pressure cooker and tubing, or you can use one of the more common home methods of extraction like solvents.

## Steam Distillation

Steam distillation uses a source of steam piped into the distillation unit at a high pressure. The steam passes through the plant material and exits into a condenser unit. The product in the condenser unit is the plant essence or essential oil.

Steam distillation units can be purchased or you can make your own steam distillation unit from a pressure cooker, tubing, and capture jar. These unites are somewhat complex and you will want to review commercial distillation units and homemade distillation unit creation instructions before attempting to make a unit of your own.

## Hydro-Distillation

Hydro-distillation is extraction accomplished by covering plant materials in water. You can envision it as being similar to making a soup. The water is heated to produce a steam that contains the plant essence. The steam is captured and used in therapeutics. This method works well for tougher materials like nuts, wood, and roots.

Hydro-distillation units are similar to standard steam distillation units and can be purchased for in home use. There are also many instructions available free on the internet that tell you how to make your own hydro-distillation unit.

## Tray Distillation

Tray distillation is much like the process you would use to steam vegetables for food. The plant material is placed into a sieve like pan. The sieve is then placed over another pan filled with water. A tightly fitting lid with a tube leading out of it is placed on top. The water is boiled so the steam passes through the plant material. The steam extracts the oils from the plant and carries it upward to the tube. The tube captures the concentrated liquid and pipes it to a holding unit. This method of distillation works best for soft plant materials. These units are also available for purchase or can be made following some simple instructions available free through an internet search.

## Simmer Extraction

You can simmer extract compounds from plant products. This method of extraction does use more heat and runs the danger of destroying the very compounds you want to protect, but it is a quick and simple method of extracting essential oils at home.

You will select the base oil you want to use for your simmer. The type of oil you select will depend largely on the ultimate use you will make of your essential oils. If you are using the oils in skin care, massage treatments, or other topical preparations then you will want to select oil that is compatible with your skin type. Jojoba oil is often a good choice if you are unsure of what oils will work well for you because it is similar to the body's own natural oils. If you will use your oils in aromatherapy treatments, you will want to select neutral oil that diffuses well.

Prepare your plant materials by chopping, grinding, or pounding the plant parts. Once again, the more parts of the plant you expose to the oils, the better the extraction results you will achieve.

Put the prepared plant parts in the pot you will use for heating. Some people like to use a crock-pot while others prefer to use a saucepan. Either will yield approximately the same results so the choice is a matter of personal preference.

Add enough of the selected carrier oil to cover the plant materials.

Cover the pan with a tight fitting lid.

Most people find they have better results and improve the likelihood of success if they use a water bath to heat the oils. Select a pan that is larger and deeper than the pan you have chosen for your plant & oil mixture. Fill this pan with 2-3 inches of water. Place the plant & oil pan into the water bath pan.

Heat the oil and plant mixture to a temperature between 100° and 125°. Do not overheat the oil bath because you will cook the plants instead of extracting the compounds.

Allow the mixture to simmer for 3 to 4 hours, stirring occasionally. You should take care not to reduce the oil amount when you stir the plants by allowing oils to escape. You want to minimize evaporation.

When you mixture has finished simmering, remove it from the heat source. You can strain the plant materials from the oil immediately or allow the plant & oil mixture to continue to steep. Some plants can steep for weeks and retain some active compounds while others will yield all of the available compounds during the heating process. You will need to get to know the plant materials you have selected in order to decide when you have extracted the maximum benefit from the plant. It is important to experiment to learn how the plant parts will react to different processes. Generally, the softer the plant materials, the more quickly they yield the compounds.

It is recommended that you use rubber gloves to protect your skin when working with essential oils. The stronger the essential oils, the more likely they are to cause a reaction.

Strain the oils through cheesecloth. Squeeze any remaining oil out of the plant materials. Discard the leftover plant materials.

You can repeat the process with new plant materials and the oil you gathered from the first extraction. Each repeated extraction with the same oil will increase the potency of the finished product.


## Solvent Extraction

Some plant essences cannot survive the heat distillation methods. These will require cold extraction. You can use a solvent to extract essential oils through cold methods.

Select the plant materials that contain the highest amount of active scent compounds. Chop, grind, or bruise the materials as appropriate for the types of plant parts you have selected. Place the chopped and bruised plant material on a tray with perforations. A dehydrator tray works well. Place the tray over a capture pan.

You will use a solvent like grain alcohol or hexane to extract matter from the plant. The solvent will extract everything that is dissolvable in the plant including waxes, pigments, and the aromatic oils.

You can use the solvent as a wash. To do this, you must have a capture pan that sits below the perforated plant tray. Pour the solvent over the plant materials. Remove the resulting liquid from the capture tray and pour it over the plant products again. Continue this process until the wash produces little or no new extraction.

You can also use the solvent as a bath. To do this, you must have a capture pan that allows the perforated tray to sit inside of it. Place the plant materials on the perforated tray. Sit the tray inside the capture pan. Pour the solvent over the plants until they are just covered. Allow the bath to sit, stirring occasionally. The length of time you must allow the bath to sit will depend on the plant material. Each plant material will give up the essences at a different pace. You can agitate the plant product occasionally to speed the process. When you believe that there is no longer any matter left to be extracted, remove the plant materials from the bath. Strain any remaining solid matter from the liquid.

When you have removed the solid matter, place the liquid into a container and seal it. The liquid should not completely fill the container. You should keep at least ¼ of the space in the container empty to allow for expansion.

Allow the mixture to rest for a day or two. You will note that the materials separate. You should be able to view three layers.

You will have an opaque or thick layer of impurities. This layer will either fall to the bottom of the jar or lay on the top of the mixture.

The solvent alcohol will appear neutral.

You will see a layer that contains the oil essences. This layer will not appear as polluted as the impurity layer or as clear as the alcohol layer. This is your essential oil layer.

When your layers have formed, carefully lift the jar without agitating the layers. Loosen the lid to prevent breakage as the materials expand. Place the jar in the freezer. The oils and impurities will freeze. The alcohol will not freeze.

Place the entire frozen mass on a straining board. If the materials have frozen to the jar, you can gently separate them with a stainless steel knife.

The alcohol will drain away. Capture the alcohol in another jar as it strains away. You will want to freeze the alcohol again to gather any remaining oils that did not separate during the first freeze.

If the oils and impure layer are next to each other, use a knife to separate the usable oils from the impurities. Discard the impurities.

Place the frozen mass of oils onto a cheesecloth spread over a capture bowl or jar. As the mixture thaws, the oils will strain into the bowl. Anything that remains in the cheesecloth is plant material that was missed during the first straining. This can be discarded. The oils that strain into the bowl are the essential oils. Place the finished essential oils into your final storage jars.

The alcohol that you set aside earlier should be returned to the freezer for a second time. Any oils that remain in the solvent will freeze.

When the oils have frozen, remove the jar from the freezer and strain it through cheesecloth spread over an empty capture bowl. The alcohol will drain through the cheesecloth leaving the frozen oil behind. You can discard the alcohol or save it for use in your next extraction. Do not use the alcohol to extract the oils from a different type of plant material unless you have considered the active compounds of both types of plant materials.

195

The frozen oil parts should be allowed to thaw into another jar. The cheesecloth will filter any residual plant solids that remain. Add the captured oils to the essential oil jar you created during the first separation.

Store the essential oils in a cool, dark area for maximum shelf life.

### Cold Pressing

Cold pressing works well for citrus peels and other plant parts whose oils can be released by scoring the plant product. You will score the plant, press the body and capture the oils being released.

## External Use of Plant Products

Many plant products are used in traditional topical preparations. There are numerous ways of using plant products in external preparations. You can use plant products in cleaners, washes, ointments, salves, creams, poultices, lotions and so forth. Almost any topical preparation you purchase at the store can be made from scratch using natural ingredients.

There are numerous natural product recipe guides available, including my Green & Natural book series that include simple recipes that you can create to replace almost every product you use. You can also create your own custom topical preparations using the plants detailed in the compendium.

The following explanations will help you to gain a fundamental picture of some of the most common topical preparations and the steps necessary to create them yourself.

## Fomentation & Compress

A fomentation is the external use of strong herbal infusions.

If you are using soft plant parts, you will follow the infusion instructions but allow the plant parts to steep for a longer period than you would when creating a drinkable infusion.

If you are using hard plant parts, you will follow the instructions from making a decoction but reduce the fluid to 1/3 or even ¼ of the original fluid amount.

Once the infusion or decoction has reached the desired strength, you will soak a clean cloth in the liquid. Cotton and wool are common fabric choices for fomentations. The saturated cloth is then applied to the affected part.

You should use most fomentations while they are still hot. In general, you want the fomentation to be as hot as can be handled. When the cloth cools, saturate it in the fluid again and reapply it to the affected area. You may want to use two cloths. One is applied while the other is soaking in the hot liquid.

Most fomentations can be wrapped in clean plastic and an elastic bandage to help retain the heat and to keep moisture from getting all over everything nearby. The clean plastic should be on the outside of the fomentation, not the area that will touch your body.

You will continue to apply the fomentation according to the instructions of the plant parts you are using and condition you are treating. The time usage of a fomentation could range from less than an hour to a couple of days. Gently re-heat the fomentation when it becomes too cool to use.

Some conditions do not lend themselves to heat. If the patient, condition, or other reason makes hot heat undesirable, the fluid can be used as a cool compress. You will follow the same instructions as you would when making a fomentation, but you will allow the mixture to cool before applying it to the skin. When the compress becomes too warm, you will exchange it for a fresh, cool cloth.

## Poultice

A poultice is made by chopping, bruising, or grating plant parts into smaller parts and applying them directly to an injured, inflamed, or problem area. The size of the plant parts used will vary depending on the instructions relating to the specific plant, malady, and treatment.

Some poultices are made by cutting the plant so that the internal parts are exposed and applying the product directly to the skin. An example of this type of poultice is the use of an aloe leaf to sooth a burn.

Other poultice recommendations require you to nearly powder the plant parts and mix the product with a small amount of water to form a paste.

The method of application will depend on the plant product and condition you are trying to alleviate.

Some poultices are hot preparations. A hot poultice is most often used to increase blood flow, alleviate pain, reduce inflammation, and relax muscles.

Hot poultices can be made by adding hot water to the ground plant parts to form a paste and applying the paste to the affected area.

A few plant parts should be directly heated before applying them to the area to be treated. You should use caution when heating plant parts because overheating can destroy beneficial compounds.

The most common method of making a hot poultice is to layer the plant parts on the area to be treated and then cover the area with a moist, hot cloth. This application method helps to increase the heat and lengthen the time of the treatment. The cloth is moistened and heated, usually using the microwave or the steam from a pan of boiling water. The cloth is exchanged for a warm one as it cools.

Some poultices are cold preparations. Cold poultices are traditionally used to draw heat or toxins from an area, reduce congestion, and as a counter to hot poultices in cases of painful inflammation. Common uses of a cold poultice are in treating skin sores, ulcers, wounds, and skin conditions like eczema.

When creating a cold poultice, you will wet the plant parts with room temperature to icy cold fluid as indicated by the plant parts being used and condition being treated. The cold compress is then applied directly to the area being treated.

Poultices occasionally call for a plant part that is irritating to the skin. If the necessary plant parts include skin irritants, you should use a thin layer of cloth between the skin and the poultice. This will not allow for concentrated absorption of beneficial compounds but it will protect the skin from damage while still providing some benefit.

It is important to remember that using plant parts as a topical preparation still delivers the compounds of the plant into the body. The skin is the largest organ in the body and it readily absorbs compounds that are placed into direct contact with it. You can overuse a poultice.

## Ointment
An ointment is made by blending powdered plant parts, plant decoctions, plant extracts, or plant oils into a base. Ointments generally contain oils, thickeners, hardeners, and plant parts. Ointments do not usually contain water.

When making ointments you will need a base, the preferred plant parts, and sterile containers. You may also choose to use a thickening agent, hardener, and preservative depending on the type of application, storage length, and slip desired in the product.

The base or carrier can be a liquid substance like almond oil, jojoba, or Vitamin E oil or semi liquid like cocoa butter or lanolin. These carriers each have properties, benefits and side effects of their own. You will want to consider the potential effects of the carrier when making your selection.

The oily, liquid carriers are commonly used in massage lotions and for creating topical pain-relief rubs. These can be made into a thicker ointment by incorporating a thickening agent and a hardener into the recipe.

The semi-solid carriers like cocoa butter tend to be used in products meant for application in a thin layer like in skin conditioning preparations. These can still be blended with thickening agents and hardeners but it is often not necessary.

Depending on the use of your finished product, the recipe may benefit from a hardener. The need for a hardener depends on the application method you plan for your product. The most common hardeners are waxes like beeswax and paraffin wax.

Some ointments will be used very quickly and are designed to treat a short-term issue. Others may be used over a period of weeks or months. If you plan to use the ointment over a period of weeks, you will want to add a preservative. Some plants have natural preservative properties while others will require enhancement. You should review the compendium to decide what type of preservative will work best with your particular recipe.

Most ointments are oil based. You will want select the appropriate oil base for your particular need. You will also find that using powdered or oil extracted plant components makes blending the ointment easier. Water based extractions or infusions do not blend as easily and may require the additional of an emulsifier.

Use a water bath to heat any carrier oil, thickening agents and hardener you plan to incorporate into your recipe. You should not heat the plant parts because heat may destroy the beneficial components.

When the carrier oil, thickener and hardening agents are warmed to a liquid state, whip them into the plant materials you have prepared and then immediately pour the resulting mixture into a clean tub, jar, or tube.

Seal the filled container and add the appropriate label.

Depending on the exact ingredients you have used, you may need to shake the mixture before each use to re-blend the ingredients. Ointments that contain thickeners and hardeners will not need to be shaken as much as those that do not.

## Labeling

If you are only making one type of plant product, you will probably remember what is in the jar or bag, but chances are good you will not be able to stop with just one product. Once you realize how easy and satisfying making your own natural products can be, you will probably make many different products intended for many different uses, making labeling an important part of the process.

There is certain information that I find invaluable

Date Started
Plants Included
Plant parts used
Amount
Base – oils, alcohol, vinegar, etc
Amount
Date Completed – Storage Date
Expiration Date

You will want to continue to explore the many, many uses of plant products. This guide gives you a wide range of products you can make and use today. My compendium provides an in-depth look at a larger variety of traditional plants used by herbalists. Scientific and natural research is constantly being done to fine tune our knowledge of the potential of plants. There are many, many sources of plant knowledge, recipes, and product creation guides available. I hope that this guide has given you a healthy knowledge base and a basic understanding of the potential uses of the plants you see every day. Feel free to drop me a note telling me about your new discoveries, recipes you love, or just to say hi! There is nothing more satisfying than sharing my love of plants and nature with a fellow creator.

## Glossary

Abortifacient – A substance that is capable of inducing an abortion

Adoptogenic – A substance that has a normalize effect against changes brought about by stressors

Acid – A chemical that produces a pH of less than 7 in water. Having a low pH.

Adjective - Adjective dyes are those dyes that require use of a mordant to bind the color to the fiber.

Alkali – A chemical that produces a pH of more than 7. Having a high pH.

Alopecia – Baldness. The partial or complete loss of hair.

Alum (aluminum sulfate) - Alum is a naturally occurring basic mordant.

Alum (aluminum acetate) - A naturally occurring common mordant.

Amenorrhea – Absence of menstruation.

Analgesic - A pain-killing drug or medicine.

Aniline - Aniline dyes or basic dyes are a class of synthetic dyes derived from coal tar that produce brilliant colors but poor colorfastness.

Anodyne - A pain-killing drug or medicine.

Antibacterial – A substance that is active against bacteria.

Anticonvulsant – A substance used to reduce or prevent convulsions

Anti-emetic - A substance that reduces or prevents nausea or vomiting.

Antifungal – A substance that is used to alleviate or prevent fungal infections.

Antihistamine - A substance that inhibits the physiological effects of histamine. A histamine is the chemical released by the body during an allergic reaction.

Anti-Inflammatory – A substance used to reduce inflammation.

Anti-Microbial- A substance that kills or inhibits the growth of microorganisms

Anti-Oxidant – Molecule that inhibits the oxidation of other molecules.

Anti-Periodic – A substance used to treat malarial-type symptoms or to present the recurrence of malarial like symptoms.

Anti-Parasitic – A substance used to treat or prevent parasitic infestations.

Anti-Septic – A substance capable of preventing or treating infection by inhibiting the growth of microorganisms.

Anti-Spasmodic - A substance that suppresses muscle spasms.

Anti-Tussive – A substance used to suppress or relieve coughing.

Anti-Viral – A substance that prevents or treats viral infections by killing a virus or that suppresses its ability to replicate.

Aphrodisiac – A substance that stimulates sexual desire.

Aromatic – A substance having a pleasant and distinctive smell that is used as a treatment.

Aroma Therapy – Aromatic plant extracts or essential oils to cause a physical or psychological effect in treatments.

Aspergillus - A type of common molds that cause food spoilage and potentially disease.

Astringent - Substance that causes the contraction of body tissues.

Bleeding – Color rinsing out of a dyed textile.

Botanical Name – The Latin name give to a species of plant to distinguish it from other plants.

Bursitis – A condition where there is inflammation in the bursa – elbow, knee, shoulder.

Cardiac - Relating to the heart

Carminative – Substance that relieves flatulence.

Cathartic - A purgative substance.

Chalogogue - A substance that stimulates the secretion of bile from the gallbladder.

Chrome – (Potassium Dichromate) Chrome is a naturally occurring common mordant.
Citric Acid – Acid found in many plant products but most common to citrus fruits. Citric Acid is used to neutralize high pH.

Coagulant - A substance that causes blood to clot or coagulate

Colorant - Substance that colors something usually food, cosmetics, or textile products.

Colorfastness – A measure of how resistant a dye material is to fading.

Common Name – The non-specific name used for everyday reference to a plant

Comminution – The action of reducing a material or substance. When processing plants the act of reducing the size of the plant parts by cutting, grinding, or pounding

Conjunctivitis – An infection or irritation causing inflammation, itching, and redness of the white part of the eye.

COPD – Chronic Obstructive Pulmonary Disease involving constriction of the airways and difficulty breathing.

Copper (copper sulphate) – Copper is a naturally occurring mordant used to give green casts to textiles.

Copperas – Term used for iron ore (ferrous sulfate) used to depress the colors of a dye bath.

Cream of Tarter (potassium bitartrate) - A naturally occurring color modifier. Cream of Tarter is not a stand-alone mordant but acts in tandem with other mordants.

Decoction – The result of concentration the essence of a substance or plant part by heating or boiling.

Demulcent – A substance that soothes inflammation and protects irritated internal tissues.

Depurative – Substance that facilitates the removal of impurities or cleansing of bodily fluids.

Detoxification - Process of removing toxic substances or qualities from matter.

Diaphoretic – A substance that induces perspiration.

Digestive –

Diosgenin – A steroid compound used in the synthesis of steroid hormones.

Diuretic – A substance causing increased passing of urine.

Dram – A unit of measurement equaling approximately 1/16 of a dry weight ounce in

US measurement 1/8 of a fluid ounce in Apothecary measurement.

Dye – Color-bearing organic compounds that penetrate fiber or other matter.

Dyebath – A solution of colorant and water used to color textiles.

Dyestuff – Any raw material that releases dye.

Dysmenorrheal – Menstruation with excessive pain involving abdominal and lower back cramping.

Emetic - Substance that causes vomiting.

Emmenagogue – Substance that stimulates or increases menstrual flow.

Emollient – Substance that has a softening or soothing affect on the skin.

Estrogenic – A substance acting like, relating to, or caused by estrogen.

Expectorant – A substance that promotes the secretion of mucus from the air passages.

Expression - The process of forcibly separating liquids from solids.

Febrifuge – Substance used to reduce fever.

Fluid extract – A type of fluid-solid substance obtained from plant matter through water or alcohol processing

Fugitive Color – Color that is prone to fading when exposed to sunlight or washing.

Galactogogue - Substance that stimulates milk secretion.

Glycosides – A compound formed from a simple sugar and another compound by the replacement of a hydroxyl in the sugar molecule.

Gram-Positive Bacteria – A class of bacterial that are stained dark blue or violet by gram staining including bacteria such as pneumococci, staphylococci, and streptococci.

Gram Negative Bacteria - A class of bacterial that do not retain the stain used in gram staining including bacteria such as e. coli, shingella, salmonella.

Hallucinogenic – A psychoactive substance capable of producing hallucinations or altered sensory experiences.

Hepatic - Of or relating to the liver.

Hydration - The process of combining with or giving water.

Hypoallergenic – A substance unlikely to cause an allergic reaction.

Hypoglycemic – A condition indicated by low blood sugar.

Hypotensive – A condition of abnormally low blood pressure.

Histamine - The chemical released by the body during an allergic reaction.

Immunostimulant - Substance that stimulate the immune system to fight infection.

Infusion – Aqueous – A drink or extract made by soaking plant parts in water.

Infusion – Oil – A drink, extract, or product made by soaking plant parts in oil.

Insecticide - Substance used for killing insects.

Interferon - A protein released in response to a virus that has the ability to inhibit virus reproduction.

Iron Ore (ferrous sulfate) used to mute or darken the colors of a dye bath.

Laxative – Substance that stimulates or facilitates evacuation of the bowels

Lighfastness - A measure of a dye products resistance to fading from light exposure.

Lipase – An enzyme that facilitates the breakdown of fats to fatty acids and glycol to other alcohols.

Lye (sodium hydroxide) – A caustic substance used to shift pH.

Maceration – Softening plant materials by soaking or steeping in a liquid. To separate the compounds by soaking or steeping

Menorrhagia – Abnormally heavy menstrual bleeding.

Menstruum - A solvent or mix of solvents.

Microphage – A cell found in the tissues or at the site of an infection that takes in foreign material.

Mordant – A substance that combines with a dye or stain to fix the colorant into a material.

Muscle Relaxant – A substance that reduces muscle tone or contractibility.

Narcotic – A psychoactive substance affecting mood or behavior.

Natural Dye – Dye derived from animal, mineral, or plant matter.

Natural Fiber – A fiber obtained from an animal, mineral, or plant source.

Nervine – A psychoactive substance that calms the nerves.

Nutritive – Substance that providing nourishment. Nutritious.

Over Dye – The act of placing one dye over another to alter the finished tone.

Percolation - The extraction of soluble components by passing the liquid through a filtering medium.

pH – A scale for measuring the acidity or alkalinity of a substance. A pH of 7 is neutral. Low pH is acidic. High pH is alkaline.

Pharynx – The membrane lined cavity behind the nose and mouth that connects them to the esophagus.

Phytoestrogen - Compounds found in plants that can mimic the effects of estrogen.

Pleurae – The membranes lining the thorax and enveloping the lungs.

Pleurisy – An inflammation of the pleurae that causes pain when breathing.

Polysaccharide – A carbohydrate that is a compound of sugar molecules bonded together.

Proof Spirit – A mixture of alcohol and water containing 50% alcohol by volume standard in the US.

Purgative – A substance that is strongly laxative in effect.

Pulmonary – Relating to the pulmonary system.

Phytosterol – A group of naturally occurring steroid plant compounds.

Reactive Dye – A class of synthetic dyes that are used to dye natural fibers that traditionally resist taking color.

Reparative – A substance that helps to repair.

Rhinitis – Inflammation of the mucus membrane of the nose.

Rubefacient – A substance whose external application produces increased circulation or redness of the skin.

Saponins – A class of steroid and terpenoid glycosides that are used in detergents and foam when shaken with water.

Sciatica – Nerve pain caused by compression of a spinal nerve in the lower back that affects the back, hip, or leg.

Sedative – Substance that causes a calming or sleep-inducing effect.

Squalene – An oily liquid that is the precursor to sterols.

Sterols – Naturally occurring unsaturated steroid alcohols.

Steroidal - Relating to steroid hormones or their effects.

Stimulant – A substance that raises levels of physiological or nervous activity in the body.

Styptic – A substance that causes bleeding to stop.

Substantive Dyes – Dyes that produce lasting color without the use of a mordant.

Succus – The juice several liquids in the body commonly termed digestive juices but also the juice of fresh plant material.

Sudorific – Relating to or causing sweating.

Tannin – A naturally occurring component of some plant products used as a mordant. It aids some dyes in being self-mordanting and shifts colors to a browner tone.

Tin (stannous chloride) - A metallic salt used as a brightening mordant.

Tincture – A substance made by dissolving plant materials in alcohol.

Vasodilator – Substance that causes dilation of blood vessels.

Vermifuge – Substance that destroys parasites.

Viscosity – The resistance of a liquid to movement and flow.

Washfastness - A measure of how resistant a dye product is to fading over time due to exposure to water or soap.

# References

Full reference list from a compendium of beneficial herbs and oils.
Personal observations, experimentations, and family notes Laurie Pippen

A. Abdul Rahuman, Geetha Gopalakrishnan, P. Venkatesan and Kannappan Geetha (2008). "Isolation and identification of mosquito larvicidal compound from Abutilon indicum (Linn.) Sweet". Parasitology Research 102

A. Ngan & R. Conduit (2011). "A double-blind, placebo-controlled investigation of the effects of Passiflora incarnata (passionflower) herbal tea on subjective sleep quality". Phytotherapy Research 25

Abbott, I. A. (1996). Ethnobotany of seaweeds: clues to uses of seaweeds. Hydrobiologia.

Adhami, VM; Aziz, MH; Mukhtar, H; Ahmad, N (2003). "Activation of prodeath Bcl-2 family proteins and mitochondrial apoptosis pathway by sanguinarine in immortalized human HaCaT keratinocytes". Clinical cancer research 9

Agrawal, K. (1992). Biochemical pharmacology of blood and bloodforming organs. Berlin: Springer-Verlag.

Agarwal R, Gupta SK, Agrawal SS, Srivastava S, Saxena R (2008). "Oculohypotensive effects of foeniculum vulgare in experimental models of glaucoma". Indian J. Physiol. Pharmacol. 52

Ahmad, Nihal; Gupta, Sanjay; Husain, Mirza M.; Heiskanen, Kaisa M.; Mukhtar, Hasan (2000). "Differential Antiproliferative and Apoptotic Response of Sanguinarine for Cancer Cells versus Normal Cells". Clinical Cancer Research 6

Aiyer HS, Kichambare S, Gupta RC 2008. Prevention of oxidative DNA damage by bioactive berry components. Nutritional Cancer. 60

Ajai K. Chemical composition of the essential oil from fresh leaves of Melaleuca leucadendron L. from north India. Journal of Essential Oil-Bearing Plants. CABI Abstracts.

Akatsuka, I. (1990). Introduction to applied phycology. The Hague: SPB Academic Pub. bv.

Akihisa, Toshihiro; Higo, Naoki; Tokuda, Harukuni; Ukiya, Motohiko; Akazawa, Hiroyuki; Tochigi, Yuichi; Kimura, Yumiko; Suzuki, Takashi et al. (2007). "Cucurbitane-type triterpenoids from the fruits of Momordica charantia and their cancer chemopreventive effects". Journal of Natural Products 70

Allaby, M. (1998). A dictionary of plant sciences (2nd ed.). New York: Oxford University Press.

Allahverdiyev, A; Duran, N; Ozguven, M; Koltas, S (2004). "Antiviral activity of the volatile oils of L. Against virus type-2". Phytomedicine 11

Almajano, M. Pilar; Carbó, Rosa; Jiménez, J. Angel López; Gordon, Michael H. (2008). "Antioxidant and antimicrobial activities of tea infusions". Food Chemistry 108

Amer A. Repellency effect of forty-one essential oils against Aedes, American Chemical Society.Biology of Plants 2005

Anderson T, Foght J (2001). "Weight loss and delayed gastric emptying following a South American herbal preparation in overweight patients". J Hum Nutr Diet 14

Anopheles and Culex mosquitos. Parasitol Res. 2006

American Journal of Botany. (n.d.) from http://www.amjbot.org

American Journal of Clinical Nutrition. (n.d.). Retrieved June 19, 2014, from http://ajcn.nutrition.org/content/by/year

Andrade, G; E Esteban, L Velasco, MJ Lorite, EJ Bedmar (1997). "Isolation and identification of N2-fixing microorganisms from the rhizosphere of Capparis spinosa (L.).". Plant and Soil (Kluwer Academic Publishers) 197

Angier, B. (1978). Field guide to medicinal wild plants. Harrisburg, Pa.: Stackpole Books.

"Antimicrobial activity of Calendula officinalis petal extracts against fungi, as well as Gram-negative and Gram-positive clinical pathogens". Complement Ther Clin Pract 18

Aphrodisiac activity of methanol extract of leaves of Passiflora incarnata Linn. in mice". Phytotherapy Research 17

Appa Rao MVR; Srinivas K, Koteshwar Rao T. "The effect of Mandookaparni (Centella asiatica) on the general mental ability (medhya) of mentally retarded children". J. Res Indian Med. 1973

Arrigoni-Blank Mde F , Oliveira RL , Mendes SS , et al. Seed germination, phenology, and antiedematogenic activity of Peperomia pellucida (L.) H. B. K. BMC Pharmacol . 2002

Aronson, J. (2009). Meyler's side effects of herbal medicines. Amsterdam: Elsevier. Auf'mkolk, M.; Ingbar, J. C.; Kubota, K.; Amir, S. M.; Ingbar, S. H. (1985). "Extracts and Auto-Oxidized Constituents of Certain Plants Inhibit the Receptor-Binding and the Biological Activity of Graves' Immunoglobulins". Endocrinology 116

Austin, DF (2004). Florida Ethnobotany. Boca Raton, FL: CRC Press.

Australian journal of herbal medicine. (n.d.). Concord West, N.S.W.: National Herbalists Association of Australia.

Avadhani, Mythili et al.; The Sweetness and Bitterness of Sweet Flag [Acorus calamus L.] – A Review; Research Journal of Pharmaceutical, Biological and Chemical Sciences, Volume 4, Issue 2

Awad, Rosalie; Muhammad, Asim; Durst, Tony; Trudeau, Vance L.; Arnason, John T. (2009). "Bioassay-guided fractionation of lemon balm (Melissa officinalisL.) using anin vitromeasure of GABA transaminase activity". Phytotherapy Research 23

Aziba PI , Adedeji A , Ekor M , Adeyemi O (2001). "Analgesic activity of Peperomia pellucida aerial parts in mice". Fitoterapia 72

Babykutty, S.; Padikkala, J.; Sathiadevan, P. P.; Vijayakurup, V.; Azis, T. K.; Srinivas, P.; Gopala, S. (2008). "Apoptosis induction of Centella asiatica on human breast cancer cells". African journal of traditional, complementary, and alternative medicines : AJTCAM / African Networks on Ethnomedicines 6

Badar, VA; Thawani, VR; Wakode, PT; Shrivastava, MP; Gharpure, KJ; Hingorani, LL; Khiyani, RM (2005). "Efficacy of Tinospora cordifolia in allergic rhinitis". Journal of Ethnopharmacology 96

Bailey DG, Dresser GK (2004). "Interactions between grapefruit juice and cardiovascular drugs". Am J Cardiovasc Drugs

Bailey, L.H.; Bailey, E.Z.; the staff of the Liberty Hyde Bailey Hortorium. 1976. Hortus third: A concise dictionary of plants cultivated in the United States and Canada. Macmillan, New York.

Balakumbahan, R.; K. Rajamani and K. Kumanan (29 December 2010). Acorus calamus. Journal of Medicinal Plants Research 4 (25): 2740–2745. Retrieved 14 May 2011.

Barnard, Edward S. & Yates, Sharon Fass, ed. (1998). "Trees". Reader's Digest North American Wildlife: Trees and Nonflowering Plants. The Reader's Digest Association, Inc.

Barnes, J., & Anderson, L. (2002). Herbal medicines: A guide for healthcare professionals. (2nd ed.). London: Pharmaceutical Press.

Bakshi N., Kumar P., Sharma M. "Antidermatophytic activity of some alkaloids from Solanum dulcamara." Indian Drugs. 45

Barton, DL; Soori, GS; Bauer, BA; Sloan, JA; Johnson, PA; Figueras, C; Duane, S; Mattar, B et al. (2010). "Pilot study of Panax quinquefolius (American ginseng) to improve cancer-related fatigue: a randomized, double-blind, dose-finding evaluation: NCCTG trial N03CA.". Supportive care in cancer : official journal of the Multinational Association of Supportive Care in Cancer 18

Bastos JF. Moreira IJ. Ribeiro TP. Medeiros IA. Antonioli AR. De Sousa DP. Santos MR. Hypotensive and vasorelaxant effects of citronellol, a monoterpene alcohol, in rats. Basic & Clinical Pharmacology & Toxicology. 106. 2010

Bayma JD , Arruda MS , Müller AH , Arruda AC , Canto WC . A dimeric ArC 2 compound from Peperomia pellucida . Phytochemistry . 2000

Beal, J. (1981). Natural products as medicinal agents: Plenary lectures of the International Research Congress on Medicinal Plant Research, Strasbourg, July 1980. Stuttgart: Hippokrates Verlag.

Bean, W. J. (1970). Trees and Shrubs Hardy in the British Isles. John Murray, London.

Beloin, N.; Gbeassor, M.; Akpagana, K.; Hudson, J.; De Soussa, K.; Koumaglo, K.; Arnason, J. T. (2005). "Ethnomedicinal uses of Momordica charantia (Cucurbitaceae) in Togo and relation to its phytochemistry and biological activity". Journal of Ethnopharmacology 96

Benedek B., Geisz N., Jäger W., Thalhammer T., Kopp B. Choleretic effects of yarrow (Achillea millefolium s.l.) in the isolated perfused rat liver. Phytomedicine 2006

Benedek, Birgit; Kopp, Brigitte (2007). "Achillea millefolium L. S.l. Revisited: Recent findings confirm the traditional use". Wiener Medizinische Wochenschrift 157

Bensky. Clavey. Stoger. (2004). Gamble Chinese Herbal Medicine

Bensky, Dan; Andrew Gamble, Steven Clavey, Erich Stöger (2004). Chinese Herbal Medicine: Materia Medica, 3rd Edition. Eastland Press.

Bent S, Kane C, Shinohara K, et al (February 2006). "Saw palmetto for benign prostatic hyperplasia". N. Engl. J. Med. 354

Blevi, V., & Sween, G. (1993). Aromatherapy. New York: Avon Books.

Balchin, M. (2006). Aromatherapy Science: A guide for healthcare professionals. London [u.a.: Pharmaceutical Press.

Bhatnagar M. Sisodia SS. Antisecretory and antiulcer activity of Asparagus racemosus Willd. against indomethacin plus phyloric ligation-induced gastric ulcer in rats. Journal of Herbal Pharmacotherapy. 6

Bialonska D, Kasimsetty SG, Khan SI, Ferreira D (11 November 2009). "Urolithins, intestinal microbial metabolites of Pomegranate ellagitannins, exhibit potent antioxidant activity in a cell-based assay". J Agric Food Chem 57

Bilušić Vundać V., Brantner A.H., Plazibat M. "Content of polyphenolic constituents and antioxidant activity of some Stachys taxa" Food Chemistry 2007 104

Blamey, M. & Grey-Wilson, C. (1989). Flora of Britain and Northern Europe. Hodder & Stoughton.

Blanco MM, Costa CA, Freire AO, Santos JG, Costa M (March 2009). "Neurobehavioral effect of essential oil of Cymbopogon citratus in mice". Phytomedicine

Bloomfield, H. (1998). Healing anxiety with herbs. New York, NY: HarperCollins.

Blumenthal, M. (2000). Herbal medicine: Expanded Commission E monographs ; herb monographs, based on those created by a Special Expert Committee of the German Federal Institute for Drugs and Medical Devices (1.st ed.). Newton, Mass.: Integrative Medicine Communications.

Boaz M, Leibovitz E, Bar Dayan Y, Wainstein J (2011). "Functional foods in the treatment of type 2 diabetes: olive leaf extract, turmeric and fenugreek, a qualitative review". Func Foods Health Dis 1

Bojo AC , Albano-Garcia E , Pocsidio GN (1994). "The antibacterial activity of Peperomia pellucida (L.) HBK (Piperaceae)". Asia Life Sci 3: 35–44.

^ Ragasa CY , Dumato M , Rideout JA (1998). "Antifungal compounds from Peperomia pellucida". ACGC Chem Res Commun 7

Bopana N. Saxena S. Asparagus racemosus--ethnopharmacological evaluation and conservation needs. [Review] [77 refs] Journal of Ethnopharmacology. 110

Böttger, Stefan; Melzig, Matthias F. (2011). "Triterpenoid saponins of the Caryophyllaceae and Illecebraceae family". Phytochemistry Letters 4

Boyer, Jeanelle; Liu, RH; Rui Hai Liu (May 2004). "Apple phytochemicals and their health benefits". Cornell University, Ithaca, New York 14853-7201 USA: Department of Food Science and Institute of Comparative and Environmental Toxicology 3

Boyle, P; Robertson, Lowe F, Roehrborn C (Apr 2004). "Updated meta analysis of clinical trials of Serenoa repens extract in the treatment of symptomatic benign prostatic hyperplasia". BJU Int 93

Bradley (1992). British Herbal Compendium 1. Bournemouth, England: British Herbal Medicine Association.

Bradwejn, J.; Zhou, Y.; Koszycki, D.; Shlik, J. (2000). "A double-blind, placebo-controlled study on the effects of Gotu Kola (Centella asiatica) on acoustic startle response in healthy subjects". Journal of clinical psychopharmacology 20

Bramati, Lorenzo; Minoggio, Markus; Gardana, Claudio; Simonetti, Paolo; Mauri, Pierluigi; Pietta, Piergiorgio (2002). "Quantitative Characterization of Flavonoid Compounds in Rooibos Tea (Aspalathus linearis) by LC–UV/DAD". Journal of Agricultural and Food Chemistry 50

Braun, L., & Cohen, M. (2006). Herbs and Natural Supplements Inkling an Evidence-Based Guide. London: Elsevier Health Sciences APAC.

Bremness, L. (1988). The complete book of herbs. New York: Viking Studio Books.

Bressler R (2006). "Grapefruit juice and drug interactions. Exploring mechanisms of this interaction and potential toxicity for certain drugs". Geriatrics 61

Brickell, C. (1994). The Royal Horticultural Society gardeners' encyclopedia of plants and flowers (Rev. ed.). London: Dorling Kindersley.

Brinkhause, B., Lindner, M., et al., "Chemical, Pharmacological and Clinical Profile of The East Asian Medical Plant 2000

British pharmacopoeia 1975. (1975). London: H.M.S.O.

British pharmacopoeia 2013. (2013). London: H.M.S.O.

Brown, D. (1996). Aromatherapy. Lincolnwood, Ill.: NTC Pub.

Brunke, E. (1986). Progress in essential oil research: Proceedings of the International Symposium on Essential Oils, Holzminden/Neuhaus, Federal Republic of Germany, September 18-21, 1985. Berlin: W. de Gruyter.

Bui LT, Nguyen DT, Ambrose PJ (2006). "Blood pressure and heart rate effects following a single dose of bitter orange". The Annals of Pharmacotherapy 40

Burdette JE, Liu J, Chen SN, Fabricant DS, Piersen CE, Barker EL, Pezzuto JM, Mesecar A, Van Breemen RB, Farnsworth NR, Bolton JL (2003). "Black cohosh acts as a mixed competitive ligand and partial agonist of the serotonin receptor". J. Agric. Food Chem. 51

Burk D.R., Cichacz Z.A., Daskalova S.M. Aqueous extract of Achillea millefolium L. (Asteraceae) inflorescences suppresses lipopolysaccharide-induced inflammatory responses in RAW 264.7 murine macrophages. Journal of Medicinal Plant Research 2010

Caceres, A. "Plants used in Guatemala for the treatment of gastrointestinal disorders. 1. Screening of 84 plants against enterobacteria." J. Ethnopharmacol. 1990

Canning S, Waterman M, Orsi N, Ayres J, Simpson N, Dye L (March 2010). "The efficacy of Hypericum perforatum (St John's wort) for the treatment of premenstrual syndrome: a randomized, double-blind, placebo-controlled trial". CNS Drugs 24

Carson, C. F.; Hammer, K. A.; Riley, T. V. (2006). "Melaleuca alternifolia (Tea Tree) Oil: a Review of Antimicrobial and Other Medicinal Properties". Clinical Microbiology Reviews 19

Cassileth, B. (1998). The alternative medicine handbook: The complete reference guide to alternative and complementary therapies. New York: W.W. Norton.

Castleman, M., & Hendler, S. (1991). The healing herbs: The ultimate guide to the curative power of nature's medicines. Emmaus, Pa.: Rodale Press.

Castner, J., & Timme, S. (1998). A field guide to medicinal and useful plants of the Upper Amazon. Gainesville, FL: Feline Press.

Castro, M. (1991). The complete homeopathy handbook: A guide to everyday health care. New York: St. Martin's Press.

Cataldo, A., Gasbarro, V., et al., "Effectiveness of the Combination of Alpha Tocopherol, Rutin, Melilotus, and Centella asiatica in The Treatment of Patients With Chronic Venous Insufficiency", Minerva Cardioangiology, 2001

Ceccarelli N., Curadi M., Picciarelli P., Martelloni L., Sbrana C., Giovannetti M. "Globe artichoke as a functional food" Mediterranean Journal of Nutrition and Metabolism 2010

Cecchini C, Cresci A, Coman MM, et al. (June 2007). "Antimicrobial activity of seven hypericum entities from central Italy". Planta Med. 73

Cerda JJ, Robbins FL, Burgin CW, Baumgartner TG, Rice RW (September 1988). "The effects of grapefruit pectin on patients at risk for coronary heart disease without altering diet or lifestyle". Clin Cardiol 11

Chaiyana W., Okonogi S."Inhibition of cholinesterase by essential oil from food plant". Phytomedicine. 2012.

Chan A, Graves V, Shea TB, A For prevention of dementia: (2006). Journal of Alzheimer's Disease 9

Chan E (1993). "Displacement of bilirubin from albumin by berberine". Biology of the Neonate 63

Chan, E.W.C. et al. (2009). "Effects of different drying methods on the antioxidant properties of leaves and tea of ginger species". Food Chemistry 113

Chan Y.-S., Cheng L.-N., Wu J.-H., Chan E., Kwan Y.-W., Lee S.M.-Y., Leung G.P.-H., Yu P.H.-F., Chan S.-W.,"A review of the pharmacological effects of Arctium lappa (burdock)" [Article in Press] Inflammopharmacology 2010

Chen, G, Sun, W-B, & Sun, H. (2007). Ploidy variation in Buddleja L. (Buddlejaceae) in the Sino - Himalaya region and its biogeographical implications. Botanical Journal of the Linnean Society. 2007

Chen R., Liu Z., Zhao J., Chen R., Meng F., Zhang M., Ge W. "Antioxidant and immunobiological activity of water-soluble polysaccharide fractions purified from Acanthopanax senticosu" Food Chemistry 2011

Chevallier, A. (1996). The encyclopedia of medicinal plants. New York: DK Pub.

Chevallier, A. (2000). Natural health encyclopedia of herbal medicine (2nd American ed.). New York: DK Pub.

Cheung SC, Szeto YT, Benzie IF (March 2007). "Antioxidant protection of edible oils". Plant Foods Hum Nutr 62

Chiang, Y. M.; Lo, C. P.; Chen, Y. P.; Wang, S. Y.; Yang, N. S.; Kuo, Y. H.; Shyur, L. F. (2005). "Ethyl caffeate suppresses NF-κB activation and its downstream inflammatory mediators, iNOS, COX-2, and PGE2in vitroor in mouse skin". British Journal of Pharmacology 146

Chidrawar, VR; Patel, KN; Sheth, NR; Shiromwar, SS; Trivedi, P (2011). "Antiobesity effect of Stellaria media against drug induced obesity in Swiss albino mice". Ayu 32

Chiej, R. (1984). The Macdonald encyclopedia of medicinal plants. London: Macdonald.

Chinese Materia Medica (1998). Beijing University of Traditional Chinese Medicine

Chittenden, F. (1951) RHS Dictionary of Plants plus Supplement. Oxford University Press.

Chopra, R. (1956). Glossary of Indian medicinal plants,. New Delhi: Council of Scientific & Industrial Research.

Chopra, R., & Chopra, R. (1969). Supplement to glossary of Indian medicinal plants. New Delhi: Publications and Information Directorate.

Chopra, R. (1992). Second supplement to Glossary of Indian medicinal plants with active principles. New Delhi: Publications & Information Directorate, CSIR.

Chopra, R. N.; Nayar, S. L.; Chopra, I. C. Glossary of Indian Medicinal Plants. 1986. New Delhi: Council of Scientific and Industrial Research.

Choudhary M.I., Jalil S., Todorova M., Trendafilova A., Mikhova B., Duddeck H. Inhibitory effect of lactone fractions and individual components from three species of the Achillea millefolium complex of Bulgarian origin on the human neutrophils respiratory burst activity. Natural Product Research 2007

Chui C.H., Gambari R., Lau F.Y., Teo I.T.N., Ho K.P., Cheng G.Y.M., Ke B., Higa T., Kok H.L., Chan A.S.C., Tang J.C.O."Anti-cancer potential of traditional Chinese herbal medicines and microbial fermentation products." Minerva Biotecnologica. 17. 2005.

Clarke, D. L. (1988). W. J. Bean Trees and Shrubs Hardy in the British Isles, Supplement. John Murray

Clement, Charles R.; de Cristo-Araújo, Michelly; d'Eeckenbrugge, Geo Coppens; Alves Pereira, Alessandro; Picanço-Rodrigues, Doriane (6 January 2010). "Origin and Domestication of Native Amazonian Crops". Diversity 2

Compendium of medicinal plants. (2004). Delhi, India: National Institute of Industrial Research.

Commission E monographs. (1998). American Botanical Council.

Committee on Comparative Toxicity of Naturally Occurring Carcinogens, Board on Environmental Studies and Toxicology, Commission on Life Sciences, and National Research Council (1996). Carcinogens and anticarcinogens in the human diet: a comparison of naturally occurring and synthetic substances. National Academy Press, Washington, D.C.

Conti B., Canale A., Bertoli A., Gozzini F., Pistelli L. Essential oil composition and larvicidal activity of six Mediterranean aromatic plants against the mosquito Aedes albopictus (Diptera: Culicidae). Parasitology Research 2010

Coombes, A. (1985). Dictionary of plant names. Portland, Or.: Timber Press.

Coon JT, Ernst E. Andrographis paniculata: a systematic review of safety and efficacy, Planta, 2004

Coon, J. (1977). The dictionary of useful plants. Emmaus: Roodale Press.

Culpepers British Herbal - Pub. William Nicholson and Son - C. 1905 (re-print of the 1653 original)

Cummings, D., & Holmes, A. (n.d.). The medicinal gardening handbook: A complete guide to growing, harvesting, and using healing herbs.

Dasanayake, Ananda P.; Silverman, Amanda J.; Warnakulasuriya, Saman (2010). "Maté drinking and oral and oro-pharyngeal cancer: A systematic review and meta-analysis". Oral Oncology 46

Davidson, A. (1999). The Oxford companion to food. Oxford: Oxford University Press.

Davis & Company Parke (1909). Manual of therapeutics. Parke, Davis & Co.

Davydov M, Krikorian AD. (October 2000). "Eleutherococcus senticosus (Rupr. & Maxim.) Maxim. (Araliaceae) as an adaptogen: a closer look". Journal of Ethnopharmacology 72

de Mesquita, M., et al. "Cytotoxic activity of Brazilian Cerrado plants used in traditional medicine against cancer cell lines." J Ethnopharmacol. 2009

de Lourdes Arruzazabala, M.; Molina, V.; Más, R.; Carbajal, D.; Marrero, D.; González, V.; Rodriguez, E. (2007). "Effects of coconut oil on testosterone-induced prostatic hyperplasia in Sprague-Dawley rats". Journal of Pharmacy and Pharmacology 59

Dedhia RC, McVary KT (June 2008). "Phytotherapy for lower urinary tract symptoms secondary to benign prostatic hyperplasia". J. Urol. 179 (6): 2119–2125.

Dekosky, S. T.; Williamson, J. D.; Fitzpatrick, A. L.; Kronmal, R. A.; Ives, D. G.; Saxton, J. A.; Lopez, O. L.; Burke, G. et al. (2008). "Ginkgo biloba for Prevention of Dementia: A Randomized Controlled Trial". Journal of the American Medical Association 300

Devi, P. U.; Ganasoundari, A. (March 1999). "Modulation of glutathione and antioxidant enzymes by Ocimum sanctum and its role in protection against radiation injury". Indian Journal of Experimental Biology 37

Dew, Tristan P.; Day, Andrea J.; Morgan, Michael R. A. (2005). "Xanthine Oxidase Activity in Vitro: Effects of Food Extracts and Components". Journal of Agricultural and Food Chemistry 53

Dhama, K., & Dhama, S. (1994). Homoeopathy: The complete handbook. New Delhi: UBS ' Distributors. Complete Homeopathy Handbook 1996 Castro Dictionary catalog of the National Agricultural Library, 1862-1965. (1967). New York: Rowman and Littlefield.

Djavan B, Fong YK, Chaudry A, et al. (2005). "Progression delay in men with mild symptoms of bladder outlet obstruction: a comparative study of phytotherapy and watchful waiting". World J Urol 23 (4): 253–6.

Dos, Santos-Neto, Ll; De, Vilhena, Toledo, Ma; Medeiros-Souza, P; De, Souza, Ga (December 2006). "The use of herbal medicine in Alzheimer's disease-a systematic review" (Free full text). Evidence-based complementary and alternative medicine : eCAM 3

Drugs and Supplements. (n.d.). Retrieved from http://www.mayoclinic.org/drugs-supplements

Duke, J. (1992). Handbook of edible weeds. Boca Raton: CRC Press.

Duke, J. (2000). The green pharmacy herbal handbook: Your comprehensive reference to the best herbs for healing. Emmaus, Pa.: Rodale Reach

Duke. J. A. and Ayensu. E. S. Medicinal Plants of China. Reference Publications, Inc. 1985

Dumitru, Alina F.; Shamji, Mohamed; Wagenmann, Martin; Hindersin, Simone; Scheckenbach, Kathrin; Greve, Jens; Klenzner, Thomas; Hess, Lorenzo et al. (2011). "Petasol butenoate complex (Ze 339) relieves allergic rhinitis–induced nasal obstruction more effectively than desloratadine". Journal of Allergy and Clinical Immunology 127

Ebadi, M. (2002). Pharmacodynamic basis of herbal medicine. Boca Raton, Fla.: CRC Press.

Ebadi, M., & Ebadi, M. (2008). Desk reference of clinical pharmacology (2nd ed.). Boca Raton: CRC Press.

Ebrahimi, Sedigheh; Soheil Ashkani Esfahani, Azizollah Poormahmudi. (2011). "Investigating the efficacy of Zizyphus jujuba on neonatal jaundice". Iranian Journal of Pediatrics 21

Edes, R. (1883). Therapeutic handbook of the United States pharmacopoeia: Being a condensed statement of the physiological and toxic action, medicinal value, methods of administration and doses of the drugs and preparations in the latest edition of the U.S. pharmacopoeia ... New York: William Wood and.

El Bardai S, Lyoussi B, Wibo M, Morel N (May 2001). "Pharmacological evidence of hypotensive activity of Marrubium vulgare and Foeniculum vulgare in spontaneously hypertensive rat". Clin. Exp. Hypertens. 23

Elsabagh, Sarah; Hartley, David E.; Ali, Osama; Williamson, Elizabeth M.; File, Sandra E. (2005). "Differential cognitive effects of Ginkgo biloba after acute and chronic treatment in healthy young volunteers". Psychopharmacology 179

Erichsen-Brown, Charlotte (1989). Medicinal and Other Uses of North American Plants: A Historical Survey with Special Reference to the Eastern Indian Tribes. Dover Publications

Erika Svangård, Ulf Göransson, Zozan Hocaoglu, Joachim Gullbo, Rolf Larsson,, Per Claeson and Lars Bohlin, 2004. "Cytotoxic Cyclotides from Viola tricolor" Journal of Natural Products 67

Estrogen-like activity of ginsenoside Rg1 derived from Panax notoginseng". The Journal of Clinical Endocrinology and Metabolism 87

Ettefagh K.A., Burns J.T., Junio H.A., Kaatz G.W., Cech N.B., "Goldenseal (Hydrastis canadensis L.) Extracts Synergistically Enhance the Antibacterial Activity of Berberine via Efflux Pump Inhibition", Planta Medica 2010

Evans, P. (1961). A modern herbal. San Francisco: Porpoise Bookshop.

A Modern Herbal 1931 Grieve

Ewing, G. (1971). Topics in chemical instrumentation; a volume of reprints from the Journal of chemical education. Easton, Pa.: Chemical Education Pub.

Facciola, S. (1998). Cornucopia II: A source book of edible plants. Vista, CA: Kampong Publications.

Farag RS. Chemical and biological evaluation of the essential oils of different Melaleuca species. Phytother Res. Jan2004;18(1):30-35.

Lee CK. A new norlupene from the leaves of Melaleuca leucadendron. J Nat Prod.

Farnsworth, N. R.; Draus, F. J.; Sager, R. W.; Bianculli, J. A. (2006). "Studies on Vinca major L. (Apocynaceae) I. Isolation of perivincine". Journal of the American Pharmaceutical Association 49

Fehske, Christian J.; Leuner, Kristina; Müller, Walter E. (2009). "Ginkgo biloba extract (EGb761®) influences monoaminergic neurotransmission via inhibition of NE uptake, but not MAO activity after chronic treatment". Pharmacological Research 60

Fern, K. Plants for a Future: Edible and Useful Plants for a Healthier World. Hampshire: Permanent Publications, 1997.

Fernández S, Wasowski C, Paladini AC, Marder M (2004). "Sedative and sleep-enhancing properties of linarin, a flavonoid-isolated from Valeriana officinalis". Pharmacol Biochem Behav 77

Figueirinha A. Cruz MT. Francisco V. Lopes MC. Batista MT. Anti-inflammatory activity of Cymbopogon citratus leaf infusion in lipopolysaccharide-stimulated dendritic cells: contribution of the polyphenols. Journal of Medicinal Food. 13

Figueroa A, Sanchez-Gonzalez MA, Wong A, Arjmandi BH (2012). "Watermelon extract supplementation reduces ankle blood pressure and carotid augmentation index in obese adults with prehypertension or hypertension". American journal of hypertension 25

Filip, Rosana; Lotito, Silvina B.; Ferraro, Graciela; Fraga, Cesar G. (2000). "Antioxidant activity of Ilex paraguariensis and related species". Nutrition Research 20

Foster, S., & Duke, J. (1990). A field guide to medicinal plants: Eastern and central North America. Boston: Houghton Mifflin.

Francois, G., et al. "Antimalarial and cytotoxic potential of four quassinoids from Hannoa chlorantha and Hannoa klaineana, and their structure-activity relationships." Int. J. Parasitol. 1998

Fu, P.P., Yang, Y.C., Xia, Q., Chou, M.C., Cui, Y.Y., Lin G., "Pyrrolizidine alkaloids-tumorigenic components in Chinese herbal medicines and dietary supplements", Journal of Food and Drug Analysis, Vol. 10, No. 4, 2002

Fugh-Berman, Adriane (2000). "Herb-drug interactions". The Lancet 355

Furst, Peter T. (1976). Hallucinogens and Culture. Chandler & Sharp.

Gadang, V; Gilbert, W; Hettiararchchy, N; Horax, R; Katwa, L; Devareddy, L (2011). "Dietary bitter melon seed increases peroxisome proliferator-activated receptor-γ gene expression in adipose tissue, down-regulates the nuclear factor-κB expression, and alleviates the symptoms associated with metabolic syndrome". Journal of medicinal food 14

Gadow, A.Von; Joubert; E.; Hansmann, C.F. (1997). "Comparison of the antioxidant activity of rooibos tea (Aspalathus linearis) with green, oolong and black tea". Food Chemistry 60

Gaginella, T. (1997). Biochemical pharmacology as an approach to gastrointestinal disorders: Basic science to clinical perspectives (1996) : IUPHAR GI Pharmacology Symposium. Dordrecht: Kluwer Academic.

Ganzera M, Aberham A, Stuppner H (May 2006). "Development and validation of an HPLC/UV/MS method for simultaneous determination of 18 preservatives in grapefruit seed extract". J. Agric. Food Chem. 54

Gautam M. Saha S. Bani S. Kaul A. Mishra S. Patil D. Satti NK. Suri KA. Gairola S. Suresh K. Jadhav S. Qazi GN. Patwardhan B. Immunomodulatory activity of Asparagus racemosus on systemic Th1/Th2 immunity: implications for immunoadjuvant potential. Journal of Ethnopharmacology. 121

Grae, I. (1974). Nature's colors; dyes from plants. New York: Macmillan.

Gray, A., & Sullivant, W. (1848). A manual of the botany of the northern United States from New England to Wisconsin and south to Ohio and Pennsylvania inclusive: (the mosses and liverworts by Wm. S. Sullivant,) arranged according to the natural system. Boston: J. Munroe.

Geller SE, Shulman LP, van Breemen RB, et al. (2009). "Safety and efficacy of black cohosh and red clover for the

management of vasomotor symptoms: a randomized controlled trial". Menopause (New York, N.Y.) 16

Genders R. Scented Flora of the World. Robert Hale. London. 1994

Gentry EJ, Jampani HB, Keshavarz-Shokri A, et al. (October 1998). "Antitubercular natural products: berberine from the roots of commercial Hydrastis canadensis powder. Isolation of inactive 8-oxotetrahydrothalifendine, canadine, beta-hydrastine, and two new quinic acid esters, hycandinic acid esters-1 and -2". Journal of Natural Products 61

Germplasm Resources Information Network. United States Department of Agriculture. 1997-05-22. Retrieved 2010-04-12.

Ghalayini IF, Al-Ghazo MA, Harfeil MN 2011. Prophylaxis and therapeutic effects of raspberry (Rubus idaeus) on renal stone formation in Balb/c mice. Int Braz J Urol. 37

Ghosh, P. C., et al. "Antitumor plants. IV. Constituents of Simarouba versicolor." Lloydia. 1977

Ghosh S, Sharma AK, Kumar S, Tiwari SS, Rastogi S, Srivastava S, Singh M, Kumar R, Paul S, Ray DD, Rawat AK "In vitro and in vivo efficacy of Acorus calamus extract against Rhipicephalus (Boophilus) microplus." Parasitol Res. 2011

Gião MS, Pestana D, Faria A, Guimarães JT, Pintado ME, Calhau C, Azevedo I, Malcata FX., 2010. Effects of extracts of selected medicinal plants upon hepatic oxidative stress. Journal Medicinal Food. 13

Gibbs A, Green C, Doctor VM. (1983). "Isolation and anticoagulant properties of polysaccharides of Typha Augustata and Daemonorops species". Thromb Res. 32

Gilani A.H., Bashir S., Khan A.-u."Pharmacological basis for the use of Borago officinalis in gastrointestinal, respiratory and cardiovascular disorders". Journal of Ethnopharmacology. 114

Giles M., Ulbricht C., Khalsa K.P.S., DeFranco Kirkwood C., Park C., Basch E., "Butterbur: An evidence-based systematic review by the natural standard research collaboration Journal of Herbal Pharmacotherapy 2005

God J, Tate PL, Larcom LL 2010. Red raspberries have antioxidant effects that play a minor role in the killing of stomach and colon cancer cells. Nutritional Research. 30

Godevac D, Tesević V, Vajs V, Milosavljević S, Stanković M., 2009. Antioxidant properties of raspberry seed extracts on micronuclei distribution in peripheral blood lymphocytes. Food Chem 47

Godowski, KC (1989). "Antimicrobial action of sanguinarine". The Journal of clinical dentistry 1

Golshahi H., Ghasemi E., Mehranzade E. (2011). "Antibacterial activity of Ocimum sanctum extract against E. coli, S. aureus and P. aeruginosa". Clinical Biochemistry. Conference: 12th Iranian Congress of Biochemistry, ICB and 4th International Congress of Biochemistry and Molecular Biology 44

Goodner, K.L. et al.; Mahattanatawee, K; Plotto, A; Sotomayor, J; Jordan, M (2006). "Aromatic profiles of Thymus hyemalis and Spanish T. vulgaris essential oils by GC-MS/GC-O". Industrial Crops and Products 24

Gregory PJ, Sperry M, Wilson AF (January 2008). "Dietary supplements for osteoarthritis". Am Fam Physician 77

Grieve, M. (1971). A modern herbal; the medicinal, culinary, cosmetic and economic properties, cultivation and folk-lore of herbs, grasses, fungi, shrubs, & trees with all their modern scientific uses,. New York: Dover Publications.

Griffith, J.Q.; J.F. Couch, M. A. Lindauer (1944). "Effect of Rutin on Increased Capillary Fragility". Proc Soc Exp Biol Med March 55

Grover, J. K.; Yadav, S. P. (2004). "Pharmacological actions and potential uses of Momordica charantia: A review". Journal of Ethnopharmacology 93

Grubben, G.J.H. & Denton, O.A. (2004) Plant Resources of Tropical Africa 2. Vegetables. PROTA Foundation, Wageningen; Backhuys, Leiden; CTA, Wageningen

Grujic-Jovanovic S., Skaltsa H.D., Marin P., Sokovic M. "Composition and antibacterial activity of the essential oil of six Stachys species from Serbia" Flavour and Fragrance Journal 2004 19

Gualtiero Simonetti (1990). Stanley Schuler, ed. Simon & Schuster's Guide to Herbs and Spices. Simon & Schuster, Inc.

Gualtiero Simonetti (1990). Stanley Schuler, ed. Simon & Schuster's Guide to Herbs and Spices. Simon & Schuster, Inc.

Guenther, E. (1949). The essential oils. New York: D. Van Nostrand.

Guo LY. Hung TM. Bae KH. Shin EM. Zhou HY. Hong YN. Kang SS. Kim HP. Kim YS.,"Anti-inflammatory

effects of schisandrin isolated from the fruit of Schisandra chinensis Baill." European Journal of Pharmacology. 591

Guo, R; Pittler, MH; Ernst, E (2007). "Herbal medicines for the treatment of allergic rhinitis: A systematic review". Annals of allergy, asthma & immunology : official publication of the American College of Allergy, Asthma, & Immunology 99

Gurudeeban, S.; Satyavani K., Ramanathan T. (2010). "Bitter Apple (Citrullus colocynthis): An Overview of Chemical Composition and Biomedical Potentials". Asian Journal of Plant Sciences 9

H. J. D. Dorman and S. G. Deans (2000). "Antimicrobial agents from plants: antibacterial activity of plant volatile oils". Journal of Applied Microbiology 88

H. Kohno, Y. Yasui, R. Suzuki, M. Hosokawa, K. Miyashita, T. Tanaka (2004), Dietary seed oil rich in conjugated linolenic acid from bitter melon inhibits azoxymethane-induced rat colon carcinogenesis through elevation of colonic PPAR γ expression and alteration of lipid composition. International Journal of Cancer, volume 110

Ha H.H., Park S.Y., Ko W.S., Kim Y. "Gleditsia sinensis thorns inhibit the production of NO through NF-B suppression in LPS-stimulated macrophages. Journal of Ethnopharmacology. 2008. 118

Hage-Sleiman, R; Mroueh, M; Daher, CF (2011). "Pharmacological evaluation of aqueous extract of Althaea officinalis flower grown in Lebanon". Pharmaceutical biology 49

Hager TJ, Howard LR, Liyanage R, Lay JO, Prior RL (February 2008). "Ellagitannin composition of blackberry as determined by HPLC-ESI-MS and MALDI-TOF-MS". Journal of Agricultural and Food Chemistry 56

Halvorsen BL, Carlsen MH, Phillips KM, et al. (July 2006). "Content of redox-active compounds (ie, antioxidants) in foods consumed in the United States". The American Journal of Clinical Nutrition 84

Hamamelitannin from Witch Hazel (Hamamelis virginiana) Displays Specific Cytotoxic Activity against Colon Cancer Cells. Susana Sánchez-Tena, Maria L. Fernández-Cachón, Anna Carreras, M. Luisa Mateos-Martín, Noelia Costoya, Mary P. Moyer, Maria J. Nuñez, Josep L. Torres and Marta Cascante, J. Nat. Prod.

Hammer, K; Carson, C; Riley, T; Nielsen, J (2006). "A review of the toxicity of Melaleuca alternifolia (tea tree) oil". Food and Chemical Toxicology 44

Hanelt, Peter; Büttner, R.; Mansfeld, Rudolf; Kilian, Ruth (2001). Mansfeld's Encyclopedia of Agricultural and Horticultural Crops. Springer.

Hannan JM. Marenah L. Ali L. Rokeya B. Flatt PR. Abdel-Wahab YH. Insulin secretory actions of extracts of Asparagus racemosus root in perfused pancreas, isolated islets and clonal pancreatic beta-cells. Journal of Endocrinology. 192

Harborne, J. (1996). Dictionary of plant toxins. Chichester: Wiley.

Harper, Douglas; Online Etymological Dictionary; http://www.etymonline.com/index

Harrison, Lorraine (2012). RHS Latin for gardeners. United Kingdom: Mitchell Beazley.

Haskell CF, Kennedy DO, Wesnes KA, Milne AL, Scholey AB (January 2007). "A double-blind, placebo-controlled, multi-dose evaluation of the acute behavioral effects of guaraná in humans". J. Psychopharmacol. (Oxford) 21

Hartwell, Jonathan L. (1971). Bioactive Plants "Plants used against cancer. A survey". Lloydia

Hausen, B. M. (1993). "Centella asiatica (Indian pennywort), an effective therapeutic but a weak sensitizer". Contact Dermatitis 29 (

Hecht SS, Carmella SG, Murphy SE (1 October 1999). "Effects of watercress consumption on urinary metabolites of nicotine in smokers." Cancer Epidemiol Biomarkers

Heinonen, M (2007). "Antioxidant activity and antimicrobial effect of berry phenolics--a Finnish perspective". Molecular nutrition & food research 51

Heinrich, Clark (2002). Magic Mushrooms in Religion and Alchemy. Rochester: Park Street Press.

Heisy, Rod M. (May 1990). "Allelopathic and Herbicidal Effects of Extracts from Tree of Heaven". American Journal of Botany 77

Henrotin Y, Clutterbuck AL, Allaway D, et al. (February 2010). "Biological actions of curcumin on articular chondrocytes". Osteoarthr. Cartil. 18

Hensel, Andreas; Maas, Mareike; Sendker, Jandirk; Lechtenberg, Matthias; Petereit, Frank; Deters, Alexandra; Schmidt, Thomas & Stark, Timo (2011). "Eupatorium perfoliatum L.: Phytochemistry, traditional use and current applications". Journal of Ethnopharmacology

Herbal therapy, medicinal plants, and natural products: An IPA compilation. (1999). Bethesda, MD: American Society of Health-System Pharmacists.

Herbs and natural supplements: An evidence based guide. (n.d.) Mosby Sydney, Australia.

Hess AM, Sullivan DL (2005). "Potential for toxicity with use of bitter orange extract and guarana for weight loss". The Annals of pharmacotherapy 39

Heywood VH. 1993 "Flowering plants of the world." Oxford University Press, New York

Hillier & Sons. (1977). Hilliers' Manual of Trees and Shrubs, 4th Edition. David & Charles, Newton Abbot, England.

Hirota, N. and Hiroi, M., 1967. 'The later studies on the camphor tree, on the leaf oil of each practical form and its utilisation', Perfumery and Essential Oil Record 58

Hirsch, Pamela; Gladstar, Rosemary (2000). Planting the future: saving our medicinal herbs. Rochester, Vt: Healing Arts Press

Hoa NK, Phan DV, Thuan ND, Ostenson CG (April 2009). "Screening of the hypoglycemic effect of eight Vietnamese herbal drugs". Methods & Findings in Experimental & Clinical Pharmacology 31

Hoffmann, Medical Herbalism: Principles and Practices, Healing Arts Press, 2003

Holliday, P. (1989). A dictionary of plant pathology. Cambridge [England: Cambridge University Press.

Holzl J, Godau P. (1989). "Receptor binding studies with Valeriana officinalis on the benzodiazepine receptor". Planta Medica 55

Hong B; Ji YH; Hong JH; Nam KY; Ahn TY A double-blind crossover study evaluating the efficacy of korean red ginseng in patients with erectile dysfunction: a preliminary report. J Urol. 2002

Huang L.-Z., Huang B.-K., Ye Q., Qin L.-P. "Bioactivity-guided fractionation for anti-fatigue property of Acanthopanax senticosus" Journal of Ethnopharmacology 2011

Huang Yuan, Dong Qi, Qiao Shan-Yi. Studies on the Chemical Constituents From Stellaria media (II). Pharmaceutical Journal of Chinese People's Liberation Army, 2007-03 (abstract) (Article in Chinese)

Hughes, R. Elwyn; Ellery, Peter; Harry, Tim; Jenkins, Vivian; Jones, Eleri (1980). "The dietary potential of the common nettle". Journal of the Science of Food and Agriculture 31

Hunt EJ, Lester CE, Lester EA, Tackett RL. (June 2001). "Effect of St. John's wort on free radical production". Life Sci. 69

Hutchens, A. (1992). A handbook of native American herbs. Boston: [New York]

Huxley, A., ed. (1992). New RHS Dictionary of Gardening. Macmillan

Huyen VT, Phan DV, Thang P, Hoa NK, Ostenson CG (May 2010). "Antidiabetic effect of Gynostemma pentaphyllum tea in randomly assigned type 2 diabetic patients". Hormone & Metabolic Research 42

Iacobellis, N S. et al. (2005). "Antibacterial Activity of Cuminum cyminum L. and Carum carvi L. Essential Oils". Journal of Agricultural and Food Chemistry 53

Index herbariorum. (1990). Bronx, N.Y.: Published and distributed for International Association for Plant Taxonomy by New York Botanical Gardens.

Indian journal of natural products. (1985). Sagar, India: [Indian Society of Pharmacognosy].

ISHS Acta Horticulturae 306: International Symposium on Medicinal and Aromatic Plants, XXIII IHC

Isolation and purification of baicalein, wogonin and oroxylin A from the medicinal plant Scutellaria baicalensis by high-speed counter-current chromatography. Hua-Bin Li and Feng Chen, Journal of Chromatography A, 2005, Volume 1074

Ital J Biochem. 1988. Effect of the triterpenoid fraction of Centella asiatica on macromolecules of the connective matrix in human skin fibroblast cultures. Tenni R, Zanaboni G, De Agostini MP, Rossi A, Bendotti C, Cetta G.

Izzo A.A. Ernst E. (2001). "Interactions Between Herbal Medicines and Prescribed Drugs: A Systematic Review". Drugs (Adis International) 61

J. Östman; M. Britton, eds. (2004), "4.7.3 Alternative Medicine Methods Used to Treat Obesity", Treating and Preventing Obesity: An Evidence Based Review, Wiley-VCH.

Jarald E., Nalwaya N., Sheeja E., Ahmad S., Jamalludin S. (2010). "Comparative study on diuretic activity of few

medicinal plants in individual form and in combination form". Indian Drugs 47

Jedlicková Z. Antibacterial properties of the Vietnamese cajeput oil and ocimum oil in combination with antibacterial agents. J Hyg Epidemiol Microbiol Immunol.

Jeong-Kyu KIM, Chang-Soo KANG, Jong-Kwon LEE, Young-Ran KIM, Hye-Yun HAN, Hwa Kyung YUN (2005). "Evaluation of Repellency Effect of Two Natural Aroma Mosquito Repellent Compounds, Citronella and Citronellal". Entomological Research 35

Jiang J.-G., Huang X.-J., Chen J., Lin Q.-S., "Comparison of the sedative and hypnotic effects of flavonoids, saponins, and polysaccharides extracted from Semen Ziziphus jujube" Natural Produ ct Research 2007 21

Jigna Parekh, Nehal Karathia, Sumitra Chanda (2006). "Screening of some traditionally used medicinal plants for potential antibacterial activity". Indian Journal of Pharmaceutical Sciences 68

Jing, M. et al. (1987). "Study on the mechanism of Valeriana officinalis for infantile viral diarrhea". Yunnan J. Traditional Chin. Med. 8

Jordan P; Wheeler S. (2001). The ultimate mushroom book. Hermes House.

Joseph I. Boullata and Angela M. Nace (2000). "Safety Issues with Herbal Medicine: Common Herbal Medicines". Pharmacotherapy 20

Joubert, E; Gelderblom, W.C.A.; Louw, A.; De Beer, D. (2008). "South African herbal teas: Aspalathus linearis, Cyclopia spp. And Athrixia phylicoides—A review". Journal of Ethnopharmacology 119

Jung HA, Su BN, Keller WJ, Mehta RG, Kinghorn AD (March 2006). "Antioxidant xanthones from the pericarp of Garcinia mangostana (Mangosteen)". Journal of Agricultural and Food Chemistry 54

Jung S.M., Schumacher H.R., Kim H., Kim M., Lee S.H., Pessler F. "Reduction of urate crystal-induced inflammation by root extracts from traditional oriental medicinal plants: Elevation of prostaglandin D2levels" Arthritis Research and Therapy 2007 9

Junwei J. Zhu, Christopher A. Dunlap, Robert W. Behle, Dennis R. Berkebile, Brian Wienhold. (2010). Repellency of a wax-based catnip-oil formulation against stable flies. Journal of Agricultural and Food Chemistry, 58

Kade, F.; Miller, W. (1993). "Dose-dependent effects of Ginkgo biloba extraction on cerebral, mental and physical efficiency: a placebo controlled double blind study". British journal of clinical research 4.

Kamal-Eldin A, Moazzami A, Washi S (January 2011). "Sesame seed lignans: potent physiological modulators and possible ingredients in functional foods & nutraceuticals". Recent Pat Food Nutr Agric 3

Kamaldeep Dhawan, Suresh Kumar, Anupam Sharma (2001). "Anti-anxiety studies on extracts of Passiflora incarnata Linneus [sic]". Journal of Ethnopharmacology 78

Kamaldeep Dhawan & Anupam Sharma (2002). "Antitussive activity of the methanol extract of Passiflora incarnata leaves". Fitoterapia 73

Kamaldeep Dhawan, Suresh Kumar & Anupam Sharma (2003). "Antiasthmatic activity of the methanol extract of leaves of Passiflora incarnata". Phytotherapy Research 17

Kamat JP. Boloor KK. Devasagayam TP. Venkatachalam SR. Antioxidant properties of Asparagus racemosus against damage induced by gamma-radiation in rat liver mitochondria. Journal of Ethnopharmacology. 71

Kamdem D. P., Gage, D. A. (1995). "Chemical Composition of Essential Oil from the Root Bark of Sassafras albidum". Journal of Organic Chemistry 61

Kang IJ, Lee MH (July 2006). "Quantification of para-phenylenediamine and heavy metals in henna dye". Contact Dermatitis 55

Kanwar, Anubha Singh ; Bhutani, Kamlesh Kumar "Effects of Chlorophytum arundinaceum, Asparagus adscendens and Asparagus racemosus on Pro-inflammatory Cytokine and Corticosterone Levels Produced by Stress" . BIOSIS Previews Phytotherapy Research. 24

Kapasakalidis, PG; Rastall, RA; Gordon, MH (2006). "Extraction of polyphenols from processed black currant (Ribes nigrum L.) residues". Journal of Agricultural and Food Chemistry 54

Katsaridis, V.; Papagiannaki C., Aimar E. (2009). "Embolization of brain arteriovenous malformations for cure: because we could and because we should". American Journal of Neuroradiology 30

Katzenschlager, R, Evans, A; Manson, A; Patsalos, PN; Ratnaraj, N; Watt, H; Timmermann, L; Van Der Giessen, R et al. (2004). "Mucuna pruriens in Parkinson's disease: a double blind clinical and pharmacological study". Journal of Neurology, Neurosurgery & Psychiatry 75

Kaufman, PB; Duke, JA; Brielmann, H; Boik, J; Hoyt, JE (1997). "A comparative survey of leguminous plants as sources of the isoflavones, genistein and daidzein: Implications for human nutrition and health". Journal of alternative and complementary medicine 3 Kaunitz, H. (1986). "Medium chain triglycerides (MCT) in aging and arteriosclerosis". Journal of Environmental Pathology, Toxicology and Oncology : official organ of the International Society for Environmental Toxicology and Cancer 6

Kennedy, D. O.; Little, W; Scholey, AB (2004). "Attenuation of Laboratory-Induced Stress in Humans After Acute Administration of Melissa officinalis (Lemon Balm)". Psychosomatic Medicine 66

Khan MR , Omoloso AD . Antibacterial activity of Hygrophila stricta and Peperomia pellucida . Fitoterapia . 2002

Khonkarn R. Okonogi S. Ampasavate C. Anuchapreeda S. Investigation of fruit peel extracts as sources for compounds with antioxidant and antiproliferative activities against human cell lines. Food & Chemical Toxicology. 48

Kilham, C. (2000). Tales from the Medicine Trail: Tracking Down the Health Secrets of Shamans, Herbalists, Mystics, Yogis, and Other Healers. [Emmaus PA]: Rodale Press.

Kim, H.; Song, M-J.; Potter, D. (2005). "Medicinal efficacy of plants utilized as temple food in traditional Korean Buddihsm". Journal of Ethnopharmacology 104

Kim, H. J.; Chang, E. J.; Cho, S. H.; Chung, S. K.; Park, H. D.; Choi, S. W. (2002). "Antioxidative activity of resveratrol and its derivatives isolated from seeds of Paeonia lactiflora". Bioscience, biotechnology, and biochemistry 66

Kim, M. H.; Nugroho, A.; Choi, J.; Park, J. H.; Park, H. J. (2011). "Rhododendrin, an analgesic/anti-inflammatory arylbutanoid glycoside, from the leaves of Rhododendron aureum". Archives of Pharmacal Research 34

Kim SJ. Min HY. Lee EJ. Kim YS. Bae K. Kang SS. Lee SK. 'Growth inhibition and cell cycle arrest in the G0/G1 by schizandrin, a dibenzocyclooctadiene lignan isolated from Schisandra chinensis, on T47D human breast cancer cells." Phytotherapy Research. 24

King, J., & Felter, H. (1898). King's American dispensatory (18th ed.). Cincinnati: Ohio Valley

Klepser TB, Klepser ME (1999). "Unsafe and potentially safe herbal therapies". Am J Health-Syst Pharm 56

Ko HC, Wei BL, Chiou WF. The effect of medicinal plants used in Chinese folk medicine on RANTES, Ethnopharmacol, 2006

Koh, H., & Chua, T. (2009). A guide to medicinal plants an illustrated, scientific and medicinal approach. Singapore: World Scientific Pub.

Kraemer, H. (1910). A text-book of botany and pharmacognosy, intended for the use of students of pharmacy, as a reference book for pharmacists, and as a handbook for food and drug analysts, (4th rev. and enl. ed.). Philadelphia & London: J.B. Lippincott Company.

Krafczyk, Nicole; Woyand, Franziska; Glomb, Marcus A. (2009). "Structure-antioxidant relationship of flavonoids from fermented rooibos". Molecular Nutrition & Food Research 53

Krochmal, A., & Krochmal, C. (1984). A field guide to medicinal plants (Updated Times Books pbk. ed.). New York, N.Y.: Times Books.

Kang IJ, Lee MH (July 2006). "Quantification of para-phenylenediamine and heavy metals in henna dye". Contact Dermatitis 55

Kulkarni AP, Mahal HS, Kapoor S, Aradhya SM (February 21, 2007). "In vitro studies on the binding, antioxidant, and cytotoxic actions of punicalagin". J Agric Food Chem 55

Kumar, S. (1998). A complete clinical handbook for every day practice. New Delhi: Indian Books & Periodicals.

Kumar S., Singh Y. V., & Singh, M. (2005). "Agro-History, Uses, Ecology and Distribution of Henna (Lawsonia inermis L. syn. Alba Lam)". Henna: Cultivation, Improvement, and Trade. Jodhpur: Central Arid Zone Research Institute.

Kunkel SD, Elmore CJ, Bongers KS, Ebert SM, Fox DK, et al. (2012) Ursolic Acid Increases Skeletal Muscle and Brown Fat and Decreases Diet-Induced Obesity, Glucose Intolerance and Fatty Liver Disease. PLoS ONE 7

Kurkin VA, Dubishchev AV, Ezhkov VN, Titova IN, Avdeeva EV (2006). "Antidepressant activity of some phytopharmaceuticals and phenylpropanoids". Pharmaceutical Chemistry Journal 40

L. Kumar P., Sharma B., Bakshi N.,"Biological activity of alkaloids from Solanum dulcamara". Natural Product Research. 23. 2009.

Larrosa M, González-Sarrías A, Yáñez-Gascón MJ, Selma MV, Azorin-Ortuño M, Toti S, Tomás-Barberán F, Dolara P, Espín JC (19 July 2009). "Anti-inflammatory properties of a pomegranate extract and its metabolite urolithin-A in a colitis rat model and the effect of colon inflammation on phenolic metabolism." J Nutr Biochem 21

Lauro, Gabriel J.; Francis, F. Jack (2000). Natural Food Colorants Science and Technology. IFT Basic Symposium Series. New York: Marcel Dekker.

Galindo-Cuspinera, V; Westhoff, DC; Rankin, SA (2003). "Antimicrobial properties of commercial annatto extracts against selected pathogenic, lactic acid, and spoilage microorganisms". Journal of food protection 66

Lawrence, B. M., 1995. 'Progress in essential oils', Perfumer and Flavorist,

"Leaf Extract Treatment During the Growth Spurt Period Enhances Hippocampal CA3 Neuronal Dendritic Arborization in Rats". Evid Based Complement Alternat Med: 2006.

Lee do Y. Choo BK. Yoon T. Cheon MS. Lee HW. Lee AY. Kim HK. Anti-inflammatory effects of Asparagus cochinchinensis extract in acute and chronic cutaneous inflammation. Journal of Ethnopharmacology. 121

Lee HJ. Jeong HS. Kim DJ. Noh YH. Yuk DY. Hong JT. Inhibitory effect of citral on NO production by suppression of iNOS expression and NF-kappa B activation in RAW264.7 cells. Archives of Pharmacal Research. 31

Lee IA, Joh EH, Kim DH, "Arctigenin Isolated from the Seeds of Arctium lappa Ameliorates Memory Deficits in Mice." Planta Med. 2011

Lee M.-Y., Shin I.-S., Seo C.-S., Ha H., Shin H.-K."Antiasthmatic effects of Gleditsia sinensis in an ovalbumin-induced murine model of asthma". International Journal of Toxicology. 30. 2011

Lee S.-J., Park K., Ha S.-D., Kim W.-J., Moon S.-K. " Gleditsia sinensis thorn extract inhibits human colon cancer cells: The role of ERK1/2, G2/M-phase cell cycle arrest and p53 expression". Phytotherapy Research. 24

Lee, Seung-Joo et al.; Umano, K; Shibamoto, T; Lee, K (2005). "Identification of volatile components in basil (Ocimum basilicum L.) and thyme leaves (Thymus vulgaris L.) and their antioxidant properties". Food Chemistry 91

Lee, YJ; Jin, YR; Lim, WC; Park, WK; Cho, JY; Jang, S; Lee, SK (2003). "Ginsenoside-Rb1 acts as a weak phytoestrogen in MCF-7 human breast cancer cells". Archives of pharmacal research 26

Leite JR, Seabra Mde L, Maluf E, et al. (July 1986). "Pharmacology of lemongrass (Cymbopogon citratus Stapf). III. Assessment of eventual toxic, hypnotic and anxiolytic effects on humans". J Ethnopharmacol 17

Leos-Rivas C., Verde-Star M.J., Torres L.O., Oranday-Cardenas A., Rivas-Morales C., Barron-Gonzalez M.P., Morales-Vallarta M.R., Cruz-Vega D.E. In vitro amoebicidal activity of borage (Borago officinalis) extract on entamoeba histolytica. Journal of Medicinal Food. 14. 2011.

Lesca, P. (1983). Protective effects of ellagic acid and other plant phenols on benzo[a]pyrene-induced neoplasia in mice.

Lewis K (April 2001). "In search of natural substrates and inhibitors of MDR pumps". Journal of Molecular Microbiology and Biotechnology 3

Lewis, WH and Elvin-Lewis, MPF (2003). Medical botany: plants affecting human health. Hoboken, New Jersey; John Wiley & Sons

Li, C. (1974). Chinese herbal medicine. Washington: U.S. Dept. of Health, Education, and Welfare, Public Health Service, National Institutes of Health.

Li, C. (2003). Chinese herbal medicine. San Diego, Calif.: Book Tree.

Li, Tao; Zhang, Hao (2008), "Identification and Comparative Determination of Rhodionin in Traditional Tibetan Medicinal Plants of Fourteen Rhodiola Species by High-Performance Liquid Chromatography-Photodiode Array Detection and Electrospray Ionization-Mass Spectrometry", Chemical & Pharmaceutical Bulletin 56

Li W.-H., Zhang X.-M., Tian R.-R., Zheng Y.-T., Zhao W.-M., Qiu M.-H.,"A new anti-HIV lupane acid from Gleditsia sinensis Lam.". Journal of Asian Natural Products Research. 9. 2007

Lichtenthäler R, Rodrigues RB, Maia JG, Papagiannopoulos M, Fabricius H, Marx F (Feb 2005). "Total oxidant scavenging capacities of Euterpe oleracea Mart. (Açaí) fruits". Int J Food Science Nutrition 56

Lim, T. K. (2013). Edible medicinal and non-medicinal plants. Dordrecht: Springer.

Lin JK, Chen YC, et al. "Suppression of protein kinase C and nuclear oncogene expression as possible molecular mechanism of cancer chemoprevention by apigenin and curcumin", J Cell Biochem

Lin RD, Mao YW, Leu SJ, Huang CY, Lee MH.,"The immuno-regulatory effects of Schisandra chinensis and its

constituents on human monocytic leukemia cells." Molecules. 2011

Lis-Balchin M., Hart S. and Simpson E. (2001). Buchu (Agathosma betulina and A. crenulata, Rutaceae) essential oils: their pharmacological action on guinea-pig ileum and antimicrobial activity on microorganisms. J Pharm Pharmacol.

Liu W. Huang XF. Qi Q. Dai QS. Yang L. Nie FF. Lu N. Gong DD. Kong LY. Guo QL. Asparanin A induces G(2)/M cell cycle arrest and apoptosis in human hepatocellular carcinoma HepG2 cells. Biochemical & Biophysical Research Communications. 381

Loewenfeld, C., & Back, P. (1980). Britain's wild larder. North Pomfret, Vt.: David & Charles.

Lohakachornpan P. Chemical compositions and antimicrobial activities of essential oil from Melaleuca leucadendron var. minor. Thai J Pharma Sci. 2001

Longe, J. (2005). The Gale encyclopedia of alternative medicine (2nd ed.). Detroit: Thomson Gale.

Loudon, J. (1866). Loudon's encyclopaedia of plants; comprising the specific character, description, culture, history, application in the arts, and every other desirable particular respecting all the plants indigenous to cultivated in, or introduced into Britain. (New impression. ed.). London: Longmans, Green

Lowther, Granville; William Worthington. The Encyclopedia of Practical Horticulture: A Reference System of Commercial Horticulture, Covering the Practical and Scientific Phases of Horticulture, with Special Reference to Fruits and Vegetables.

Lu, G.; Lu G, Edwards CG, Fellman JK, Mattinson DS, Navazio J. (February 2003). "Biosynthetic origin of geosmin in red beets (Beta vulgaris L.).". Journal of Agricultural and Food Chemistry (abstract) (American Chemical Society) 12

Luczak, S; Swiatek, L; Daniewski, M (1989). "Phenolic acids in herbs Lysimachia nummularia L. And L. Vulgaris L". Acta poloniae pharmaceutica 46

Lynas, L. (1972). Medicinal and food plants of the North American Indians: A bibliography. Bronx, N.Y.: Library of New York Botanical Garden.

M. M. Lolitkar and M. R. Rajarama Rao (1962), Note on a Hypoglycaemic Principle Isolated from the fruits of Momordica charantia. Journal of the University of Bombay, volume 29

Mabey, Richard; 'Plants with a Purpose: A guide to the everyday use of wild plants', William Collins, Fontana, Glasgow, 1977

MacGregor FB, Abernethy VE, Dahabra S, Cobden I, Hayes PC (1989). "Hepatotoxicity of herbal remedies". British Medical Journal 299

Mahadevan, S.; Park, Y. (2007). "Multifaceted Therapeutic Benefits of Ginkgo biloba L.: Chemistry, Efficacy, Safety, and Uses". Journal of Food Science 73

Major Apoptosis-Inducing Components of Bitter Gourd". Journal of Agricultural and Food Chemistry 56

Mandal SC. Kumar C K A. Mohana Lakshmi S. Sinha S. Murugesan T. Saha BP. Pal M. Antitussive effect of Asparagus racemosus root against sulfur dioxide-induced cough in mice. Fitoterapia. 71

Manniche, Lisa; An Ancient Egyptian Herbal, pg. 74; American University in Cairo Press; Cairo; 2006

Marc Spehr; Günter Gisselmann, Alexandra Poplawski, Jeffrey A. Riffell, Christian H. Wetzel, Richard K. Zimmer, Hanns Hatt (2003). "Identification of a Testicular Odorant Receptor Mediating Human Sperm Chemotaxis". Science 299 (5615): 2054.

Marnewick, Jeanine L.; Rautenbach, Fanie; Venter, Irma; Neethling, Henry; Blackhurst, Dee M.; Wolmarans, Petro; Macharia, Muiruri (2011). "Effects of rooibos (Aspalathus linearis) on oxidative stress and biochemical parameters in adults at risk for cardiovascular disease". Journal of Ethnopharmacology 133

Marzouk, B.; Haloui E., Akremi N., Aouni M., Marzouk Z., Fenina N. (2012). "Antimicrobial and anticoagulant activities of Citrullus colocynthis Schrad. leaves from Tunisia (Medenine)". African Journal of Pharmacy and Pharmacology 6

Matlwaska (2002). "Flavonoid compounds in the flowers of Abutilon indicum (Linn.) Sweet". Acia Poloniac Pharmaceutic - Drug Research 59

Matsumoto T., Hosono-Nishiyama K., Yamada H. , "Antiproliferative and apoptotic effects of butyrolactone lignans from Arctium lappa on leukemic cells" Planta Medica 2006

May, G., et al. "Antiviral activity of aqueous extracts from medicinal plants in tissue cultures." Arzneim-Forsch 1978

Mazza, M.; Capuano, A.; Bria, P.; Mazza, S. (2006). "Ginkgo biloba and donepezil: a comparison in the

treatment of Alzheimer's dementia in a randomized placebo-controlled double-blind study". European Journal of Neurology 13

McCabe, Melvina; Gohdes, Dorothy; Morgan, Frank; Eakin, Joanne; Sanders, Margaret; Schmitt, Cheryl (2005). "Herbal Therapies and Diabetes Among Navajo Indians". Diabetes Care 28

McCaleb, R., & Leigh, E. (2000). The encyclopedia of popular herbs: Your complete guide to the leading medicinal plants. Roseville, CA: Prima Pub.

McClain, M. (2001). The biogeochemistry of the Amazon Basin. New York: Oxford University Press.

McCutcheon A.R., Stokes W.R., Thorson L.M., Ellis S.M., Hancock R.E.W., Towers G.H.N. Anti-mycobacterial screening of British Columbian medicinal plants. International Journal of Pharmacognosy 1997 35

McDaniel, S.; Goldman, GD (2002). "Consequences of Using Escharotic Agents as Primary Treatment for Nonmelanoma Skin Cancer". Archives of Dermatology 138

McDougall GJ, Ross HA, Ikeji M, Stewart D. 2008. Berry extracts exert different antiproliferative effects against cervical and colon cancer cells grown in vitro. Journal Agricultural Food Chem. 56

McGuffin, M. American Herbal Products Association's botanical safety handbook. American Herbal Products Association.

McKay, Diane L.; Blumberg, Jeffrey B. (2007). "A review of the bioactivity of south African herbal teas: Rooibos (Aspalathus linearis) and honeybush (Cyclopia intermedia)". Phytotherapy Research 21

McKenna, D., & Jones, K. (2011). Botanical Medicines the Desk Reference for Major Herbal Supplements. (Second ed.). New York: Routledge.

Mears, R., & Hillman, G. (2007). Wild food. London: Hodder & Stoughton.

Medeiros RM, de Figueiredo AP, Benício TM, Dantas FP, Riet-Correa F (February 2008). "Teratogenicity of Mimosa tenuiflora seeds to pregnant rats". Toxicon 51

Medicinal Herbs Article list, How to use wild herbs, herb pictures,. (n.d.). Retrieved from http://www.altnature.com/gallery/

MedlinePlus - Health Information from the National Library of Medicine. (n.d.). Retrieved from http://www.nlm.nih.gov/medlineplus/

Mill Goetz P. "Demonstration of the psychotropic effect of mother tincture of Zizyphus jujuba" Phytotherapie 2009

Mills E et al. (2005). "Impact of African herbal medicines on antiretroviral metabolism". AIDS 19

Mills, S. (1985). The dictionary of modern herbalism: A comprehensive guide to practical herbal therapy. New York: Thorsons Pub. Group

Mills, S., & Bone, K. (2000). Principles and practice of phytotherapy: Modern herbal medicine. Edinburgh: Churchill Livingstone.

Miyase T., Yamamoto R., Ueno A.,"Phenylethanoid glycosides from Stachys officinalis" Phytochemistry 1996 43

Moorman, D. (1998). Native American ethnobotany. Portland, Or.: Timber Press.

Mondal, S.; Varma, S.; Bamola, V. D.; Naik, S. N.; Mirdha, B. R.; Padhi, M. M.; Mehta, N.; Mahapatra, S. C. (2011). "Double-blinded randomized controlled trial for immunomodulatory effects of Tulsi (Ocimum sanctum Linn.) leaf extract on healthy volunteers". Journal of Ethnopharmacology 136

Moore, M. (1990). Los Remedios: Traditional Herbal Remedies of the Southwest. Santa Fe, NM: Museum of New Mexico Press.

Mori, S.; Ishikawa, C.; Nakachi, S.; Mori, N. (2011). "Anti-adult T-cell leukemia effects of Bidens pilosa". International Journal of Oncology 38

Mosquito larvicidal activity of oleic and linoleic acids isolated from Citrullus colocynthis (Linn.) Schrad A. Abdul Rahuman, P. Venkatesan and Geetha Gopalakrishnan, Parasitology Research, 2008

Muganza, D., et al. "In vitro antiprotozoal and cytotoxic activity of 33 ethonopharmacologically selected medicinal plants from Democratic Republic of Congo." J Ethnopharmacol. 2012

Mukherjee P.K., Kumar V., Mal M., Houghton P.J. "Acorus calamus: Scientific validation of ayurvedic tradition from natural resources"Pharmaceutical Biology 2007

Muñoz V , Sauvain M , Bourdy G , et al. A search for natural bioactive compounds in Bolivia through a multidisciplinary approach: Part III. Evaluation of the antimalarial activity of plants used by Alteños Indians . J Ethnopharmacol 2000

NDL/FNIC Food Composition Database. (n.d.). Retrieved from http://ndb.nal.usda.gov/

Naftali T., Feingelernt H., Lesin Y., Rauchwarger A., Konikoff F.M. "Ziziphus jujuba extract for the treatment of chronic idiopathic constipation: A controlled clinical trial" Digestion 2008

Nahrstedt A, Butterweck V (September 1997). "Biologically active and other chemical constituents of the herb of Hypericum perforatum L". Pharmacopsychiatry 30

Nascimento, Gislene G. F.; Locatelli, Juliana; Freitas, Paulo C.; Silva, Giuliana L. (2000). "Antibacterial activity of plant extracts and phytochemicals on antibiotic-resistant bacteria". Brazilian Journal of Microbiology 31

Nathan, P. J.; Tanner, S.; Lloyd, J.; Harrison, B.; Curran, L.; Oliver, C.; Stough, C. (2004). "Effects of a combined extract of Ginkgo biloba and Bacopa monniera on cognitive function in healthy humans". Human Psychopharmacology 19

National Agricultural Library Digital Collections. (n.d.). Retrieved from http://naldc.nal.usda.gov/naldc/home.xhtml National Center for Complementary and Alternative Medicine

National Library of Medicine - National Institutes of Health. (n.d.). Retrieved from http://www.nlm.nih.gov

Natural carcinogenic products, EK Weisburger – Environmental Science & Technology, 1979 – ACS Publications

Newton KM, Reed SD, LaCroix AZ, Grothaus LC, Ehrlich K, Guiltinan J (2006). "Treatment of vasomotor symptoms of menopause with black cohosh, multibotanicals, soy, hormone therapy, or placebo: a randomized trial". Annals of Internal Medicine 145

Nielsen, IL; Haren, GR; Magnussen, EL; Dragsted, LO; Rasmussen, SE (2003). "Quantification of anthocyanins in commercial black currant juices by simple high-performance liquid chromatography. Investigation of their pH stability and antioxidative potency". Journal of Agricultural and Food Chemistry 51

Nishanta Rajakaruna, Cory S. Harris and G.H.N. Towers (2002). "Antimicrobial Activity of Plants Collected from Serpentine Outcrops in Sri Lanka". Pharmaceutical Biology 40

Niwano, Y.; et al., Keita; Yoshizaki, Fumihiko; Kohno, Masahiro; Ozawa, Toshihiko (2011). "Extensive screening for herbal extracts with potent antioxidant properties". Journal of Clinical Biochemistry and Nutrition 48

Noosidum A. Excito-repellency properties of essential oils from Melaleuca leucadendron L, Litsea cubeba (Lour.) Persoon and Litsea salicifolia (Nees) on Aedes aegypti (L.) mosquitoes. J Vector Ecol. 2008

Norris, LE; Collene, AL; Asp, ML; Hsu, JC; Liu, LF; Richardson, JR; Li, D, et al. (2009 Sep). "Comparison of dietary conjugated linoleic acid with safflower oil on body composition in obese postmenopausal women with type 2 diabetes mellitus.". The American journal of clinical nutrition 90

Noureddini M., Rasta V.-R. Analgesic Effect of aqueous extract of Achillea millefolium L. on rat's formalin test. Pharmacologyonline 2008

Nuntanakorn P, Jiang B, Yang H, Cervantes-Cervantes M, Kronenberg F, Kennelly EJ (2007). "Analysis of polyphenolic compounds and radical scavenging activity of four American Actaea species". Phytochem Anal 18

Obolskiy D, Pischel I, Siriwatanametanon N, Heinrich M (2009). "Garcinia mangostana L. (mangosteen): A phytochemical and pharmacological review". Phytother Res 23

Ody, P. (2000). Complete guide to medicinal herbs (2nd American ed.). New York: Dorling Kindersley.

Ogihara, Y. (2003). Sho-saiko-to: Scientific evaluation and clinical applications. London: Taylor & Francis.

Ogra, R. K. et al.; Indian calamus (Acorus calamus L.): not a tetraploid; Current Science, Vol. 97, No. 11, 10 December 2009; Current Science Association; Bangalore

Okabe, H.; Miyahara, Y.; Yamauci, T. (1982). "Studies on the constituents of Momordica charantia L. Chemical Pharmacology Bulletin 30

O'Neill, M. J., et al. "Plants as sources of antimalarial drugs, Part 6. Activities of Simarouba amara fruits." J. Ethnopharmacol. 1988

Online Medical Dictionary. University of Newcastle upon Tyne Centre for Cancer Education. n.d.

Ott, J. (1976). Hallucinogenic Plants of North America. Berkeley, CA: Wingbow Press.

Oyebanji (2011). "Phytochemistry and in vitro anti-oxidant activities of Stellaria media, Cajanus cajan and Tetracera potatoria methanolic extracts". Journal of Medicinal Plants Research 5

Pak K.C., Lam K.Y., Law S., Tang J.C.O. "The inhibitory effect of Gleditsia sinensis on cyclooxygenase-2 expression in human esophageal squamous cell carcinoma." International Journal of Molecular Medicine. 23

Pakistan encyclopaedia planta medica: A joint research project of Hamdard Foundation Pakistan and H.E.J. Research Institute of Chemistry. (1986). Karachi: Hamdard.

Pan, JG; Xu, ZL; Ji, L (1992). "Chemical studies on essential oils from 6 Artemisia species". Zhongguo Zhong yao za zhi 17

Papoutsi Z. Kassi E. Tsiapara A. Fokialakis N. Chrousos GP. Moutsatsou P. (2005). "Evaluation of estrogenic/antiestrogenic activity of ellagic acid via the estrogen receptor subtypes ERalpha and ERbeta". Journal of Agricultural & Food Chemistry 53

Parry, E. (1921). The chemistry of essential oils and artificial perfumes, (4th ed.). London: Scott, Greenwood and Son.

Parry J, Su L, Moore J et al. (May 2006). "Chemical compositions, antioxidant capacities, and antiproliferative activities of selected fruit seed flours". J. Agric. Food Chem. 54

Patel, D. K.; Prasad S.K., Kumar R., Hemalatha S. (2012). "An overview on antidiabetic medicinal plants having insulin mimetic property". Asian Pacific Journal of Tropical Biomedicine 2

Peng, X; Zhao, Y; Liang, X; Wu, L; Cui, S; Guo, A; Wang, W (2006). "Assessing the quality of RCTs on the effect of beta-elemene, one ingredient of a Chinese herb, against malignant tumors". Contemporary clinical trials 27

Perry, Ek; Pickering, At; Wang, Ww; Houghton, P; Perry, Ns (Winter 1998). "Medicinal plants and Alzheimer's disease: Integrating ethnobotanical and contemporary scientific evidence". Journal of alternative and complementary medicine (New York, N.Y.) 4

Phillips, R., & Rix, M. (2002). The botanical garden the definitive reference with more than 2000 photographs. Buffalo, NY: Firefly Books.

Phillips, R., & Rix, M. (2002). The botanical garden: Volume 1 [trees and shrubs]. London: Macmillan. Phillips / Rix

Phillips, R., & Rix, M. (2002). The botanical garden: Volume 2, [perennials and annuals]. London: Macmillan. Phillips / Rix

Physicians' desk reference 2011 (65th ed.). (2010). Montvale, N.J.: Physicians' Desk Reference.

Piacente, S; Carbone, V., Plaza, A., Zampelli, A. & Pizza, C. (2002). "Investigation of the Tuber Constituents of Maca (Lepidium meyenii Walp.)". Journal of Agricultural and Food Chemistry 50

Plant Guide. United States Department of Agriculture Natural Resources Conservation Service. May 30, 2002.

Plants, L. (2000). Proceedings of the National Seminar on the Frontiers of Research and Development in Medicinal Plants: September 16-18, 2000. Lucknow, India: Central Institute of Medicinal and Aromatic Plants.

Platt R (2000). "Current concepts in optimum nutrition for cardiovascular disease". Prev Cardiol 3

Plotkin MJ, Balick MJ (Apr 1984). "Medicinal uses of South American palms". J Ethnopharmacol 10

Polyphenolic Constituents of Fruit Pulp of Euterpe oleracea Mart. (Açai palm). S. Gallori, A. R. Bilia, M. C. Bergonzi, W. L. R. Barbosa and F. F. Vincieri, Chromatographia, 2004

Popovici M., Pârvu A.E., Oniga I., Toiu A., Tămaş M., Benedec D. Effects of two Achillea species tinctures on experimental acute inflammation. Farmacia 2008

Potrich F.B., Allemand A., da Silva L.M., dos Santos A.C., Baggio C.H., Freitas C.S., Mendes D.A.G.B., Andre E., de Paula Werner M.F., Marques M.C.A. Antiulcerogenic activity of hydroalcoholic extract of Achillea millefolium L.: Involvement of the antioxidant system. Journal of Ethnopharmacology 2010

Pownall TL, Udenigwe CC, Aluko RE (2010). "Amino acid composition and antioxidant properties of pea seed ( Pisum sativum L.) enzymatic protein hydrolysate fractions". Journal of Agricultural and Food Chemistry

Prager N, Bickett K, French N,Marcovici G (2002). "A randomized, double-blind, placebo-controlled trial to determine the effectiveness of botanically derived inhibitors of 5-a-reductase in the treatment of androgenetic alopecia". J Altern Complement Ther 8

Prakash, P.; Gupta, N. (April 2005). "Therapeutic uses of Ocimum sanctum Linn (Tulasi) with a note on eugenol and its pharmacological actions: A short review". Indian Journal of Physiology and Pharmacology 49

Premila, M. (2006). Ayurvedic herbs: A clinical guide to the healing plants of traditional Indian medicine. New York: Haworth Press.

Qiao, C.-Y., Jin-Hua Ran, Yan Li and Xiao-Quan Wang (2007): Phylogeny and Biogeography of Cedrus (Pinaceae) Inferred from Sequences of Seven Paternal Chloroplast and Maternal Mitochondrial DNA Regions. Annals of Botany

Qingdi Q. Li, Gangduo Wang, Manchao Zhang, Christopher F. Cuff, Liang Huang, Eddie Reed (2009). "β-Elemene, a novel plant-derived antineoplastic agent, increases cisplatin chemosensitivity of lung tumor cells by triggering apoptosis". Oncology Reports 22

Qiu SX, Dan C, Ding LS, Peng S, Chen SN, Farnsworth NR, Nolta J, Gross ML, Zhou P (2007). "A triterpene glycoside from black cohosh that inhibits osteoclastogenesis by modulating RANKL and TNFα signaling pathways". Chemistry & Biology 14

Rabbani GH, Butler T, Knight J, Sanyal SC, Alam K (May 1987). "Randomized controlled trial of berberine sulfate therapy for diarrhea due to enterotoxigenic Escherichia coli and Vibrio cholerae". The Journal of Infectious Diseases 155

Rai, V.; Mani, U.V.; Iyer, U.M. (1997). "Effect of Ocimum sanctum Leaf Powder on Blood Lipoproteins, Glycated Proteins and Total Amino Acids in Patients with Non-insulin-dependent Diabetes Mellitus". Journal of Nutritional and Environmental Medicine 7

Randløv C, Mehlsen J, Thomsen CF, Hedman C, von Fircks H, Winther K (March 2006). "The efficacy of St. John's Wort in patients with minor depressive symptoms or dysthymia—a double-blind placebo-controlled study". Phytomedicine 13

Rani, S.; Khan, S.A.; Ali, M. (2010). "Phytochemical investigation of the seeds of Althea officinalis L". Natural Product Research 24

Rastogi, R. (1990). Compendium of Indian medicinal plants. Lucknow: Central Drug Ray RB, Raychoudhuri A, Steele R, Nerurkar P., Bitter Melon (Momordica charantia) Extract Inhibits Breast Cancer Cell Proliferation by Modulating Cell Cycle Regulatory Genes and Promotes Apoptosis. Cancer Res. 2010

Rehder, A. 1940, reprinted 1977. Manual of cultivated trees and shrubs hardy in North America exclusive of the subtropical and warmer temperate regions. Macmillan publishing Co., Inc, New York.

Research Institute and Publications & Information Directorate, New Delhi.

Reutera, J.; C. Huykea, H. Scheuvensa, M. Plochc, K. Neumannd, T. Jakobb, C. M. Schemppa (2008). "Skin tolerance of a new bath oil containing St. John's wort extract". Skin pharmacology and physiology 21 Rahman, A., et al. "Anti-tuberculosis activity of quassinoids." Chemical Pharmacology Bulletin. 1997.

Rhoads, Ann F., Timothy A. Block, and Anna Anisko (Illustrator). The Plants of Pennsylvania: An Illustrated Manual, Second edition (2007). University of Pennsylvania Press.

Riddle, John M. (1999). Eve's Herbs: A History of Contraception and Abortion in the West. Harvard University Press.

Riehemann, K; Behnke, B; Schulze-Osthoff, K (1999). "Plant extracts from stinging nettle (Urtica dioica), an antirheumatic remedy, inhibit the proinflammatory transcription factor NF-kappaB". FEBS letters 442

Rinaldi, S. Silva, D. O. Bello, F. Alviano, C S. Alviano, D S. Matheus, ME. Fernandes, P D. (2009). Characterization of the antinociceptive and anti-inflammatory activities from Cocos nucifera L. (Palmae). Journal of Ethnopharmacology 122

Ritchie, F. (1999). Handbook of edible wild plants and weeds. Springfield, Or.: Ritchie Unlimited Publications.

Rivera-Arce E, Chávez-Soto MA, Herrera-Arellano A et al. (February 2007). "Therapeutic effectiveness of a Mimosa tenuiflora cortex extract in venous leg ulceration treatment". J Ethnopharmacol 109

Rivera-Arce E, Gattuso M, Alvarado R et al. (September 2007). "Pharmacognostical studies of the plant drug Mimosae tenuiflorae cortex". J Ethnopharmacol 113

Rodrigues, Eliana & Carlini, E.A. (2006): Plants with possible psychoactive effects used by the Krahô Indians, Brazil. Revista Brasileira de Psiquiatria

Roodenrys, S.; Booth, D.; Bulzomi, S.; Phipps, A.; Micallef, C.; Smoker, J. (2002). "Chronic effects of Brahmi (Bacopa monnieri) on human memory". Neuropsychopharmacology 27

Rose, J. (1987). Jeanne Rose's modern herbal. New York, N.Y.: Perigee Books.

Rosengarten, Frederic, Jr. (2004). The Book of Edible Nuts. Dover Publications.

Ross, I. (1999). Medicinal plants of the world: Chemical constituents, traditional, and modern medicinal uses. Totowa, N.J.: Humana Press.

Ross, J. (2003). Combining Western herbs and Chinese medicine: Principles, practice, and materia medica. Seattle, Wash.: Greenfields Press.

Roy, K.; Thakur M., Dixit V.K. (2007). "Effect of Citrullus colocynthis on hair growth in albino rats". Pharmaceutical Biology 45

Royal Horticultural Society; http://apps.rhs.org.uk/plantselector/

Said, O., Khalil, K. Fulder, S. and Azaizeh, H. Ethnopharmacological Survey of the Medicinal herbs in Israel, the Golan Heights and the West Bank Region. Journal of Ethnopharmacology, 83

Sairam K. Priyambada S. Aryya NC. Goel RK.Gastroduodenal ulcer protective activity of Asparagus racemosus: an experimental, biochemical and histological study. Journal of Ethnopharmacology. 86

Sale C, Harris RC, Delves S, Corbett J (May 2006). "Metabolic and physiological effects of ingesting extracts of bitter orange, green tea and guarana at rest and during treadmill walking in overweight males". Int J Obes (Lond) 30

Salunkhe, D.K., J.K. Chavan, R.N. Adsule, and S.S. Kadam. (1992). World Oilseeds – Chemistry, Technology, and Utilization. Springer.

Samorini, Giorgio (2002). Animals and psychedelics: the natural world and the instinct to alter consciousness.

Sayyah, M.; Saroukhani, G.; Peirovi, A.; Kamalinejad, M. (August 2003). "Analgesic and anti-inflammatory activity of the leaf essential oil of Laurus nobilis Linn". Phytother Res 17

Schafferman, D.; Beharav A., Shabelsky E., Yaniv Z (1998). "Evaluation of Citrullus colocynthis, a desert plant native in Israel, as a potential source of edible oil". Journal of Arid Environments 40

Schauss A.G., Wu X., Prior R.L., Ou B., Huang D., Owens J., Agarwal A., Jensen G.S., Hart A.N., Shanbrom E. (2006). "Antioxidant capacity and other bioactivities of the freeze-dried amazonian palm berry, Euterpe oleraceae Mart. (acai)". J Agric Food Chem 54

Schnitzler, P; Schuhmacher, A; Astani, A; Reichling, J (2008). "Melissa officinalis oil affects infectivity of enveloped herpesviruses". Phytomedicine 15

Scholey, A B (2003). "Modulation of Mood and Cognitive Performance Following Acute Administration of Single Doses of Melissa Officinalis (Lemon Balm) with Human CNS Nicotinic and Muscarinic Receptor-Binding Properties". Neuropsychopharmacology 28

Schubert SY, Lansky EP, Neeman I (July, 1999). "Antioxidant and eicosanoid enzyme inhibition properties of pomegranate seed oil and fermented juice flavonoids". J Ethnopharmacol 66

Schultz, Gretchen; Peterson, Chris; Coats, Joel (2006). "Natural Insect Repellents: Activity against Mosquitoes and Cockroaches".

Schulz, V. (2004). Rational phytotherapy: A reference guide for physicians and pharmacists (5th ed.). Berlin: Springer.

Seal S, Chatterjee P, Bhattacharya S, Pal D, Dasgupta S, et al. (2012) Vapor of Volatile Oils from Litsea cubeba Seed Induces Apoptosis and Causes Cell Cycle Arrest in Lung Cancer Cells. PLoS ONE 7

Seden K. Dickinson L. Khoo S. Back D.. Grapefruit-drug interactions. [Review]. Drugs. 2010. 70.

Sheeja K, Shihab PK, Kuttan G. Antioxidant and inflammatory modulating activities of the plant Andrographis paniculata Nees, Immunopharmacol Immunotoxicol. 2006.

Seeram NP, Aronson WJ, Zhang Y et al. (September 2007). "Pomegranate ellagitannin-derived metabolites inhibit prostate cancer growth and localize to the mouse prostate gland". J. Agric. Food Chem. 55

Semiz, A, Sen A. (February 2007). "Antioxidant and chemoprotective properties of Momordica charantia L. (bitter melon) fruit extract". African Journal of Biotechnology 6

Seeram, NP (2008). "Berry fruits: compositional elements, biochemical activities, and the impact of their intake on human health, performance, and disease". Journal of Agricultural and Food Chemistry 56

Seidl, P. (1995). Chemistry of the Amazon: Biodiversity, natural products, and environmental issues : Developed from the First International Symosium on Chemistry and the Amazon sponsored by the Associação Brasileira de Química, American Chemical Semiz, A, Sen A. (February 2007). "Antioxidant and chemoprotective properties of

Momordica charantia L. (bitter melon) fruit extract". African Journal of Biotechnology 6

Seo SW et al. (Jan 2011). "Protective effects of Curcuma longa against cerulein-induced acute pancreatitis and pancreatitis-associated lung injury". Int J Mol Med 27

Sharma K. Bhatnagar M. Kulkarni SK. "Effect of Convolvulus pluricaulis Choisy and Asparagus racemosus Willd on learning and memory in young and old mice: a comparative evaluation." Indian Journal of Experimental Biology. 48

Sharma, P.; Kulshreshtha, S.; Sharma, A.L. (1998). "Anti-cataract activity of Ocimum sanctum on experimental cataract". Indian Journal of Pharmacology 30

Sharma U. Saini R. Kumar N. Singh B. Steroidal saponins from Asparagus racemosus. Chemical & Pharmaceutical Bulletin. 57

Shi J, Yu J, Pohorly JE, Kakuda Y (2003). "Polyphenolics in grape seeds-biochemistry and functionality". Journal Medicinal Food 6

Shibib, BA; Khan, LA; Rahman, R (May 15). "Hypoglycemic activity of Coccinia indica and Momordica charantia in diabetic rats: depression of the hepatic gluconeogenic enzymes glucose-6-phosphatase and fructose-1,6-bisphosphatase and elevation of both liver and red-cell shunt enzyme glucose-6-phosphate dehydrogenase". Biochem J. 292

Shin HR, Kim JY, Yun TK, Morgan G, Vainio H (2000). "The cancer-preventive potential of Panax ginseng: a review of human and experimental evidence". Cancer Causes Control 11

Shukla, A.; Rasik, A. M.; Jain, G. K.; Shankar, R.; Kulshrestha, D. K.; Dhawan, B. N. (1999). "In vitro and in vivo wound healing activity of asiaticoside isolated from Centella asiatica". Journal of Ethnopharmacology 65

Shukla PK, Khanna VK, Ali MM, Maurya R, Khan MY, Srimal RC. "Neuroprotective effect of Acorus calamus against middle cerebral artery occlusion-induced ischaemia in rat" Hum Exp Toxicology 2006.

Silva FL, Fischer DC, Tavares JF, Silva MS, de Athayde-Filho PF, Barbosa-Filho JM.,"Compilation of secondary metabolites from Bidens pilosa L." Molecules, 2011

Simic, M; Kundaković, T; Kovacević, N (September 2003). "Preliminary assay on the antioxidative activity of Laurus nobilis extracts". Fitoterapia 74

Simon PW (1997). Plant Pigments for Color and Nutrition.

Singh, A.; Singh, S. K. (2009). "Evaluation of antifertility potential of Brahmi in male mouse". Contraception 79

Singh GK. Garabadu D. Muruganandam AV. Joshi VK. Krishnamurthy S. Antidepressant activity of Asparagus racemosus in rodent models. Pharmacology, Biochemistry & Behavior. 91

Sinisalo, Marjatta; Enkovaara, Anna-Liisa; Kivistö, Kari T. (2010). "Possible hepatotoxic effect of rooibos tea: A case report". European Journal of Clinical Pharmacology 66

Small, E., & Catling, P. (1999). Canadian medicinal crops. Ottawa: NRC Research Press.

Society, Centro de Tecnologia Mineral, and Instituto Nacional de Pesquisas da Amazonia Manaus, Amazonas, Brazil, November 21-25, 1993. Washington, DC:

Smith, A, (1997). A Gardener's Handbook of Plant Names: Their Meanings and Origins. Dover Publications

Smith, P; MacLennan, K; Darlington, CL (1996). "The neuroprotective properties of the Ginkgo biloba leaf: a review of the possible relationship to platelet-activating factor (PAF)". Journal of Ethnopharmacology 50

Stuart, M. (1981). The Encyclopedia of herbs and herbalism. New York: Crescent Books

South, G., & Whittick, A. (1987). Introduction to phycology. Oxford [Oxfordshire: Blackwell Scientific Publications.

Stablein JJ. Melaleuca tree and respiratory disease. Ann Allergy Asthma Immunol. 2002

Standley, L; Winterton, P; Marnewick, JL; Gelderblom, WC; Joubert, E; Britz, TJ (2001 Jan). "Influence of processing stages on antimutagenic and antioxidant potentials of rooibos tea.". Journal of Agricultural and Food Chemistry 49

Stough, C.; Downey, L. A.; Lloyd, J.; Silber, B.; Redman, S.; Hutchison, C.; Wesnes, K.; Nathan, P. J. (2008). "Examining the nootropic effects of a special extract of Bacopa Monniera on human cognitive functioning: 90 day double-blind placebo-controlled randomized trial". Phytotherapy Research 22

Streloke, M. et al.; Ascher, K. R. S.; Schmidt, G. H.; Neumann, W. P. (1989). "Vapor pressure and volatility of β-asarone, the main ingredient of an indigenous stored-product insecticide, Acorus calamus oil". Phytoparasitica 17

Sturtevant, WC (1955). The Mikasuki Seminole: Medical Beliefs and Practices. Ann Arbor, MI: University Microfilms.

Stuttgart: Georg Thieme Verlag. Biology and chemistry of active natural substances: International symposium, Bonn, July 17-22, 1990, plenary lectures. (1991).

Suanarunsawat, T.; Boonnak, T.; Na Ayutthaya, W. D.; Thirawarapan, S. (2010). "Anti-hyperlipidemic and cardioprotective effects of Ocimum sanctum L. fixed oil in rats fed a high fat diet". Journal of Basic and Clinical Physiology and Pharmacology 21

Suh SO, Kroh M, Kim NR, Joh YG, Cho MY. (2002). "Effects of red ginseng upon postoperative immunity and survival in patients with stage III gastric cancer". American Journal of Chinese Medicine. 30

Sultan S, Spector J, Mitchell RM (December 2006). "Ischemic colitis associated with use of a bitter orange-containing dietary weight-loss supplement". Mayo Clinic Proceedings 81

Sun, Meng; Lou, Wei; Chun, Jae Yeon; Cho, Daniel S.; Nadiminty, Nagalakshmi; Evans, Christopher P. et al. (2010). "Sanguinarine Suppresses Prostate Tumor Growth and Inhibits Survivin Expression". Genes & Cancer 1

Szapary, PO; Wolfe, ML; Bloedon, LT; Cucchiara, AJ; Dermarderosian, AH; Cirigliano, MD; Rader, DJ (2003). "Guggulipid Ineffective for Lowering Cholesterol". JAMA 290

T. Ogasawara, k.Chiba, m.Tada in (Y. P. S. Bajaj ed ). 1988. Medicinal and Aromatic Plants, Volume 10. Springer, Taati, Majid; Masoud Alirezaei, Mohamad Hadi Moshkatalsadat, Bahram Rasoulian, Mehrnoush Moghadasi, Farzam Sheikhzadeh, Ali Sokhtezari. (2011). "Protective effects of Ziziphus jujuba fruit extract against ethanol-induced hippocampal oxidative stress and spatial memory impairment in rats". Journal of Medicinal Plants Research 5

Tan, NH; Fung, SY; Sim, SM; Marinello, E; Guerranti, R; Aguiyi, JC (2009). "The protective effect of Mucuna pruriens seeds against snake venom poisoning". Journal of Ethnopharmacology 123

Tanacetum Balsamita L: A Medicinal Plant. M.J. Pérez-Alonso, A. Velasco-Negueruela, A. Burzaco

Tang J., Wang C.K., Pan X., Yan H., Zeng G., Xu W., He W., Daly N.L., Craik D.J., Tan N."Isolation and characterization of cytotoxic cyclotides from Viola tricolor" Peptides 2010

Tang SY, Gruber J, Wong KP, Halliwell B (April 2007). "Psoralea corylifolia L. inhibits mitochondrial complex I and proteasome activities in SH-SY5Y cells". Ann. N. Y. Acad. Sci. 1100: 486–96.

Tang W.K., Chui C.H., Fatima S., Kok S.H., Pak K.C., Ou T.M., Hui K.S., Wong M.M., Wong J., Law S., Tsao S.W., Lam K.Y., Beh P.S., Srivastava G., Ho K.P., Chan A.S., Tang J.C. "Inhibitory effects of Gleditsia sinensis fruit extract on telomerase activity and oncogenic expression in human esophageal squamous cell carcinoma." International journal of molecular medicine. 19. 2007.

Tannin-Spitz, T; Grossman S., Dovrat S., Gottlieb H.E., Bergman M. (2007). "Growth inhibitory activity of cucurbitacin glucosides isolated from Citrullus colocynthis on human breast cancer cells". Biochemical Pharmacology 73

Tatsis, EC; Boeren, S; Exarchou, V; Troganis, AN; Vervoort, J; Gerothanassis, IP (2007). "Identification of the major constituents of Hypericum perforatum by LC/SPE/NMR and/or LC/MS". Phytochemistry 48

Taur D.J., Patil R.Y.,"Mast cell stabilizing, antianaphylactic and antihistaminic activity of Coccinia grandis fruits in asthma". Chinese Journal of Natural Medicines. 9

Taylor, Frederick R. (2011). "Nutraceuticals and Headache: The Biological Basis". Headache: the Journal of Head and Face Pain 51

Taylor LG (2005). The healing power of rainforest herbs: a guide to understanding and using herbal medicinals. Garden City Park, NY: Square One Publishers.

Teschke, R; Bahre, R (2009). "Severe hepatotoxicity by Indian Ayurvedic herbal products: A structured causality assessment". Annals of hepatology 8.

Teucher, T; Obertreis, B; Ruttkowski, T; Schmitz, H (1996). "Cytokine secretion in whole blood of healthy subjects following oral administration of Urtica dioica L. Plant extract". Arzneimittel-Forschung 46

Thakur M. Chauhan NS. Bhargava S. Dixit VK. A comparative study on aphrodisiac activity of some ayurvedic herbs in male albino rats. Archives of Sexual Behavior. 38

The Organic Gardener's Handbook of Natural Pest and Disease, Fern Marshall Bradley, Barbara W. Ellis, Deborah L. Martin,

The pharmacopœia of the United States of America: (the United States pharmacopœia). (12th revision (U.S.P. XII) / ed.). (1942). Washington, D.C.: Published by the Board of Trustees

The Pharmacopoeia of the United States of America (The United States pharmacopoeia) 19th rev. (1974). Rockville, Md.: United States Pharmacopeial Convention.

The use of herbal medicines by people with cancer: A qualitative study. (2009). BioMed Central.

"Therapeutic effect of arctiin and arctigenin in immunocompetent and immunocompromised mice infected with influenza" Biological and Pharmaceutical Bulletin 2010

Thierer, John W.; Niering, William A., and Olmstead, Nancy C. (2001) National Audubon Society Field Guide to North American Wildflowers, Eastern Region, Revised Edition. Alfred A. Knopf

Thompson LU, Chen JM, Li T, Strasser-Weippl K, Goss PE (2005). "Dietary flaxseed alters tumor biological markers in postmenopausal breast cancer". Clinical Cancer Research 11

Thomson, W. (1978). Healing Plants: A modern herbal. London: Macmillan.

Tipton, K. (1979). Neurochemistry and biochemical pharmacology. Baltimore: University Park Press.

Tiwari M, Dwivedi UN, Kakkar P. 2010. Suppression of oxidative stress and pro-inflammatory mediators by Cymbopogon citratus D. Stapf extract in lipopolysaccharide stimulated murine alveolar macrophages. Food Chemistry Toxicology

Toiu A. Muntean E. Oniga I. Vostinaru O. Tamas M. " Pharmacognostic research on Viola tricolor L. (Violaceae)." Revista Medico-Chirurgicala a Societatii de Medici Si Naturalisti Din Iasi. 1

Toiu A. Parvu AE. Oniga I. Tamas M."Evaluation of anti-inflammatory activity of alcoholic extract from Viola tricolor.", Revista Medico-Chirurgicala a Societatii de Medici Si Naturalisti Din Iasi. 11

Trease, G. (1952). A Text-Book of Pharmacognosy ... Sixth edition. Pp. viii. 821. Baillière, Tindall & Cox: London.

Tsch, C. (2005). The encyclopedia of psychoactive plants: Ethnopharmacology and its applications. Rochester, Vt.: Park Street Press.

Tsuda H; Ohshima Y; Nomoto H et al. (2004). "Cancer prevention by natural compounds". Drug Metabolism and Pharmacokinetics 19

Tulyaganov, T. S.; Nigmatullaev, A. M. (2000). Chemistry of Natural Compounds 36

Tutin, T. (1976). Flora Europaea. Cambridge: Cambridge University Press.

Ukiya M, Akihisa T, Yasukawa K et al. Anti-inflammatory, anti-tumor-promoting, and cytotoxic activities of constituents of pot marigold (Calendula officinalis) flowers. (2006).

Umek, A; Kreft, S; Kartnig, T; Heydel, B (1999). "Quantitative phytochemical analyses of six hypericum species growing in slovenia". Planta medica 65 UN Food & Agriculture Organisation | Online references | cyclopaedia.net. (n.d.). Retrieved from http://www.cyclopaedia.info/UN-Food-and-Agriculture-Organisation

Valdes, A., et al. "In vitro anti-microbial activity of the Cuban medicinal plants Simarouba glauca DC, Melaleuca leucadendron L and Artemisia absinthium L." Mem Inst Oswaldo Cruz. 2008

Valeriote, F. A., et al. "Anticancer activity of glaucarubinone analogues." Oncol Res. 1998

Vaughan, J.G.; Geissler, C.A. (1997). The New Oxford Book of Food Plants. Oxford University Press.

Veronese ML, Gillen LP, Burke JP, Dorval EP, Hauck WW, Pequignot E, Waldman SA, Greenberg HE. Exposure-dependent inhibition of intestinal and hepatic CYP3A4 in vivo by grapefruit juice. Journal of Clinical Pharmacology. 2003;43

Visarata, N.; Ungsurungsie, M. (1981). "Extracts from Momordica charantiaL". Pharmaceutical Biology 19

Volz, S. M., and S. S. Renner (Volz and Renner) 2009. Phylogeography of the ancient Eurasian medicinal plant genus Bryonia (Cucurbitaceae) inferred from nuclear and chloroplast sequences. Taxon 58

von Woedtke T, Schlüter B, Pflegel P, Lindequist U, Jülich WD (June 1999). "Aspects of the antimicrobial efficacy of grapefruit seed extract and its relation to preservative substances contained". Pharmazie 54

Vukics V. Kery A. Guttman A."Analysis of polar antioxidants in Heartsease (Viola tricolor L.) and Garden pansy (Viola x wittrockiana Gams.)". Journal of Chromatographic Science. 46

Waako PJ, Gumede B, Smith P, Folb PI (May 2005). "The in vitro and in vivo antimalarial activity of Cardiospermum halicacabum L. and Momordica foetida Schumch. Et Thonn". J Ethnopharmacol 99

Wada L, Ou B (June 2002). "Antioxidant activity and phenolic content of Oregon caneberries". Journal of Agricultural and Food Chemistry 50

Wagh S., Vidhale N.N. (2010). "Antimicrobial efficacy of Boerhaavia diffusa against some human pathogenic bacteria and fungi". Biosciences Biotechnology Research Asia 7

Wagner, Hildebert (1999). Immunomodulatory agents from plants. Birkhäuser.

Wang C., Xia Y.F. Gao Z.Z., Lu D., Dai Y. "Inhibition of mast cell degranulation by saponins from Gleditsia sinensis-structure-activity relationships." Natural Product Communications. 4. 2009

Wang JJ, Shi QH, Zhang W, Sanderson BJ (2012). "Anti-skin cancer properties of phenolic-rich extract from the pericarp of mangosteen (Garcinia mangostana Linn.)". Food Chemistry Toxicology 50

Wang, Lu et al. (2009). "Ultrasonic nebulization extraction coupled with headspace single drop microextraction and gas chromatography–mass spectrometry for analysis of the essential oil in Cuminum cyminum L". Analytica Chimica Acta 647

Wang ZT, Ng TB, Yeung HW, Xu GJ (December 1996). "Immunomodulatory effect of a polysaccharide-enriched preparation of Codonopsis pilosula roots". Gen. Pharmacol. 27 Warrier, P. K.; V. P. K. Nambiar, C. Ramankutty, R. Vasudevan Nair (1996). Indian medicinal plants. Orient Blackswan.

Weber HA, Zart MK, Hodges AE, et al. (December 2003). "Chemical comparison of goldenseal (Hydrastis canadensis L.) root powder from three commercial suppliers". Journal of Agricultural and Food Chemistry 51 Weber W, Vander Stoep A, McCarty RL, Weiss NS, Biederman J, McClellan J (June 2008). "A Randomized Placebo Controlled Trial Of Hypericum perforatum For Attention Deficit Hyperactivity Disorder In Children And Adolescents". JAMA 299

Webster, D.E.; J. Lu, S.-N. Chen, N.R. Farnsworth and Z. Jim Wang (2006). "Activation of the μ-opiate receptor by Vitex agnus-castus methanol extracts: Implication for its use in PMS". Journal of Ethnopharmacology 106

Weerasinghe, Priya; Hallock, Sarathi; Brown, Robert E.; Loose, David S.; Buja, L. Maximilian (2012). "A model for cardiomyocyte cell death: Insights into mechanisms of oncosis". Experimental and Molecular Pathology

Weinmann, S; Roll, S; Schwarzbach, C; Vauth, C; Willich, SN (2010). "Effects of Ginkgo biloba in dementia: systematic review and meta-analysis". BMC geriatrics 10 Weisskopf. Schaffner. Jundt. Sulser. Wyler. Tullberg-Reinert. Planta Medica 2005

Wells, A., Edwards, E.D., Houston, W. W. K., Lepidoptera: Hesperioidea, Papilionoidea, Volume 31, CSIRO, 2001.

Wheatley D (2004). "Triple-blind, placebo-controlled trial of Ginkgo biloba in sexual dysfunction due to antidepressant drugs". Hum Psychopharmacol 19.

Wilt TJ, Ishani A, Rutks I, MacDonald R (2000). "Phytotherapy for benign prostatic hyperplasia". Public Health Nutr 3

Winston, David & Maimes, Steven. "Adaptogens: Herbs for Strength, Stamina, and Stress Relief," Healing Arts Press, 2007.

Whitford AC (1941). "Textile fibers used in eastern aboriginal North America". Anthropological Papers of the American Museum of Natural History 38

Wichtl, Max,Herbal drugs and phytopharmaceuticals: a handbook,2004

Wild Medicinal Plants: What to Look For, When to Harvest, How to Use 2002 Schneider / Mellichamp

William Thomas Fernie, Herbal Simples Approved for Modern Uses of Cure, 3rd enlarged ed. Bristol: Wright, 1914

Williamson, E. (2009). Stockley's herbal medicines interactions a guide to the interactions of herbal medicines, dietary supplements and nutraceuticals with conventional medicines. London: Pharmaceutical Press.

Wilt T, Ishani A, Mac Donald R (2002). "Serenoa repens for benign prostatic hyperplasia". In Tacklind, James. Cochrane Database Syst Rev (3): CD001423.

Winston & Kuhn's Herbal Therapy & Supplements: A Scientific and Traditional Approach 2007 Kuhn / Winston

Witkowska-Banaszczak E., Bylka W., Matlawska I., Goślińska O., Muszyński Z. ,"Antimicrobial activity of Viola tricolor herb". Fitoterapia 2005

Wong AHC, Smith M, Boon HS (1998). "Herbal remedies in psychiatric practice". Arch Gen Psychiatry 55

Wright CI, Van-Buren L, Kroner CI, Koning MM (October 2007). "Herbal medicines as diuretics: a review of the scientific evidence". J Ethnopharmacol 114

Wright SC. Maree JE. Sibanyoni M. Treatment of oral thrush in HIV/AIDS patients with lemon juice and lemon grass (Cymbopogon citratus) and gentian violet. Phytomedicine. 16. 2009.

Wyk, B., & Wink, M. (2004). Medicinal plants of the world: An illustrated scientific guide to important medicinal plants and their uses. Portland: Timber Press.

Xie L.-H., Ahn E.-M., Akao T., Abdel-Hafez A.A.-M., Nakamura N., Hattori M."Transformation of arctiin to estrogenic and antiestrogenic substances by human intestinal bacteria" Chemical and Pharmaceutical Bulletin 2003

Xu XM, Li L, Chen M., "Studies on the chemical constituents of Schisandra pubescens". Zhong Yao Cai. 2009

Xu Y.J., Han C.J., Xu S.J., Yu X., Jiang G.Z., Nan C.H. "Effects of Acanthopanax senticosus on learning and memory in a mouse model of Alzheimer's disease and protection against free radical injury to brain tissue" Neural Regeneration Research 2008

Yamada, K.; Hung, P.; Park, T. K.; Park, P. J.; Limb, B. O. (2011). "A comparison of the immunostimulatory effects of the medicinal herbs Echinacea, Ashwagandha and Brahmi". Journal of Ethnopharmacology 137

Yemm RS, Poulton JE (June 1986). "Isolation and characterization of multiple forms of mandelonitrile lyase from mature black cherry (Prunus serotina Ehrh.) seeds". Archives of biochemistry and biophysics 247

Yeung, H. (1985). Handbook of Chinese herbs and formulas. Los Angeles, U.S.A.: H.C. Yeung.

Yeung. Him-Che. Handbook of Chinese Herbs and Formulas. 1985. Los Angeles: Institute of Chinese Medicine.

Yoo, Ki-Yeon; Hua Li, In Koo Hwang, Jung Hoon Choi, Choong Hyun Lee, Dae Young Kwon, Shi Yong Ryu, Young Sup Kim, Il-Jun Kang, Hyung-Cheul Shin, and Moo-Ho Won. (2010). "Zizyphus Attenuates Ischemic Damage in the Gerbil Hippocampus via Its Antioxidant Effect". Journal of Medicinal Food 13

Yoshikawa M, Murakami T, Kishi A et al. (2001). Medicinal flowers. III. Marigold.(1): hypoglycemic, gastric emptying inhibitory, and gastroprotective principles and new oleanane-type triterpene oligoglycosides, calendasaponins A, B, C, and D, from Egyptian Calendula officinalis. Chem Pharm

Yu, Xiuzhu; Van De Voort, Frederick R.; Li, Zhixi; Yue, Tianli (2007). "Proximate Composition of the Apple Seed and Characterization of Its Oil". International Journal of Food Engineering 3

Yuan CS, Mehendale S, Xiao Y, Aung HH, Xie JT, Ang-Lee MK (2004). "The gamma-aminobutyric acidergic effects of valerian and valerenic acid on rat brainstem neuronal activity.". Anesth Analg 98

Yun TK, Lee YS, Lee YH, Kim SI, Yun HY (2001). "Anticarcinogenic effect of Panax ginseng C.A. Meyer and identification of active compounds". Journal of Korean Medical Science 16

Zakay-Rones, Zichria; Noemi Varsano, Moshe Zlotnik, Orly Manor, Liora Regev, Miriam Schlesinger, Madeleine Mumcuoglu (1995). "Inhibition of Several Strains of Influenza Virus in Vitro and Reduction of Symptoms by an Elderberry Extract (Sambucus nigra L.) during an Outbreak of Influenza B Panama" (PDF). J Altern Complement Med 1 Zakim, D. (1985). Biochemical pharmacology and toxicology. New York: Wiley. Biochemical Pharmacology. 2011

Zarse, K., et al. "The phytochemical glaucarubinone promotes mitochondrial metabolism, reduces body fat, and extends lifespan of Caenorhabditis elegans." Horm Metab Res. 2011

Zhang XW, Li WF, Li WW, Ren KH, Fan CM, Chen YY, Shen YL (2011). "Protective effects of the aqueous extract of Scutellaria baicalensis against acrolein-induced oxidative stress in cultured human umbilical vein endothelial cells". Pharm Biol 49

Zhao F., Wang L., Liu K. "In vitro anti-inflammatory effects of arctigenin, a lignan from Arctium lappa L., through inhibition on iNOS pathway" Journal of Ethnopharmacology 2009

Zhao G, Li S, Qin GW, Fei J, Guo LH (2007). "Inhibitive effects of Fructus Psoraleae extract on dopamine transporter and noradrenaline transporter.". J Ethnopharmacol 112 (3): 498–506.

Zhou L., Li D., Wang J., Liu Y., Wu J."Antibacterial phenolic compounds from the spines of Gleditsia sinensis Lam." Natural Product Research. 21. 2007.

214

Zhao LH, Huang CY, Shan Z, Xiang BG, Mei LH (2005). "Fingerprint analysis of Psoralea corylifolia by HLPC and LC-MS". J Chromatogr B 821: 67–74.

Zhu X. Zhang W. Zhao J. Wang J. Qu W. Hypolipidaemic and hepatoprotective effects of ethanolic and aqueous extracts from Asparagus officinalis L. by-products in mice fed a high-fat diet. Journal of the Science of Food & Agriculture. 90

Zick S.M., Sen A., Feng Y., Green J., Olatunde S., Boon H."Trial of essiac to ascertain its effect in women with breast cancer (TEA-BC)" Journal of Alternative and Complementary Medicine 2006

Zillur Rahman and M. Shamim Jairajpuri. Neem in Unani Medicine. Neem Research and Development Society of Pesticide Science, India, New Delhi, 1993. Edited by N.S. Randhawa and B.S. Parmar. 2nd revised edition

Spencer, C. F., et al. "Survey of plants for antimalarial activity." Lloydia 1947

# Index

Acacia senegal ................................................... 2
Acacia tortilis ..................................................... 2
Acalypha arvensis ........................................48, 49
Achillea sibirica ............................................... 169
Acorus gramineus............................................ 152
Aegle marmelos................................................. 22
Aeruginosa ...........................................62, 69, 90, 209
Agave americana .............................................. 12
Agave parryi ...................................................... 51
Ageratum houstonianum ..................................... 5
Agrimonia pilosa................................................ 84
Agropyron repens............................................... 62
Agrostemma githago .......................................... 61
Ailanthus altissima .......................................... 158
Air purification ...............................31, 45, 50, 158
Akebia trifoliata ................................................. 7
Alchornea castaneifolia...................................... 98
Alepidea amatymbica ........................................ 94
Alisma plantago .............................................. 163
Alliaria petiolata............................................... 79
Allium sativum .................................................. 77
Allium ursinum ................................................ 164
Aloe barbadensis ............................................. 10
Aloe vera ........................................................ 10
Anacardium occidentale .................................... 50
Anchusa officinalis ............................................. 7
Andrographis paniculata ................................... 13
Anethum graveoleus .......................................... 66
Angelica sinensis............................................... 66
Aquilegia vulgaris ............................................. 60
Arctium lappa .......................... 44, 208, 211, 214
Arctostaphylos uva-ursi .................................. 161
Argyreia speciosa............................................ 167
Arisaema consanguineum................................. 152
Aristolochia clematitis........................................ 30
Aristolochia contorta ....................................... 111
Aristolochia debilis .......................................... 112
Armoracia rusticana .......................................... 92
Artemisia absinthium..............................168, 214
Artemisia annua.............................................. 169
Artemisia argyi .................................................. 5
Artemisia dracunculus..................................... 154
Artemisia scoparia........................................... 136
Artemisia tridentate ........................................ 140
Artemisia vulgaris ........................................... 116
Asperula odorata ............................................ 167
Aster tataricus................................................. 155
Astragalus membranaceus ................................. 19

Azadirachta indica .......................................... 120
Bacillus dysenteriae..............5, 40, 63, 66, 86, 136
Bacillus subtilis ............................5, 20, 50, 62, 136
Bacillus typhi............5, 8, 66, 76, 86, 116, 135, 136
Balsamorhiza sagittata...................................... 18
Baptisia tinctoria ............................................. 97
Berberis aristata ............................................... 55
Berberis canadensis .......................................... 26
Berberis microphylla.......................................... 46
Berberis vulgaris ............................................... 24
Betula pubescens .............................................. 29
Bidens pilosa...........................................128, 211, 213
Bixa orellana ................................................... 15
Bupleurum falcatum .......................................... 43
Burns ........ 15, 17, 18, 23, 47, 71, 101, 117, 133, 149
Bursera microphylla........................................... 70
Bursera simaruba ............................................. 83
Calamintha nepeta .......................................... 122
Calendula officinalis .........................47, 207, 214
Calophyllum inophyllum ................................... 153
Camellia sinensis ............................................ 155
Cannabis sativa ................................................ 49
Capsella bursa ............................................... 144
Carlina acaulis................................................. 49
Cecropia peltata ............................................... 71
Celosia argantea .............................................. 60
Centaurea cyanus ............................................ 21
Cetraria islandica ............................................. 94
Chimaphila maculata....................................... 166
Chimaphila umbellata ....................................... 34
Cichorium intybus ............................................. 54
Cinnamomum zeylanicum .................................. 57
Citrullus colocynthis..........................32, 209, 211, 213
Citrus limonum ............................................... 106
Citrus x aurantifolia......................................... 108
Cleaners ................. 1, 24, 50, 58, 72, 121, 135, 197
Cleaning ..5, 6, 8, 10, 13, 15, 26, 27, 31, 43, 44, 57,
     63, 69, 70, 84, 100, 105, 106, 107, 110, 120, 121,
     136, 139, 140, 146, 157, 159, 184
Cleansing ........................21, 45, 78, 118, 164, 203
Coccoloba uvifera ........................................... 143
Cochlearia officinalis........................................ 143
Cola acuminata .............................................. 103
Colds ............................17, 36, 43, 77, 95, 147
Commiphora myrrha ........................................ 118
Conjunctivitis.........................21, 24, 46, 55, 56, 81
Coriandrum sativum ......................................... 56
Cornus officinalis ............................................ 144

216

Corossol epineux....................................................... 82
Cucurbita foetidissima ............................................ 42
Cymbopogon citratus..... 107, 207, 209, 211, 214
Cymbopogon martinii .............................................. 124
Cyperus articulatus ................................................... 3
Decalepis hamiltonii ............................................... 152
Dendranthema x grandiflorum...................... 55
Dental ....................2, 14, 32, 58, 78, 140, 141, 165
Dictamnus albus ..................................................... 45
Digestive........4, 28, 68, 79, 104, 121, 142, 185, 206
Diphtheria ............................................................... 114
Disinfectant ........31, 43, 57, 69, 100, 123, 141, 158
Drosera rotundifolia............................................... 151
drug resistant.........................................6, 21, 57, 92
e. coli.. 5, 8, 20, 62, 69, 71, 86, 87, 96, 99, 109, 116,
    120, 121, 134, 135, 138, 143, 152, 155, 161, 167,
    170, 171, 204, 209
Echinacea angustifolia .............................68, 69
Echinacea purpurea .................................68, 69
Echinopanax horridum............................................ 65
Elaeagnus umbellata .............................................. 20
Elsholtzia ciliata ..................................................... 162
enterococcus faecium ............................................ 69
Ericameria nauseosa .............................................. 134
Erythroxylum coca.................................................. 59
Eucalyptus globulus ................................................ 71
Evodia officinalis .................................................... 72
Eye ............. 31, 47, 55, 56, 60, 62, 81, 162, 167, 203
Eyes.................... 21, 24, 36, 46, 55, 102, 127, 157
Filipendula ulmaria ................................................ 114
Forsythia suspensa................................................. 76
Fucus vesiculosus ................................................... 38
Gaillardia pinnatifida............................................... 39
Garcinia mangostana ...........113, 210, 212, 214
Gastrointestinal 6, 8, 14, 22, 30, 43, 46, 55, 65, 68,
    72, 81, 82, 98, 146, 148, 150, 208, 209
Geranium robertianum ............................................ 86
Gleditsia sinensis..........88, 209, 211, 212, 213, 214
Gram positive .................9, 16, 20, 85, 92, 96, 151
Gram-negative ...9, 16, 20, 59, 79, 85, 92, 96, 151
Gram-positive ..........7, 15, 33, 49, 50, 74, 120, 136
Grindelia robusta .................................................... 82
Gymnema sylvestre ................................................ 84
Harpagophytum procumbens ...................... 64
Hedyotis diffusa...................................................... 145
Helichrysum angustifolium...................................... 95
Herniaria glabra ..................................................... 139
Heuchera americana ............................................... 11
Hibiscus sabdariffa .................................87, 138
Houttuynia cordata ................................................ 74

Humulus lupulus ...................................................... 90
Hydnocarpus wightiana ................................... 53
Hydrastis canadensis .................81, 208, 209, 214
Hypericum perforatum ...148, 208, 212, 213, 214
Hypoxis hemerocallidea ........................................ 4
Hyssopus officinalis ............................................... 93
Illicium verum ........................................................ 149
Immune system 1, 6, 13, 18, 19, 20, 30, 31, 33, 34,
    37, 47, 48, 49, 54, 70, 75, 88, 95, 98, 104, 120,
    124, 126, 154, 157, 204
Immunity.. 17, 30, 54, 56, 68, 77, 83, 106, 109, 133,
    209, 213, 214
Imperata cylindrica ......................................... 39
Infection . 1, 5, 6, 8, 9, 10, 11, 12, 13, 18, 22, 23, 26,
    27, 28, 29, 30, 32, 36, 39, 40, 41, 42, 43, 44, 47,
    48, 50, 51, 52, 53, 54, 55, 56, 58, 59, 60, 62, 63,
    64, 65, 67, 68, 69, 70, 71, 74, 75, 76, 80, 83, 84,
    86, 87, 88, 89, 90, 91, 93, 95, 97, 98, 99, 101, 103,
    105, 106, 109, 110, 113, 114, 115, 116, 117, 118,
    119, 120, 121, 125, 126, 127, 128, 129, 131, 132,
    133, 134, 136, 138, 139, 140, 141, 142, 143, 144,
    145, 149, 150, 151, 154, 157, 158, 160, 161, 163,
    165, 166, 168, 170, 202, 203, 204, 205
Infections 2, 3, 4, 5, 6, 7, 8, 9, 10, 12, 13, 14, 15, 16,
    17, 19, 20, 21, 22, 25, 29, 30, 31, 32, 33, 34, 36,
    38, 40, 41, 44, 45, 46, 47, 48, 50, 51, 52, 53, 54,
    55, 56, 57, 58, 59, 60, 61, 62, 63, 66, 67, 68, 69,
    70, 71, 74, 75, 76, 77, 78, 79, 80, 81, 82, 83, 85,
    86, 87, 88, 89, 90, 91, 92, 93, 94, 95, 96, 98, 99,
    101, 102, 104, 105, 106, 109, 110, 111, 112, 113,
    114, 116, 117, 118, 119, 120, 121, 122, 123, 124,
    126, 128, 129, 130, 131, 132, 133, 134, 135, 136,
    138, 139, 143, 144, 145, 146, 147, 149, 151, 152,
    153, 154, 155, 156, 157, 159, 160, 161, 163, 164,
    166, 167, 169, 170, 171, 202
Influenza ... 17, 36, 43, 67, 77, 90, 95, 110, 116, 119,
    135, 156, 161, 214
Inula britannica ..................................................... 171
Inula helenium ........................................................ 69
Isatis tinctoria ....................................................... 166
Juniperus communis ................................................ 99
Larix decidua ........................................................ 104
Larrea tridentata...................................................... 52
Laurus nobilis ...................................................26, 213
Lavandula angustifolia ......................................... 105
Lavandula officinalis.............................................. 105
Lawsonia inermis .................................................85, 210
Leontopodium alpinum .......................................... 69
Lepidium sativum................................................... 77
Ligusticum porteri .................................................. 116
Ligustrum lucidum.................................................. 79

Lindera benzoin.................................................... 147
Liquidambar orientalis..................................... 150
Lomatium dissecta ........................................... 110
Lomatium dissectum......................................... 31
Lonicera japonica ............................................... 90
Lonicera periclymenum...................................... 89
Lophophora williamsii ..................................... 128
Lysimachia nummularia.........................115, 211
Lythrum salicaria .............................................. 110
Magnolia officinalis .......................................... 112
Mallotus philippensis .......................................... 96
Malus domestica ................................................ 16
Marchantia polymorpha.......................109, 110
Marrubium vulgare...................................91, 208
Melaleuca alternifolia ...................156, 208, 209
Melaleuca leucadendron ......45, 207, 209, 211,
     212, 214
Melaleuca viridiflora .............................122, 123
meningococci.................................................... 63
Mentha spicata ................................................ 146
Mentha x piperita officinalis ....................... 126
Mentha x piperita vulgaris ............................ 126
Mimosa hostilis ................................................ 100
Monarda didyma ............................................... 27
Monotropa uniflora ............................................ 97
Moringa oleifera ................................................ 67
Mouth....2, 3, 5, 9, 11, 12, 21, 25, 27, 28, 29, 31, 32,
     40, 41, 42, 47, 50, 51, 52, 56, 58, 62, 63, 64, 65,
     67, 70, 76, 80, 81, 83, 84, 85, 88, 89, 90, 93, 94,
     98, 99, 101, 102, 103, 105, 106, 110, 117, 118,
     123, 126, 127, 129, 130, 132, 138, 139, 140, 142,
     143, 144, 145, 148, 151, 153, 158, 161, 205
Mycobacterium tuberculi ................................. 8
Myrciaria dubia.................................................. 48
Myroxylon pereirae ........................................... 24
Myrtus communis .............................................. 119
Nymphaea lotus ............................................... 111
Nymphaea odorata ......................................... 132
Ocimum sanctum.......88, 208, 209, 211, 212, 213
Origanum vulgare ............................................ 124
p. aeruginosa ..................................................... 20
Paris polyphylla.................................................. 86
Pelargonium sidoides ...................................... 160
Peperomia pellucida.........................62, 207, 210
peptic ulcers ...................................................... 32
Persicaria bistorta ............................................. 32
Philonotis fontana ............................................. 16
Phytolacca acinosa ......................................... 130
Picea abies........................................................ 147
Pimpinella anisum.............................................. 13

Pimpinella major ............................................... 129
Pinus balsamea ................................................. 23
Piper methysticum............................................ 101
Pistacia lentiscus .............................................. 114
Plantago lanceolata ......................................... 42
Plantago major ................................................ 129
Pneumococci........63, 96, 111, 112, 136, 163, 204
Pneumonia......36, 40, 45, 67, 69, 90, 96, 110, 114,
     116, 119, 124, 135, 156, 161
Pogostemon cablin............................................ 125
Polygonum aviculare ....................................... 103
Polygonum multiflorum ...................................... 75
Pongamia pinnata ........................................... 132
Portulaca oleracea .......................................... 133
Prunella vulgaris ............................................... 8, 9
Prunus serotina ...........................................35, 214
pseudomonas.............5, 62, 69, 90, 135, 152, 171
Pseudomonas ...................................................... 8
Psoralea corylifolia .............................20, 213, 215
Ptelea trifoliata ................................................ 163
Pterocarpus marsupium.................................. 102
Pulicaria dysenterica ........................................ 75
Pulsatilla chinensis............................................. 22
Punica granatum .............................................. 131
Pyrola rotundifolia............................................ 165
Raphanus sativus .............................................. 134
Ravensara aromatica ...................................... 135
Rhododendron aureum........................136, 210
Rhus glabra ....................................................... 151
Rosa laevigata ................................................... 53
Rubia cordifolia ................................................. 96
Rumex acetosa ................................................ 145
Rumex crispus ................................................... 170
s. aureus ............................................................. 20
Salmonella........25, 71, 90, 120, 121, 152, 170, 204
Salvia miltiorrhiza.............................................. 135
Salvia officinalis ................................................ 139
Sanguinaria canadensis ................................... 40
Sassafras albidum.........................................141, 210
Satureja montana ............................................. 142
Scrophularia ningpoensis ............................... 123
Sedum acre...................................................... 149
Shingella.............................................25, 71, 204
Simarouba amara ............................................. 33
Simarouba glauca ......................................121, 214
Solidago virgaurea........................................... 80
Sores ....5, 8, 9, 11, 12, 13, 21, 29, 30, 31, 36, 38, 40,
     43, 44, 47, 48, 50, 51, 52, 53, 54, 55, 58, 59, 60,
     64, 65, 70, 74, 79, 80, 81, 86, 87, 89, 91, 93, 97,
     98, 99, 101, 102, 103, 105, 109, 110, 113, 114,

117, 118, 120, 121, 125, 126, 127, 128, 130, 132, 133, 134, 138, 139, 140, 141, 143, 145, 148, 150, 151, 153, 154, 157, 161, 165, 166, 168, 170, 171, 198

Spondias purpurea................................................. 99

Staphylococcus.... 5, 8, 25, 40, 48, 50, 55, 57, 61, 62, 63, 69, 71, 86, 87, 88, 90, 91, 96, 98, 99, 101, 106, 109, 111, 112, 114, 116, 120, 121, 124, 128, 135, 136, 144, 145, 151, 152, 153, 155, 160, 161, 163, 167, 170, 171, 204

Staphylococcus aureus ...5, 8, 50, 61, 62, 63, 69, 90, 109, 111, 112, 116, 120, 121, 136

Streptococci ....25, 50, 66, 116, 132, 134, 136, 152

Streptococcus ....55, 57, 69, 76, 90, 106, 110, 120, 121, 124, 151, 161

Syzygium aromaticum..................................... 58

Tabebuia avellanedae................................. 125

Tamarindus indica ....................................... 154

Taraxacum officinale.................................... 63

Tecoma stans................................................ 171

Terminalia catappa ......................................... 9

Throat....2, 3, 5, 9, 11, 12, 18, 23, 25, 27, 29, 31, 32, 41, 42, 47, 50, 51, 52, 62, 63, 64, 67, 68, 76, 80, 81, 83, 84, 85, 89, 93, 94, 98, 99, 101, 102, 103, 105, 106, 109, 110, 117, 118, 123, 127, 129, 130, 131, 132, 138, 140, 142, 143, 144, 145, 151, 153, 158, 160, 161, 165, 166, 186

Thuja occidentalis........................................ 17

Thymus vulgaris.....................................157, 211

Tinsospora cardiofolia ..................................... 83

Topical 2, 3, 4, 5, 7, 8, 11, 12, 13, 14, 17, 18, 22, 23, 24, 26, 28, 29, 30, 31, 32, 36, 38, 40, 42, 43, 44, 47, 48, 49, 50, 51, 52, 53, 55, 58, 59, 60, 61, 62, 63, 64, 65, 66, 69, 71, 74, 75, 76, 78, 79, 80, 81, 84, 86, 87, 89, 90, 91, 92, 93, 95, 96, 98, 99, 101, 102, 103, 104, 105, 106, 107, 109, 110, 113, 114, 116, 117, 118, 120, 121, 122, 123, 124, 125, 126, 127, 128, 132, 133, 134, 135, 136, 137, 138, 139, 140, 141, 142, 143, 144, 145, 146, 149, 150, 151, 152, 153, 154, 155, 156, 157, 158, 161, 163, 164, 165, 166, 168, 169, 171, 185, 192, 193, 197, 199

Tribulus terrestris .............................................. 159

Tropaeolum majus........................................... 119

Ulcers...5, 8, 9, 11, 13, 15, 17, 18, 21, 25, 29, 30, 31, 32, 36, 38, 40, 42, 43, 44, 47, 48, 50, 52, 53, 54, 55, 56, 58, 59, 60, 63, 64, 65, 72, 74, 76, 79, 80, 84, 86, 87, 89, 90, 91, 93, 97, 98, 99, 101, 102, 103, 105, 109, 110, 113, 114, 117, 118, 120, 121, 125, 126, 127, 128, 130, 132, 133, 134, 138, 139, 141, 143, 145, 148, 149, 150, 151, 153, 154, 157, 161, 165, 166, 168, 170, 171, 198

Urinary tract.4, 7, 20, 21, 29, 34, 39, 40, 41, 48, 53, 54, 59, 60, 62, 63, 80, 82, 83, 90, 92, 93, 103, 113, 114, 119, 120, 129, 133, 138, 139, 144, 145, 157, 161, 163, 165, 166, 170, 208

Usnea barbata .............................................. 160

Vaccinium angustifolium................................ 41

Vaccinium myrtillus ....................................... 28

Verbascum thapsus....................................... 117

Vinca minor.................................................. 127

Vinca rosea ................................................. 127

Vitex gaumeri ................................................ 74

Water ....2, 10, 14, 15, 16, 27, 30, 31, 32, 36, 39, 40, 45, 50, 52, 55, 67, 92, 102, 107, 111, 116, 122, 125, 127, 132, 134, 145, 153, 159, 162, 164, 171, 174, 175, 176, 177, 178, 179, 183, 184, 185, 186, 187, 188, 189, 191, 192, 193, 198, 199, 202, 204, 205, 206, 208

Wounds.....9, 10, 17, 18, 32, 34, 65, 69, 70, 94, 115, 141, 213

Wounds.3, 5, 8, 9, 10, 11, 12, 13, 15, 17, 18, 21, 22, 24, 27, 29, 30, 31, 36, 40, 42, 43, 44, 47, 48, 50, 51, 52, 53, 54, 55, 58, 59, 60, 64, 71, 74, 75, 76, 78, 79, 80, 81, 84, 86, 87, 89, 91, 93, 95, 97, 98, 99, 101, 102, 103, 105, 109, 110, 113, 114, 117, 120, 121, 125, 126, 127, 128, 130, 132, 133, 134, 135, 138, 139, 141, 143, 144, 145, 148, 149, 150, 151, 153, 154, 157, 161, 163, 164, 165, 166, 168, 170, 171, 198

Xanthium strumarium..................................... 59

Ziziphus jujuba....................................37, 212, 213

www.ingramcontent.com/pod-product-compliance
Lightning Source LLC
Chambersburg PA
CBHW081100290526
45795CB00006B/1927